TUMOR METASTASIS

Edited by **Ke Xu**

Tumor Metastasis
http://dx.doi.org/10.5772/61798
Edited by Ke Xu

Contributors

Therese Becker, Joseph Po, David Lynch, Paul De Souza, Shiang Huang, Yanjie Hu, Jin'e Zheng, Chia-Hsun Hsieh, Tao Sun, Yuan Qin, Wei-Long Zhong, Hyun Guy Kang, San Ha Kang, Anirban Kumar Mitra, Yunus Luqmani, Monerah Al Soraj, Maitham Khajah, Serdar Altınay, Martin Berger, Elina Beleva, Zhanet Grudeva-Popova, Veselin Popov

Published by InTech

Janeza Trdine 9, 51000 Rijeka, Croatia

Publishing Process Manager Andrea Koric

Technical Editor SPi Global

Cover InTech Design team

First published September, 2016

Printed in Croatia

Additional hard copies can be obtained from orders@intechopen.com

Tumor Metastasis, Edited by Ke Xu

p. cm.

Print ISBN 978-953-51-2630-0

Online ISBN 978-953-51-2631-7

For EU product safety concerns:
IN TECH d.o.o., Prolaz Marije Krucifikse Kozulić 3, 51000 Rijeka, Croatia,
info@intechopen.com or visit our website at intechopen.com.

Meet the editor

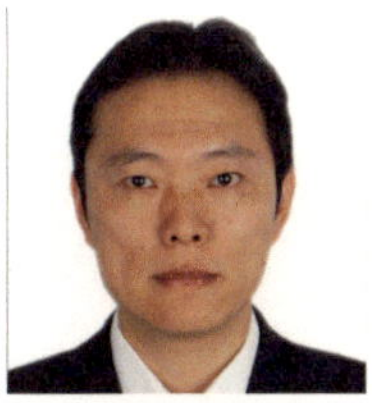

Professor Ke Xu earned his BSc in Microbiology in 1989 from Nankai University (China) and his PhD in Cell and Molecular Biology in 2001 from the University of Essex (UK). He completed his postdoctoral training at the Institute of Cancer Research (UK) and then carried out his research fellowship at Imperial College London (UK). He joined the Tianjin Lung Cancer Institute at Tianjin Medical University General Hospital (China) in 2007, studying the mechanism of metastasis and chemoresistance of lung cancer. He also develops novel anticancer drugs. Professor Ke Xu is an active member of American Association of Cancer Research, American Society for Cell Biology, Chinese Anti-Cancer Association, and Chinese Pharmaceutical Association.

Contents

Preface

Cancer is a leading cause of death nowadays; it causes more deaths than coronary heart disease. According to the latest report of the International Agency for Research on Cancer, there were estimated 14.1 million new cancer cases and 8.2 million deaths occurred in 2012 worldwide. Among all types of cancer, lung cancer remains the leading cause of cancer-related death in men, and breast cancer is the leading cause of cancer-related death in women. Although governments over the world have invested huge human and material resources on cancer prevention and cancer treatment, there are no significant improvements on it. The occurrence of cancer is still increasing. This is because of the increasing risk factors such as pollution due to urbanization and economic development, aging and growth of the population, overweight/obesity, and the lifestyle behaviors such as smoking, physical inactivity, and poor diet.

Cancer metastasis is the major cause of cancer-related death; around 90% of cancer patients die of metastasis. Tumor metastasis is a complex process; the cascade of metastasis involves several steps: loss of cellular adhesion, increased ability of migration and invasion, entry blood and lymph vessels, exit from the circulation into new site, and colonization at the distant site. This book provides broad coverage of the field of tumor metastasis.

In the first section of this book, "Tumor Metastasis," **Chapter 1** discusses the role of hemostatic system in tumor. Cancer induces hemostatic imbalance through the production and secretion of procoagulant substances, suppression of anticoagulant mechanisms, endothelial activation, and angiogenic switch. By manipulating hemostatic processes, tumor induces tolerant host environment necessary for the evasion of defense attacks, survival, and progression. **Chapter 2** reviews the role of the extracellular matrix (ECM) and how disruption of ECM dynamics may contribute to cancer. This focuses on the properties and functions of the ECM, abnormal ECM dynamics, tumor microenvironment and ECM, and the role of ECM and ECM-associated proteins in metastasis. Ovarian cancer is the most lethal of all gynecologic malignancies. Seventy percent of ovarian cancer patients present with disseminated disease at the time of diagnosis. **Chapter 3** provides an overview of ovarian cancer metastasis highlighting the unique dissemination and the underlying mechanisms of regulation of the steps involved. The role of the microenvironment in the process of metastasis is also reviewed. **Chapter 4** highlights current data on the involvement of aquaporins (AQPs) in processes associated with malignant progression and discusses possible applications of AQP-based therapy as an effective means of inhibiting cancer cells from metastasis. In **Chapter 5** Soraj et al. discuss the current state of research on characterization of extracellular vesicles (EVs) and highlight possible strategies for their use in cancer therapy. In **Chapter 6**, Al-Taee et al. investigate the modulated gene expression of PDAC cells during liver colonization. Their results show that many genes and miRNAs are modulated significantly in expression during the early stage of liver colonization and continuously thereafter. These overall changes lead to distinguish certain categories and processes participating in cancer progression. **Chapter 7** reviews various methods of minimally invasive surgery for metastatic bone tumor and emphasizes on the PMMA bone cement injection technique. It also discusses optimal customized surgical options according to patient's circumstances.

Circulating tumor cells (CTCs) are defined as tumor cells which are detached from a primary tumor or metastasis into vasculature and can be detected in the bloodstream of cancer patients. In the tumor metastasis process, CTCs play a very important role; therefore, the study of CTCs is becoming crucial in cancer management. The next section of this book is "Circulating Tumor Cells." **Chapter 8** by Hsieh et al. introduces the role of circulating tumor cells in cancer progression and the strategies for CTC isolation and enumeration. It also reviews the clinical applications and important findings in clinical trials. In **Chapter 9**, Hu et al. demonstrate the value of multiparameter flow cytometry in detecting breast cancer cells in the peripheral blood, which has higher sensitivity and higher specificity compared with RT-PCR. They also find that CTC number is related to TNM stage, metastasis, and the overall survival of patients.

In the last section on "Epithelial-Mesenchymal Transition," **Chapter 10** introduces the key role of epithelial-mesenchymal transition (EMT) in cancer and discusses different elements of EMT cascades that could be targeted and also the difficulties in translating the preclinical findings in routine clinic. **Chapter 11** explores the significance of EMT in CTC formation and the role of EMT in cancer metastasis and resistance to therapy. It also reviews the past and current limitations of evaluating EMT phenotypes in CTC isolation and analysis.

We hope that the reviews and studies described here will provide a wide-ranging forum in the tumor metastasis field. Although significant progresses are made in tumor metastasis study, the mechanism of metastasis is still not fully understood. It is believed that based on novel achievements in metastasis study, more tumor patients will benefit from the new strategies on metastasis diagnosis and treatment, in particular the targeted therapy.

Ke Xu
Tianjin Lung Cancer Institute
Tianjin Medical University General Hospital
Tianjin, China

Section 1

Tumor Metastasis

Chapter 1

Hemostatic System in Malignancy: Providing the "Soil" in Metastatic Niche Formation

Elina Beleva, Veselin Popov and
Janet Grudeva-Popova

Additional information is available at the end of the chapter

http://dx.doi.org/10.5772/64697

Abstract

Malignancy arises and progresses in tight association with changes in the tumor microenvironment and deregulation of hemostatic system. Cancer induces hemostatic imbalance through production and secretion of procoagulant substances, suppression of anticoagulant mechanisms, endothelial activation, and angiogenic switch. Cancer cells are equipped with certain coagulation signaling receptors such as tissue factor (TF) and urokinase plasminogen activator receptor (uPAR). Tissue factor: as major initiator of coagulation, TF is considered the main cause for hypercoagulability in cancer. Constitutive TF expression by cancer cells is a hallmark of malignancy rendering tumors proangiogenic and prometastatic. TF fosters metastasis through coagulation-dependent pathways leading to fibrin deposition in the evolving premetastatic niche. TF has been identified as an independent predictor for metastatic development and adverse prognosis. uPAR: Tissue overexpression of uPAR is demonstrated in almost all human cancers and is associated with advanced disease. Increased uPAR expression is driven by molecular events involving K-ras and SRC oncogenes. Transactivation of these receptors, mediated by binding to hemostatic proteins, activates intracellular signaling pathways, modulates gene expression and facilitates processes of tumor initiation, epithelial-to-mesenchymal transition, anoikis, and metastasis. By manipulating hemostatic processes, tumor induces tolerant host environment necessary for evasion of defense attacks, survival, and progression.

Keywords: hemostasis, cancer, metastasis, tissue factor, urokinase plasminogen activator

1. Introduction

Malignancy is associated with derangement of the dynamic homeostasis of hemostatic system. Associated perturbations are characterized by various clinical manifestations with some of them infrequently being indicative of an occult cancer. The interaction between the presence of hemostatic imbalance and cancer has long been recognized. Starting first with the clinical observations by the French surgeon Armand Trousseau of increased thrombotic tendency in patients with advanced gastric cancer knowledge of the interrelationship between malignancy and hemostasis has since evolved conceptually into understanding its intrinsic biology. Relationship between hemostasis and cancer is bidirectional. On the one side, it is viewed as a process where the innate defense system of hemostasis modulates cancerous development. On the other side, tumor itself manipulates hemostatic system via paracrine regulatory mechanisms and utilizes hemostatic functions to induce host tolerance for its development and evasion of immune surveillance. Knowledge of the molecular and cellular processes involved in thrombosis in cancer and their differentiation from the physiological hemostasis is essential for understanding the factors driving the increased tumor-associated prothrombotic tendency. It also allows for identifying the certain hemostatic components as determinants of the neoplastic process and their incorporation into development of antitumor strategies.

2. Tumor prothrombotic mechanisms

Factors that enhance thrombogenicity of neoplasms are complex and reflect the interaction of a variety of mechanisms that can be summarized on the basis of the classical triad suggested by Virchow: hypercoagulability, vascular endothelial injury, and stasis.

2.1. Changes in hemostasis factors

Tumor cells have the properties to qualitatively and quantitatively modify plasma and cellular components of hemostasis either directly by synthesis and secretion of procoagulant substances or indirectly by intracellular cytokine-mediated mechanisms (**Table 1**).

2.1.1. Synthesis and secretion of procoagulant substances

Production of procoagulant components by the tumor cells enhances fibrin deposition at the sites of extravasation and extracellularly within the tumor microenvironment.

Tissue factor (TF)—cellular procoagulant and the main initiator of coagulation. Under physiological conditions, procoagulant active form of TF cannot be detected in circulation and on the surface of intact endothelium [1]. TF overexpression is considered a hallmark of the malignant phenotype, identified for the first time in the description of thromboplastin properties of leukemic cells [2]. Subsequently, high activity of TF was observed in the supernatant samples from patients with promyelocytic leukemia [3]. Constitutive expression of TF on neoplastically transformed cells has been confirmed by other authors. TF was found overexpressed on tumor cell surface of a number of cancers. TF overexpression is found on the surface of microparticles or is secreted into the tumor microenvironment [3, 4]. Increased TF-dependent procoagulant activity is observed in circulating tumor cells with stem cell phenotype [5]. By inducing proinflammatory response through synthesis and secretion of tumor cytokines: IL-1β, TNF-α, vascular endothelial growth factor (VEGF), malignant cells upregulate TF expression on the surface of monocytes/macrophages, endothelium [6–9], and the degree of tissue expression of TF in the primary tumor correlates with levels of the circulating antigen [10]. Overexpression of TF has a specific biological role in mediating tumor growth and metastasis [11].

Cysteine proteinase (CP)—endopeptidase with a molecular weight of 68 KDa, whose only known substrate is f.X. CP can directly activate f.X to f.Xa without involving f.VII, and unlike other activators of f.X, CP proteolytically cleaves its molecule at several sites [12]. It has been identified in extracts from embryonic tissues (amnion and chorion), solid tumors, and leukemic blasts [13–15]. CP has not been detected in extracts from normal tissues as well as in patients in complete remission. Its expression in acute promyelocytic leukemia is inhibited by treatment with all-trans-retinoic acid, which confirms the hypothesis that undifferentiated cells express CP and upon recovery of differentiation its expression is suppressed [16].

F.VII—a cofactor of tissue factor required for its procoagulant activity. Endogenously synthesized f.VII from non-hepatic tumor cells capable of activating the coagulation via f.Xa mediates proinvasive signaling pathways [17]. Proteolytically active f.VII in combination with TF induces anti-apoptotic effects and inhibits anoikis [18].

Prothrombin/thrombin—a key proteolytic enzyme of coagulation. It is produced by different tumor types and exerts pleiotropic biological effects in the processes of angiogenesis and tumor proliferation [19]. In patients with low-grade carcinoma, f.II induces intravascular coagulation, increases tumor platelet adhesion in vitro, and the formation of metastases in vivo [20].

F.VIII: vWF—various cancers are associated with elevated levels of von Willebrand factor (vWF) and f.VIII as a consequence of tumor-induced proinflammatory cytokine response (TNF-α, IL-6) [21–25].

F.V—cofactor of f.X. By expressing f.V receptor, activity tumor cells are functionally involved in catalyzing the prothrombinase complex [26]. Increased coagulation activity in patients with breast cancer is correlated with the presence of single nucleotide polymorphisms in the gene of f.V and increased thrombotic risk [27].

F.XIII—fibrin stabilizing factor. Tumor cells from breast cancer have f.XIII-like activity. By catalyzing fibrin cross-linking and deposition, they potentiate tumor growth and metastasis [28].

Fibrinogen/fibrin—electron microscopy analysis demonstrated that fibrin is an integral component of the examined tumors [29]. Fibrin deposition potentiates formation of metastatic emboli that trap circulating tumor cells in the vascular bed and promote adhesion to the endothelium [30]. Plasma fibrinogen levels are significantly elevated in patients with multiple myeloma and breast cancer at the time of diagnosis and during follow-up compared to healthy controls [31, 32].

Procoagulant microparticles (MP)—submicron extracellular vesicles. Their procoagulant capacity is determined by the expression of negatively charged phosphatidylserine and functionally active TF [33]. Increased MP-associated procoagulant activity was detected in patients with myeloproliferative neoplasms [34]. By intracellular exchange of MP, tumor cells transfer oncogenic signal and amplify the angiogenic phenotype [35].

Heparanase—endoglucuronidase that degrades heparan sulfate. Overexpressed in almost all known malignancies but has not been detected in normal tissue adjacent to the tumor. Tumor cells secrete heparanase, which induces the expression of TF, activates directly f.X, and inactivates tissue factor pathway inhibitor [36].

2.1.2. Suppression of natural anticoagulant mechanisms

Protein C (PrC)—inactivates Va and VIIIa in the presence of thrombin, and its functions are mediated by specific endothelial receptor. PrC performs cytoprotective and antimetastatic effects independently of coagulation [37]. Association between increased incidence of thrombotic events and acquired resistance to PrC (APC), unrelated to factor V Leiden, has been observed in multiple myeloma and colorectal cancer [38, 39]. There could be mechanisms of cell resistance due to the modification of the endothelial receptor and induction of APC under the influence of tumor proinflammatory cytokines [39, 40].

Protein S—cofactor PrC whose activity can be inhibited by circulating paraproteins [24].

Antithrombin III (ATIII)—a major serpin that inactivates factors IIa, IXa, Xa, XIa, XIIa, kallikrein, plasmin. Decreased levels of ATIII are found in patients with malignant diseases and decreased survival [41, 42].

Tissue factor pathway inhibitor (TFPI)—main inhibitor of the complex TF:VIIa. Overexpression of heparanase induces increase of functionally inactive TFPI in plasma (36), a putative role of a tumor suppressor gene [43, 44].

2.1.3. Defective fibrinolysis—hypofibrinolysis

Tumor cells expressed on their cellular surface all proteins necessary for regulation of the fibrinolytic pathways. Deregulation in generating normal fibrinolytic activity was observed in patients with solid tumors and is a mechanism for the development of thrombotic tendency [45].

Plasminogen activator inhibitor-1 (PAI-1)—important regulator of plasminogen activity. PAI-1 is overexpressed in different types of tumors [21]. Genomic sequencing of hepatocytes expressing the MET oncogene demonstrated significantly increased expression of the gene for PAI-1 and COX-2 that corresponded with triple increase in levels of circulating plasma proteins [46].

Thrombin-activated fibrinolysis inhibitor (TAFI)—blocks the binding of plasminogen to fibrin. Reported elevated levels of TAFI in patients with cancer and thromboembolic events were compared to patients with acute venous thrombosis and normal controls [47, 48].

Proteinase inhibitor of fibrinolysis (α2-antiplasmin, α2-macroglobulin)—secreted in the tumor microenvironment/in high doses/in cancers with increased risk of venous thromboembolism [49]. Immunohistochemical studies demonstrate the expression of fibrinolytic inhibitors only in tumor cells, which could explain the absence of fibrinolytic activity in some tumors [50].

2.2. Endothelial activation

Blood vessels and endothelial cells play a major role in the control of the processes of hemostasis, thrombosis, and inflammation. Endothelial tromboregulation is accomplished by selective expression of mediators (autacoids and cell adhesion molecules) in response to specific agonists. The synthesized mediators are involved in all phases of the hemostasic process and regulate/maintain vascular reactivity. Intact endothelium is anticoagulant and profibrinolytic under physiologic conditions. From the perspective of the Virchow's triad, endothelium loses its tromboresistive properties upon damage—for example, stretching of the vessel wall, mechanical and chemical injury, turbulent flow, inflammation. Malignant process causes deregulation of endothelial homeostasis, which can be defined more precisely as activation rather than damage as endothelial cells alter their functional capacity and acquire new properties in the absence of violation of tissue integrity [51]. Factors of endothelial activation in the presence of malignant process include the following: (a) dysfunctional endothelium—overexpression of adhesion molecules; (b) loss of anticoagulant and acquisition of procoagulant properties; and (c) switch to proangiogenic phenotype [52].

2.2.1. Overexpression of adhesion molecules

Endothelial expression of selectins and ligands from the immunoglobulin superfamily is increased under the effect of tumor-induced cytokine and cellular interactions. Tumor-associated macrophages secrete TNF-α, IL-1, IL-6, IFN-γ, which increase the expression of adhesion molecules through activation of de novo synthesis of mRNA [22]. Increased expression of adhesion molecules ICAM-1, VCAM-1, and E-selectin mediated by NF-κB transcriptional activation was found when co-culturing endothelial and tumor cells [53]. Gene profiling of bone marrow cells from patients with multiple myeloma shows increased expression of genes BNIP3, IER3, and SEPW1. Through their silencing by small interfering RNA processes such as endothelial proliferation, adhesion and capillary formation are influenced [54].

2.2.2. Procoagulant conversion and loss of anticoagulant properties

Thrombomodulin (TM)—important endothelial cell-associated receptor that acts as direct anticoagulant. Binding of thrombin activates PrC system and inactivates the proteolytic degradation of procoagulant substrates [55]. Circulating tumor cytokines decreases TM levels causing degradation of its molecule and increased endothelial expression of TF [56]. There is inverse proportional relationship between TM expression and cellular proliferation in vivo.

Downregulated to absent TM expression is found in metastatic foci, while forced expression of TM in transgenic mouse models of squamous cell carcinoma lacking TM expression leads to a differentiated epithelial-like phenotype—effect regulated by Snail transcription factor [57]. Interference of the TM-PrC system that occurs as a result of lower TM and development of acquired resistance to PrC of cellular type is one of the factors for procoagulant conversion of endothelium.

In response to stimuli from the tumor microenvironment, antagonistic deregulation is observed in endothelial expression of the pairs of vWF/ADAMTS13, TF TFPI, PAI-1/plasminogen activators. Cytokine-activated endothelium releases high-molecular complexes of vWF, which are hyper-reactive to platelet aggregation, thrombus formation, and adhesion, whereas expression of ADAMTS13 depolymerase is suppressed [58]. Local procoagulant activity of endothelium is potentiated further by the effects of heparanase, which induces expression of TF and simultaneously dissociates its inhibitor TFPI from the endothelial cell surface [59]. And last but not least, the endothelial cells as a primary source of fibrinolytic activators participate in the induction of hypofibrilinolitic state by defective secretion of plasminogen activators in enhancing the expression of a fibrinolytic inhibitor PAI-1 [60]. Different mechanisms of microvascular dysfunction in combination with activated coagulation are the main pathogenetic factors in the development of thrombotic microangiopathy in malignancies.

2.2.3. Switch to proangiogenic phenotype

Increased angiogenic activity is due to complex processes in which fully differentiated, nonproliferating endothelial cells acquire invasive, migratory, and proliferative properties. The processes of the angiogenic switch are determined by the increased production of positive regulators of angiogenesis (VEGF, FGF2, IL-8, PIGF, FGF-β, PDGF), which originate from tumor cells—they can be mobilized from the extracellular matrix or are released by stromal cells, recruited in the tumor [61]. At the same time, many of these processes are coupled with regulatory coagulation processes. For example, endothelial growth factor VEGF, secreted by the tumor cells, increases endothelial expression of TF, which causes inverse decrease in the expression of the negative angiogenic regulator—thrombospondin [62]. Synthesis and secretion of another potent proangiogenic cytokine—interleukin-8 (IL-8) from endothelial cells —are increased, and the effect is dose dependent on the levels of fibrin deposits [63]. A similar mechanism is responsible for fibrin-induced expression of the gene for TF from umbilical vascular endothelial cells [64]. Additionally, thrombin and coagulation degradation products mediate haptotaxis of endothelial cells by selective exposure of a set of integrins. Thereby, they orientate the formation of capillaries and vasculogenesis in the direction of the angiogenic stimulus [65, 66].

Angiopoietin-1,2/Tie2 system is a key regulator of physiologic endothelial angiogenic activity, which controls the proliferation and differentiation of endothelial cells during embryonic development. Tie2 is an endothelial-specific receptor tyrosine kinase whose ligands are angiopoietin-1 (Ang-1) and angiopoietin-2 (Ang-2). Angiopoietin-1 is secreted by perivascular cells and in complex with Tie2 stabilizes the endothelium in quiescent state and potentiates the maturation of blood vessels. Angiopoietin-2 acts as an antagonist of Ang-1/Tie2. It is overexpressed during tumor angiogenesis and is responsible for pro-angiogenic endothelial conversion [67]. Tumor blood vessels express structural and functional abnormalities such as abnormal vascular permeability and increased potential for rapid growth and remodeling due to overexpression of Ang-2 [68]. Experimental data support the interdependence of the processes of procoagulant and pro-angiogenic endothelial conversion. Ang-1 inhibits overexpression of TF in HUVECs in a putative mechanism of PI3/Akt signal activation [69]. Thrombin-induced angiogenesis in an in vivo model of chorion allantoic membrane is accompanied by a double increase in expression of mRNA, encoding VEGF and Ang2 [70].

Endothelium performs a crucial role as a regulatory nexus in the processes of hemostasis and angiogenesis. The complexity of interactions allows on the one hand multiple targeting of several pathological mechanisms involved in angiogenesis and tumor progression and on the other hand mediates expression of side effects associated with the system of hemostasis.

2.3. Impaired blood flow

In the context of Virchow triad, disturbed blood flow is a predisposing factor for thrombosis. Venous stasis is most often secondary—due to external compression of local or metastatic tumor masses, adenopathy—inflammation caused by the tumor. The main mechanism involves inadequate clearance of coagulation factors and local endothelial hypoxia that induces endothelial expression of TF and platelet activating factor, increased leukocyte adhesion and platelet activation. Additional predisposing factor is the prolonged immobilization of cancer patients both in hospital and at home. Additive effect of disturbances clearance of activated coagulation factors and hypoxic endothelial damage in conditions of prolonged immobilization contribute to the development of a thrombotic process.

3. Tissue factor

Besides its major role in hemostasis, TF has been identified as an important signaling receptor in cancer biology. Ample preclinical evidence has accumulated over the past decade, implicating TF as an important effector in the processes of tumor initiation, growth, angiogenesis, and metastasis. Moreover, this has led to the development of approaches exploring TF as a potential target for anticancer therapy [71]. TF is overexpressed in many types of human tumors, including breast cancer, pancreatic cancer, gastric cancer, prostate cancer, colorectal cancer, non-small-cell lung cancer, melanoma, leukemia, lymphoma, esophageal cancer, hepatocellular carcinoma, brain glioblastoma, but not in their normal tissue counterparts [1]. TF overexpression in cancer cells has been correlated with tumor progression and unfavorable prognostic indicators such as increased angiogenesis, advanced disease stage, and resistant phenotype [72–74]. Therefore, TF overexpression in situ could be considered a biomarker for solid tumors.

Enhanced TF expression in cancer has been reported to be an oncogenic-driven event. In colorectal cancer, activation of the K-ras oncogene and loss-of-function mutation of p53 result in constitutive activation of mitogen-activated protein kinase (MAPK) and PI3K pathways leading to increased TF expression [75]. In turn, inhibition of the PI3K and MAPK by restoration of the PTEN tumor suppressor gene in glioma cells downregulates TF expression dependent on EGFR amplification [76]. In medulloblastoma cell lines, TF expression has been shown to result from mutation in the c-Met oncogene and subsequent activation of Src kinases [77]. It has been observed that a certain subset of tumor cells, known as cancer stem cells, which constitutively express activated oncogenes and are capable of undergoing multilineage differentiation, are characterized by TF abundant phenotype [5]. Moreover, enhanced TF expression is observed during the processes of epithelial-to-mesenchymal-transition, whereby epithelial cells acquire a mesenchymal, more aggressive and motile phenotype [78]. This indicates that TF is possibly involved in maintaining cancer cell self-perpetuance.

There is a structure function dependency in TF mode of action. TF plays a role in cancer progression both by initiating tumor growth and by promoting efficient tumor cell dissemination. Tumor-promoting activities of TF occur via non-hemostatic mechanism and can be attributed to the cytoplasmic domain signaling dependent mostly on the activation of the protease activated receptor 2 (PAR2). Prometastatic properties of TF can rather be coupled with its extracellular domain and the subsequent generation of thrombin, which, as a potent growth factor, exhibits further pleiotropic cellular effects.

TF-mediated signaling is critical for both physiological and pathological angiogenesis. TF deficiency in murine knockout experiments caused early embryonic lethality due to impaired vasculature development [79]. Zhang et al. demonstrated that tumors overexpressing TF become highly vascularized once implanted into mice and the observed growth induction could not be inhibited despite maximal anticoagulation [80]. It has been revealed that involvement of TF cytoplasmic domain in several transduction cascades accounts for the production by tumor cells of angiogenic cytokines and contributes to increased angiogenesis in a paracrine fashion [81]. Formation of the complex TF/VIIa leads to increase of intracellular Ca^{2+} and phosphorylation of serine residues on TF cytoplasmic tail. This triggers signaling via the G-protein coupled membrane receptor PAR2 that activates MAPK and PI3K transduction cascades, resulting in increased gene expression of the angiogenic cytokines VEGF, VEGF-C, CXCL1, Il-8, and Cyr61 [82–84]. In addition to PAR2 signaling, the cytoplasmic domain of TF can be phosphorylated independently of f.VII ligand binding by protein kinase C (PKC) resulting in the transcriptional activation of VEGF, VEGFR, TGF, and suppressed expression of anti-angiogenic molecules such as thrombospondin [85, 86]. The relationship between TF and VEGF has been extensively studied and is manifested by reciprocal co-stimulation of their expression profiles. VEGF induces TF expression by orchestrating the binding of nuclear factors NFAT and AP-1 to the promoter region of TF gene [87]. Regulation of VEGF is in turn dependent on the TF cytoplasmic domain signaling, which is demonstrated by the finding that tumor cells transfected with truncated TF cDNA lacking the cytoplasmic domain fail to produce VEGF, but preserve the TF procoagulant function [86]. Experimental ex vivo and in vivo studies have further supported the TF-VEGF interrelationship by finding increased co-expression on tumor sections and their association with increased angiogenesis and malignant potential in human tumors [73–75, 88, 89].

http://dx.doi.org/10.5772/64697

TF enhances tumor growth via TF/VIIa/PAR2 signaling. This is evidenced by studies on cancer cell lines, where overexpression of TF by cancer cells conferred growth advantage compared to cell lines expressing low levels of TF [71, 86]. Delay in primary and metastatic tumor growth was observed after specific TF/VIIa inhibition with the anticoagulant rNAPc2 but not after inhibition of f.Xa [90]. Studies on selective targeting of different domains of the complex TF:VIIa revealed that PAR2 signaling and integrin ligation is sufficient for TF tumor-promoting properties [91].

Prometastatic properties of TF can be attributed to its extracellular domain, which is required for its major role in triggering coagulation. The extracellular mutant domain (TFmut) has markedly diminished function for activation of f.X, while full-length or cytoplasmic tail-deleted TF retains its procoagulant activity [85, 92]. The expression of TF in tumors can induce downstream coagulation activation via the TF/VIIa/Xa pathway leading to fibrin and tumor stroma formation. Tumor cells become encapsulated in fibrin and platelet-rich thrombi, being protected from the host immune defense and arrest in the microcirculation. Local thrombin formation facilitates arrest of tumor cells to the vessel wall by upregulation of adhesion molecules and strengthening cell-to-cell junctions [93]. Fibrin matrix in the tumor stroma builds itself a multifunctional scaffold rich on growth factors such as platelet derived growth factor (PDGF), transforming growth factor (TGF), fibroblast growth factor (FGF), that is not only protective, but also promotes matrix-cell interactions necessary for neovascularization [94]. Thrombin, constitutively generated by the activated coagulation cascade in the tumor surrounding, mobilizes the adhesion molecules αIIbβ3-integrin, P-selectin, CD40 ligand, and enhances tumor cell interactions to platelets, endothelial cells and matrix [95–97]. Thrombin has also an important function in angiogenesis by inducing the activation of endothelial-secreted collagenase type IV, which degrades basement matrix proteins and collagen during neoangiogenesis [98]. In vivo experimental models of metastasis demonstrated dramatic increase of lung metastasis with thrombin-treated tumor cells compared with untreated cells [99].

In summary, TF-mediated effects either in a coagulation-independent mechanism via direct cytoplasmic domain signaling and TF/VIIa/PAR2 or dependent on the coagulation products induce diverse sets of cellular responses inherent to tumor cells including tumor growth, neoangiogenesis, cell migration, and metastasis. Taking into account the specific biologic role of TF in the malignant tissue, detecting circulating TF in cancer patients might be informative of active disease and ongoing processes of matrix reorganization, cell destruction, and neovascularization.

4. uPA/uPAR system

The physiologic role of fibrinolysis is dissolution of the fibrin clot and collagen degradation exerted by the action of plasmin. Generation of plasmin, the main enzyme in fibrinolysis, occurs upon activation of plasminogen by the tissue plasminogen activator (tPA) and the urokinase plasminogen activator (uPA).Therefore, function of the urokinase plasminogen activator (uPA) and its high-affinity cellular receptor (uPAR) is critical for fibrinolytic activities including targeted degradation of the basement matrix. Moreover, uPAR is motile within the cellular membrane, which allows its allocation at the cellular front of desired direction for proteolysis [100]. Under normal conditions, the process of active proteolysis is tightly controlled by the proteolytic systems.

In cancer, biology activation of uPA/uPAR system is a prerequisite for efficient focal proteolysis, adhesion, migration and enables penetrating tumor cells to invade and metastasize [101]. Extracellular matrix proteolysis acts at all stages of the metastatic cascade: detachment of tumor cells from primary site, intravasation, hematogeneous dissemination, extravasation, and metastases formation. These processes are executed by proteolytic enzymatic systems, including uPA/uPAR, matrix metalloproteinases, and cysteine proteinases, which interact synergistically and are responsible for the complex proteolytic activity of tumors [102].

The cellular receptor for the urokinase plasminogen activator (uPAR) is a key molecule for efficient pericellular proteolysis. Apart from potentiating proteolytic activity, the complex uPA/uPAR ignites series of intracellular signaling events associated with the processes of proliferation, adhesion, chemotaxis, migration, and angiogenesis. Tissue overexpression of uPA/uPAR is found in various human tumors—breast, prostate, GIT, and lung. It is associated with advanced disease and is independent adverse prognostic factor for survival [103]. Direct involvement of uPAR in processes of tumor biology characterizes it as a hallmark of the malignant invasive phenotype. Overexpression of uPAR cDNA in osteosarcoma cells increases its ability to penetrate the basal membrane [104]. Invasive potential of tumor cells in chorion-allantois membrane of chicken embryos correlates with uPAR-associated proteolytic activity [105]. Expression of uPAR gene by tumor cells is required for vascular intravasation, whereas uPAR gene expression decreases invasive potential of transformed fibroblasts in vitro [106]. Experiments with anti-uPAR inhibitory antibodies demonstrate reduction of the matric proteolytic activity [107, 108]. Levels and activity of uPAR are regulated at the transcriptional level by oncogene-controlled promoter activation. uPAR promoter region contains binding motifs for several transcriptional factors that regulate cellular differentiation, migration, and apoptosis: specific protein 1 (SP1), activator protein 1 (AP1) and activator protein 2 (AP2) [109]. uPAR basal expression is regulated proximally from SP1 transcriptional starting point. In tumor models of colorectal cancer, constitutive, and induced uPAR expression is regulated by AP1 binding motif via MAPK and c-JUN NH_2-terminal kinase (JNK) signaling [110]. AP2 binding motif is required for constitutive overexpression of uPAR promoter activity in invasive tumor cells after stimulation by the tumor promoter phorbol acetate.

The role of K-ras and SRC oncogenes in uPAR regulation has been identified. K-ras regulates uPAR mediated proteolysis by transcriptional binding of AP1 to the promoter motif. Down-regulation of promoter activity as in deletion of the AP1 binding activity has been observed in tumor clones with K-ras allelic deletion. The knockout effect is accompanied by significant reduction of uPAR expression and tumor-associated proteolysis [111]. Increased uPAR protein expression and laminin degradation parallel to c-SRC activation are observed in SW 480 cells transfected to constitutively overexpress s-SRC. Elevated uPAR expression is due to transcriptional activation secondary to increased binding of SP1 to the complementary promoter motif. This defines SP1 as distal factor of c-SRC-mediated regulation of uPAR [109]. Tissue overexpression of uPA/uPAR has been detected in many human tumors like breast, prostate, gastrointestinal, and lung cancers. Oncogenes responsible for enhancement of uPA/uPAR expression in malignant tissue include ras, jun, myc, fos, rel, and ets. uPAR expression can also be stimulated by the expression of TF and the epidermal growth factor receptor (EGFR) [112].

Factor	Coagulation function	Role in tumor biology
f.I (fibrinogen)	Formation of the hemostatic clot	Potentiates formation of metastatic emboli and enhances survival of tumor cells
f.II (prothrombin/thrombin)	Converts fibrinogen to fibrin	Growth factor, role in angiogenesis, tumor proliferation, and metastasis formation
f.III (tissue factor)	Major initiator of coagulation	Exerts proangiogenic and prometastatic effects, role in tumor growth initiation
f.VII	Cofactor for TF	Inhibition of anoikis, supports tumor invasion
f. XIII	Stabilizes fibrin	Potentiates tumor growth and metastasis
Cysteine proteinase	Direct activator of f.X has not been identified in healthy individuals	Suppressed expression by blasts upon differentiation
Heparanase	Degradation of heparan sulfate	Local invasion and metastasis
Protein C	Anticoagulant function via Va and VIIIa inactivation	Activated PrC resistance related to loss of cytoprotective and antimetastatic effects
Tissue factor pathway inhibitor	Main inhibitor of the complex TF:VIIa	Putative role of a tumor suppressor gene
Plasminogen activator inhibitor-1 (PAI-1)	Regulator of plasminogen activity	Overexpression found in various tumor types, related to MET oncogene
uPA/uPAR system	Generation of plasmin	Focal proteolysis, tumor cell invasion and migration
Thrombomodulin	Direct anticoagulant via thrombin binding and PrC activation	Forced TM expression in cancer cells lacking TM leads to differentiated phenotype via Snail

Table 1. Coagulation function vs. role in tumor biology of hemostatic factors.

Fibrinolytic system components can be identified as determinants of invasion in tumor biology and reflect the metastatic potential of tumors.

5. Conclusion

Identification of hemostatic system as a component of the tumor microenvironment would provide a research scaffold for novel determinants of tumor progression. The role of hemostatic components in the processes of tumor growth, angiogenesis, invasion, and metastasis makes them an accessible potential target for targeted therapy. Analysis of their predictive and prognostic value as surrogate biomarkers for tumor-induced events would yield development of novel tools for monitoring and antitumor strategies.

Author details

Elina Beleva*, Veselin Popov and Janet Grudeva-Popova

*Address all correspondence to: elina_beleva@yahoo.de

Department of Clinical Oncology, Medical Faculty, Medical University—Plovdiv, Plovdiv, Bulgaria

References

[1] Chu AJ. Tissue factor, blood coagulation, and beyond: an overview. Int J Inflam. 2011;2011:367284.

[2] Eisemann G, Stefanini M. Thromboplastic activity of leukemic white cells. Proc Soc Exp Biol Med. 1954;86(4):763–5.

[3] Gralnick HR, Abrell E. Studies of the procoagulant and fibrinolytic activity of promyelocytes in acute promyelocytic leukaemia. Br J Haematol. 1973;24(1):89–99.

[4] Shoji M, Hancock WW, Abe K, Micko C, Casper KA, Baine RM, et al. Activation of coagulation and angiogenesis in cancer: immunohistochemical localization in situ of clotting proteins and vascular endothelial growth factor in human cancer. Am J Pathol. 1998;152(2):399–411.

[5] Milsom C, Anderson GM, Weitz JI, Rak J. Elevated tissue factor procoagulant activity in CD133-positive cancer cells. J Thromb Haemost. 2007;5(12):2550–2.

[6] Sallah S, Wan JY, Nguyen NP, Hanrahan LR, Sigounas G. Disseminated intravascular coagulation in solid tumors: clinical and pathologic study. Thromb Haemost. 2001;86(3):828–33.

[7] Contrino J, Hair G, Kreutzer DL, Rickles FR. In situ detection of tissue factor in vascular endothelial cells: correlation with the malignant phenotype of human breast disease. Nat Med. 1996;2(2):209–15.

[8] Cozzolino F, Torcia M, Miliani A, Carossino AM, Giordani R, Cinotti S, et al. Potential role of interleukin-1 as the trigger for diffuse intravascular coagulation in acute nonlymphoblastic leukemia. Am J Med. 1988;84(2):240–50.

[9] Moore KL, Esmon CT, Esmon NL. Tumor necrosis factor leads to the internalization and degradation of thrombomodulin from the surface of bovine aortic endothelial cells in culture. Blood. 1989;73(1):159–65.

[10] Rao LV. Tissue factor as a tumor procoagulant. Cancer Metastasis Rev. 1992;11(3–4): 249–66.

[11] Rak J, Milsom C, May L, Klement P, Yu J. Tissue factor in cancer and angiogenesis: the molecular link between genetic tumor progression, tumor neovascularization, and cancer coagulopathy. Semin Thromb Hemost. 2006;32(1):54–70.

[12] Gordon SG, Mourad AM. The site of activation of factor X by cancer procoagulant. Blood Coagul Fibrinolysis. 1991;2(6):735–9.

[13] Falanga A, Alessio MG, Donati MB, Barbui T. A new procoagulant in acute leukemia. Blood. 1988;71(4):870–5.

[14] Kwaan HC, Parmar S, Wang J. Pathogenesis of increased risk of thrombosis in cancer. Semin Thromb Hemost. 2003;29(3):283–90.

[15] Gordon SG, Hasiba U, Cross BA, Poole MA, Falanga A. Cysteine proteinase procoagulant from amnion-chorion. Blood. 1985;66(6):1261–5.

[16] Falanga A, Consonni R, Marchetti M, Locatelli G, Garattini E, Passerini CG, et al. Cancer procoagulant and tissue factor are differently modulated by all-trans-retinoic acid in acute promyelocytic leukemia cells. Blood. 1998;92(1):143–51.

[17] Koizume S, Jin MS, Miyagi E, Hirahara F, Nakamura Y, Piao JH, et al. Activation of cancer cell migration and invasion by ectopic synthesis of coagulation factor VII. Cancer Res. 2006;66(19):9453–60.

[18] Sorensen BB, Rao LV, Tornehave D, Gammeltoft S, Petersen LC. Antiapoptotic effect of coagulation factor VIIa. Blood. 2003;102(5):1708–15.

[19] Nash GF, Walsh DC, Kakkar AK. The role of the coagulation system in tumour angiogenesis. Lancet Oncol. 2001;2(10):608–13.

[20] Nierodzik ML, Plotkin A, Kajumo F, Karpatkin S. Thrombin stimulates tumor-platelet adhesion in vitro and metastasis in vivo. J Clin Invest. 1991;87(1):229–36.

[21] Zwicker JI, Furie BC, Furie B. Cancer-associated thrombosis. Crit Rev Oncol Hematol. 2007;62(2):126–36.

[22] Franchini M, Montagnana M, Targher G, Manzato F, Lippi G. Pathogenesis, clinical and laboratory aspects of thrombosis in cancer. J Thromb Thrombolysis. 2007;24(1):29–38.

[23] Elice F, Jacoub J, Rickles FR, Falanga A, Rodeghiero F. Hemostatic complications of angiogenesis inhibitors in cancer patients. Am J Hematol. 2008;83(11):862–70.

[24] Auwerda JJ, Sonneveld P, de Maat MP, Leebeek FW. Prothrombotic coagulation abnormalities in patients with newly diagnosed multiple myeloma. Haematologica. 2007;92(2):279–80.

[25] Vormittag R, Simanek R, Ay C, Dunkler D, Quehenberger P, Marosi C, et al. High factor VIII levels independently predict venous thromboembolism in cancer patients: the cancer and thrombosis study. Arterioscler Thromb Vasc Biol. 2009;29(12):2176–81.

[26] VanDeWater L, Tracy PB, Aronson D, Mann KG, Dvorak HF. Tumor cell generation of thrombin via functional prothrombinase assembly. Cancer Res. 1985;45(11 Pt 1):5521–5.

[27] Tinholt M, Viken MK. Common genetic polymorphisms in the coagulation factors 5 and 10 genes are associated with risk of breast cancer and correlate with increased coagulation activity (121/3290F). Presented at the Annual Meeting of the American Society of Human Genetics, Boston, MA, October 25, 2013.

[28] Hettasch JM, Bandarenko N, Burchette JL, Lai TS, Marks JR, Haroon ZA, et al. Tissue transglutaminase expression in human breast cancer. Lab Invest. 1996;75(5):637–45.

[29] Costantini V, Zacharski LR. Fibrin and cancer. Thromb Haemost. 1993;69(5):406–14.

[30] Palumbo JS, Kombrinck KW, Drew AF, Grimes TS, Kiser JH, Degen JL, et al. Fibrinogen is an important determinant of the metastatic potential of circulating tumor cells. Blood. 2000;96(10):3302–9.

[31] van Marion AM, Auwerda JJ, Lisman T, Sonneveld P, de Maat MP, Lokhorst HM, et al. Prospective evaluation of coagulopathy in multiple myeloma patients before, during and after various chemotherapeutic regimens. Leuk Res. 2008;32(7):1078–84.

[32] Kirwan CC, McDowell G, McCollum CN, Kumar S, Byrne GJ. Early changes in the haemostatic and procoagulant systems after chemotherapy for breast cancer. Br J Cancer. 2008;99(7):1000–6.

[33] Falanga A, Tartari CJ, Marchetti M. Microparticles in tumor progression. Thromb Res. 2012;129(Suppl. 1):S132–6.

[34] Trappenburg MC, van Schilfgaarde M, Marchetti M, Spronk HM, ten Cate H, Leyte A, et al. Elevated procoagulant microparticles expressing endothelial and platelet markers in essential thrombocythemia. Haematologica. 2009;94(7):911–8.

[35] Al-Nedawi K, Meehan B, Rak J. Microvesicles: messengers and mediators of tumor progression. Cell Cycle. 2009;8(13):2014–8.

[36] Nadir Y, Brenner B. Heparanase multiple effects in cancer. Thromb Res. 2014;133(Suppl. 2):S90–4.

[37] Bouwens EA, Stavenuiter F, Mosnier LO. Mechanisms of anticoagulant and cytoprotective actions of the protein C pathway. J Thromb Haemost. 2013;11(Suppl. 1):242–53.

[38] Elice F, Fink L, Tricot G, Barlogie B, Zangari M. Acquired resistance to activated protein C (aAPCR) in multiple myeloma is a transitory abnormality associated with an increased risk of venous thromboembolism. Br J Haematol. 2006;134(4):399–405.

[39] Ferroni P, Riondino S, Portarena I, Formica V, La Farina F, Martini F, et al. Association between increased tumor necrosis factor alpha levels and acquired activated protein C resistance in patients with metastatic colorectal cancer. Int J Colorectal Dis. 2012;27(12):1561–7.

[40] Castoldi E, Rosing J. APC resistance: biological basis and acquired influences. J Thromb Haemost. 2010;8(3):445–53.

[41] Unsal E, Atalay F, Atikcan S, Yilmaz A. Prognostic significance of hemostatic parameters in patients with lung cancer. Respir Med. 2004;98(2):93–8.

[42] Dixit A, Kannan M, Mahapatra M, Choudhry VP, Saxena R. Roles of protein C, protein S, and antithrombin III in acute leukemia. Am J Hematol. 2006;81(3):171–4.

[43] Stavik B, Skretting G, Aasheim HC, Tinholt M, Zernichow L, Sletten M, et al. Downregulation of TFPI in breast cancer cells induces tyrosine phosphorylation signaling and increases metastatic growth by stimulating cell motility. BMC Cancer. 2011;11:357.

[44] Zhu B, Zhang P, Zeng P, Huang Z, Dong TF, Gui YK, et al. Tissue factor pathway inhibitor-2 silencing promotes hepatocellular carcinoma cell invasion in vitro. Anat Rec (Hoboken). 2013;296(11):1708–16.

[45] Rocha E, Páramo JA, Fernández FJ, Cuesta B, Hernández M, Paloma MJ, et al. Clotting activation and impairment of fibrinolysis in malignancy. Thromb Res. 1989;54(6):699–707.

[46] Boccaccio C, Sabatino G, Medico E, Girolami F, Follenzi A, Reato G, et al. The MET oncogene drives a genetic programme linking cancer to haemostasis. Nature. 2005;434(7031):396–400.

[47] Kaftan O, Kasapoglu B, Koroglu M, Kosar A, Yalcin SK. Thrombin-activatable fibrinolysis inhibitor in breast cancer patients. Med Princ Pract. 2011;20(4):332–5.

[48] Radu CM, Spiezia L, Campello E, Gavasso S, Woodhams B, Simioni P. Thrombin activatable fibrinolysis inhibitor in cancer patients with and without venous thromboembolism. Thromb Res. 2013;132(4):484–6.

[49] Keohane ME, Hall SW, VandenBerg SR, Gonias SL. Secretion of alpha 2-macroglobulin, alpha 2-antiplasmin, and plasminogen activator inhibitor-1 by glioblastoma multiforme in primary organ culture. J Neurosurg. 1990;73(2):234–41.

[50] Kwaan HC, Radosevich JA, Xu CG, Lastre C. Tissue plasminogen activator and inhibitors of fibrinolysis in malignant melanoma. Tumour Biol. 1988;9(6):301–6.

[51] Pober JS. Warner-Lambert/Parke-Davis award lecture. Cytokine-mediated activation of vascular endothelium. Physiology and pathology. Am J Pathol. 1988;133(3):426–33.

[52] Blann AD. Endothelial cell activation markers in cancer. Thromb Res. 2012;129(Suppl. 1):S122–6.

[53] Haddad O, Chotard-Ghodsnia R, Verdier C, Duperray A. Tumor cell/endothelial cell tight contact upregulates endothelial adhesion molecule expression mediated by NFkappaB: differential role of the shear stress. Exp Cell Res. 2010;316(4):615–26.

[54] Ria R, Todoerti K, Berardi S, Coluccia AM, De Luisi A, Mattioli M, et al. Gene expression profiling of bone marrow endothelial cells in patients with multiple myeloma. Clin Cancer Res. 2009;15(17):5369–78.

[55] Esmon CT. The roles of protein C and thrombomodulin in the regulation of blood coagulation. J Biol Chem. 1989;264(9):4743–6.

[56] Moore KL, Esmon CT, Esmon NL. Tumor necrosis factor leads to the internalization and degradation of thrombomodulin from the surface of bovine aortic endothelial cells in culture. Blood. 1989;73(1):159–65.

[57] Vega S, Morales AV, Ocaña OH, Valdés F, Fabregat I, Nieto MA. Snail blocks the cell cycle and confers resistance to cell death. Genes Dev. 2004;18(10):1131–43.

[58] Bernardo A, Ball C, Nolasco L, Moake JF, Dong JF. Effects of inflammatory cytokines on the release and cleavage of the endothelial cell-derived ultralarge von Willebrand factor multimers under flow. Blood. 2004;104(1):100–6.

[59] Nadir Y, Brenner B, Gingis-Velitski S, Levy-Adam F, Ilan N, Zcharia E, et al. Heparanase induces tissue factor pathway inhibitor expression and extracellular accumulation in endothelial and tumor cells. Thromb Haemost. 2008;99(1):133–41.

[60] Levi M, Lensing AW, Büller HR, Prandoni P, Dooijewaard G, Cuppini S, et al. Deep vein thrombosis and fibrinolysis. Defective urokinase type plasminogen activator release. Thromb Haemost. 1991;66(4):426–9.

[61] Ribatti D, Nico B, Crivellato E, Roccaro AM, Vacca A. The history of the angiogenic switch concept. Leukemia. 2007;21(1):44–52.

[62] Zhang Y, Deng Y, Luther T, Müller M, Ziegler R, Waldherr R, et al. Tissue factor controls the balance of angiogenic and antiangiogenic properties of tumor cells in mice. J Clin Invest. 1994;94(3):1320–7.

[63] Qi J, Goralnick S, Kreutzer DL. Fibrin regulation of interleukin-8 gene expression in human vascular endothelial cells. Blood. 1997;90(9):3595–602.

[64] Contrino J, Goralnick S, Qi J, Hair G, Rickles FR, Kreutzer DL. Fibrin induction of tissue factor expression in human vascular endothelial cells. Circulation. 1997;96(2):605–13.

[65] Browder T, Folkman J, Pirie-Shepherd S. The hemostatic system as a regulator of angiogenesis. J Biol Chem. 2000;275(3):1521–4.

[66] Felding-Habermann B, Ruggeri ZM, Cheresh DA. Distinct biological consequences of integrin alpha v beta 3-mediated melanoma cell adhesion to fibrinogen and its plasmic fragments. J Biol Chem. 1992;267(8):5070–7.

[67] Saharinen P, Eklund L, Alitalo K. Angiopoietins and Tie receptors. In: Figg WD, Folkman J, editors. Angiogenesis an Integrative Approach from Science to Medicine. New York: Springer Science+ Business Media, LLC; 2008.

[68] Eklund L, Olsen BR. Tie receptors and their angiopoietin ligands are context-dependent regulators of vascular remodeling. Exp Cell Res. 2006;312(5):630–41.

[69] Kim I, Oh JL, Ryu YS, So JN, Sessa WC, Walsh K, et al. Angiopoietin-1 negatively regulates expression and activity of tissue factor in endothelial cells. FASEB J. 2002;16(1):126–8.

[70] Caunt M, Huang YQ, Brooks PC, Karpatkin S. Thrombin induces neoangiogenesis in the chick chorioallantoic membrane. J Thromb Haemost. 2003;1(10):2097–102.

[71] Liu Y, Jiang P, Capkova K, et al. Tissue factor-activated coagulation cascade in the tumor microenvironment is critical for tumor progression and an effective target for therapy. Cancer Res. 2011;71:6492–502.

[72] Lwaleed B, Cooper A. Tissue factor expression and multidrug resistance in cancer: two aspects of a common cellular response to a hostile milieu. Med Hypotheses. 2000;55:470–3.

[73] Poon R, Lau C, Ho J, et al. Tissue factor expression correlates with tumor angiogenesis and invasiveness in human hepatocellular carcinoma. Clin Cancer Res. 2003;9:5339–45.

[74] Khorana A, Ahrendt S, Ryan C, et al. Tissue factor expression, angiogenesis, and thrombosis in pancreatic cancer. Clin Cancer Res. 2007;13:2870–75.

[75] Yu J, May L, Lhotak V, et al. Oncogenic events regulate tissue factor expression in colorectal cancer cells: implications for tumor progression and angiogenesis. Blood. 2005;105:1734–41.

[76] Rong Y, Belozerov V, Tucker-Burden C, et al. Epidermal growth factor receptor and PTEN modulate tissue factor expression in glioblastoma through JunD/activator protein-1 transcriptional activity. Cancer Res. 2009;69:2540–9.

[77] Provençal M, Berger-Thibault N, Labbé D, et al. Tissue factor mediates the HGF/Met-induced anti-apoptotic pathway in DAOY medulloblastoma cells. J Neurooncol. 2010;97:365–72.

[78] Milsom C, Yu J, Mackman N, et al. Tissue factor regulation by epidermal growth factor receptor and epithelial-to-mesenchymal transitions: effect on tumor initiation and angiogenesis. Cancer Res. 2008;68:10068–76.

[79] Carmeliet P, Mackman N, Moons L, et al. Role of tissue factor in embryonic blood vessel development. Nature. 1996;383(6595):73–75.

[80] Zhang Y, Deng Y, Luther T, et al. Tissue factor controls the balance of angiogenic and antiangiogenic properties of tumor cells in mice. J Clin Invest. 1994;94:1320–7.

[81] van den Berg YW, Osanto S, Reitsma PH, Versteeg HH. The relationship between tissue factor and cancer progression: insights from bench and bedside. Blood. 2012;119:924–32.

[82] Liu Y, Mueller B. Protease-activated receptor-2 regulates vascular endothelial growth factor expression in MDA-MB-231 cells via MAPK pathways. Biochem Biophys Res Commun. 2006;344:1263–70.

[83] Hjortoe G, Petersen L, Albrektsen T, et al. Tissue factor-factor VIIa–specific up-regulation of IL-8 expression in MDA-MB-231 cells is mediated by PAR-2 and results in increased cell migration. Blood. 2004;103:3029–37.

[84] Albrektsen T, Sørensen B, Hjortø G, et al. Transcriptional program induced by factor VIIa-tissue factor, PAR1 and PAR2 in MDA-MB-231 cells. J Thromb Haemost. 2007;5:1588–97.

[85] Shoji M, Abe K, Nawroth P, et al. Molecular mechanisms linking thrombosis and angiogenesis in cancer. Trends Cardiovasc Med. 1997;7:52–9.

[86] Abe K, Shoji M, Chen J, et al. Regulation of vascular endothelial growth factor production and angiogenesis by the cytoplasmic tail of tissue factor. Proc Natl Acad Sci U S A. 1999;96:8663–8.

[87] Armesilla A, Lorenzo E, Gómez del Arco P, et al. Vascular endothelial growth factor activates nuclear factor of activated T cells in human endothelial cells: a role for tissue factor gene expression. Mol Cell Biol. 1999;19:2032–43.

[88] Nakasaki T, Wada H, Shigemori C, et al. Expression of tissue factor and vascular endothelial growth factor is associated with angiogenesis in colorectal cancer. Am J Hematol. 2002;69:247–54.

[89] Shigemori C, Wada H, Matsumoto K, et al. Tissue factor expression and metastatic potential of colorectal cancer. Thromb Haemost. 1998;80:894–8.

[90] Beleva E, Grudeva-Popova J. From Virchow's triad to metastasis. JBUON. 2013;18(1): 25–33.

[91] Versteeg H, Schaffner F, Kerver M, et al. Inhibition of tissue factor signaling suppresses tumor growth. Blood. 2008;111:190–9.

[92] Ruf W, Miles D, Rehemtulla A, et al. Tissue factor residues 157–167 are required for efficient proteolytic activation of factor X and factor VII. J Biol Chem. 1992;267:22206–10.

[93] Ruf W, Mueller B. Tissue factor in cancer angiogenesis and metastasis. Curr Opin Hematol. 1996;3:379–84.

[94] Nagy J, Brown L, Senger D, et al. Pathogenesis of tumor stroma generation: a critical role for leaky blood vessels and fibrin deposition. Biochim Biophys Acta. 1989;948:305–26.

[95] Wojtukiewicz M, Tang D, Nelson K, et al. Thrombin enhances tumor cell adhesive and metastatic properties via increased alpha IIb beta 3 expression on the cell surface. Thromb Res. 1992;68:233–45.

[96] Stenberg P, McEver R, Shuman MA, et al. A platelet alpha-granule membrane protein (GMP-140) is expressed on the plasma membrane after activation. J Cell Biol. 1985;101:880–6.

[97] Henn V, Slupsky J, Grafe M, et al. CD40 ligand on activated platelets triggers an inflammatory reaction of endothelial cells. Nature. 1998;391(6667):591–4.

[98] Zucker S, Mirza H, Conner C, et al. Vascular endothelial growth factor induces tissue factor and matrix metalloproteinase production in endothelial cells: conversion of prothrombin to thrombin results in progelatinase A activation and cell proliferation. Int J Cancer. 1998;75:780–6.

[99] Nierodzik M, Kajumo F, Karpatkin S. Effect of thrombin treatment of tumor cells on adhesion of tumor cells to platelets in vitro and tumor metastasis in vivo. Cancer Res. 1992;52:3267–72.

[100] Thunø M, Macho B, Eugen-Olsen J. SuPAR: the molecular crystal ball. Dis Markers. 2009;27:157–72.

[101] Schmitt M, Harbeck N, Thomssen C, et al. Clinical impact of the plasminogen activation system in tumor invasion and metastasis: prognostic relevance and target for therapy. Thromb Haemost. 1997;78:285–96.

[102] Schmitt M, Harbeck N, Thomssen C, Wilhelm O, Magdolen V, Reuning U, et al. Clinical impact of the plasminogen activation system in tumor invasion and metastasis: prognostic relevance and target for therapy. Thromb Haemost. 1997;78(1):285–96.

[103] Korte W. Changes of the coagulation and fibrinolysis system in malignancy: their possible impact on future diagnostic and therapeutic procedures. Clin Chem Lab Med. 2000;38(8):679–92.

[104] Taniguchi T, Kakkar AK, Toddenham EG, Wlliamson RC, Lemoine NR. Enhanced expression of urokinase receptor induced through the tissue factor-factor VIIa pathway in human pancreatic cancer. Cancer Res. 1998;58(19):4461–7.

[105] Ossowski L. In vivo invasion of modified chorioallantoic membrane by tumor cells: the role of cell surface-bound urokinase. J Cell Biol. 1988;107(6 Pt 1):2437–45.

[106] Quattrone A, Fibbi G, Anichini E, Pucci M, Zamperini A, Capaccioli S, et al. Reversion of the invasive phenotype of transformed human fibroblasts by anti-messenger oligonucleotide inhibition of urokinase receptor gene expression. Cancer Res. 1995;55(1):90–5.

[107] Mohanam S, Sawaya R, McCutcheon I, Ali-Osman F, Boyd D, Rao JS. Modulation of in vitro invasion of human glioblastoma cells by urokinase-type plasminogen activator receptor antibody. Cancer Res. 1993;53(18):4143–7.

[108] Reiter LS, Kruithof EK, Cajot JF, Sordat B. The role of the urokinase receptor in extracellular matrix degradation by HT29 human colon carcinoma cells. Int J Cancer. 1993;53(3):444–50.

[109] Allgayer H. Molecular regulation of an invasion-related molecule—options for tumour staging and clinical strategies. Eur J Cancer. 2006;42(7):811–9.

[110] Gum R, Juarez J, Allgayer H, Mazar A, Wang Y, Boyd D. Stimulation of urokinase-type plasminogen activator receptor expression by PMA requires JNK1-dependent and -independent signaling modules. Oncogene. 1998;17(2):213–25.

[111] Allgayer H, Wang H, Shirasawa S, Sasazuki T, Boyd D. Targeted disruption of the K-ras oncogene in an invasive colon cancer cell line down-regulates urokinase receptor expression and plasminogen-dependent proteolysis. Br J Cancer. 1999;80(12):1884–91.

[112] Lugassy G, Klepfish A. The fibrinolytic system in cancer. In: Lugassy G, Falanga A, Kakkar AK, Rickles FR (Eds). Thrombosis and Cancer. London: Martin Dunitz; 2004. pp. 61–63.

Chapter 2

Is Extracellular Matrix a Castle Against to Invasion of Cancer Cells?

Serdar Altınay

Additional information is available at the end of the chapter

http://dx.doi.org/10.5772/64495

Abstract

Metastasis is a complicated course that involves the spread of a neoplasm to distant parts of the body from its original site. A cancer cell must complete a series of steps before it becomes a clinically detectable lesion for successful colonization in the body. These are separation from the primary tumor, invasion and penetration of their basement membranes, entry into the blood vessels and survival within blood, and entry into lymphatics. A major challenge in extracellular matrix (ECM) biology is to understand the roles of the ECM and how disruption of ECM dynamics may contribute to cancer. A noteworthy area of forthcoming cancer research will be to determine whether abnormal ECM could be an effective cancer therapeutic target. We should understand how ECM composition and organization are normally maintained and how they may be deregulated in cancer. So the aims of this chapter were to focus on extracellular matrix. Invasion and metastatic skills, properties and functions of the ECM, abnormal ECM dynamics, tumor microenvironment and ECM, details of ECM invasion, role of ECM and ECM-associated proteins in metastasis, tumor dormant and metastatic process, essential component of the niches, role of the ECM in tumor angiogenesis and lymphangiogenesis are be briefly explained in this chapter.

Keywords: extracellular matrix, niche, tumor dormancy, metastasis, cancer

1. Introduction

Extracellular matrix (ECM) was synthesized and secreted by embryonic cells starting from the early stages of its development. Our knowledge on the composition, structure, and function of ECM increased significantly in recent years. The most prominent among these is that extracellular microenvironment holds a critical importance in cellular growth, survival, differentiation, and morphogenesis [1].

The major role played by the local microenvironment or niches in the arrangement of cellular behavior is gradually accepted more and more in cancer biology [2–5]. The fact that extracellular matrix is a dynamic source in the progression of cancer became the center of attention for researchers [1, 5–7].

ECM affects negatively multiple proteases in remodeling, but it should be debated whether proteolysis constitutes a mandatory step in tissue invasion [8]. Many groups reported that the crossed structural barriers of cancer cells may be transferred to ECM only via the proteolytic pathway. Yet, others suggested that the neoplastic cells progressed toward the matrix by pushing or suppressing without proteases [9–12]. No matter what the route is, neoplastic cells invade the two major subtypes of ECM, namely basal membrane and interstitium [13–17].

2. Invasion and metastatic skills

The dissemination of tumors is a complex process occurring in a sequential series which can be named as a sequence of invasive-metastatic events (**Figure 1**). These phases are composed

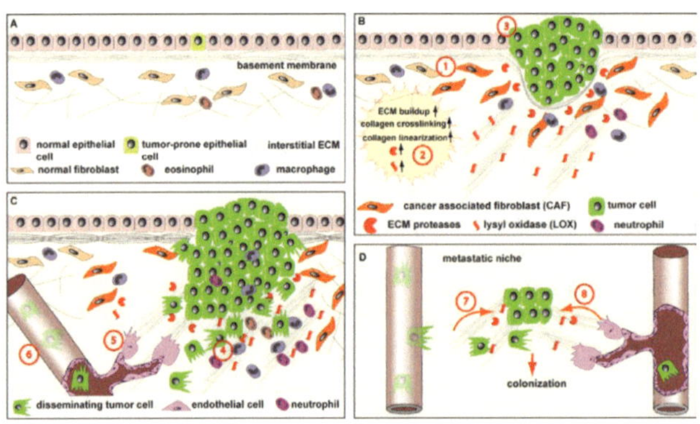

Figure 1. Abnormal ECM promotes cancer progression. (A) ECM remodeling is tightly controlled to ensure organ homeostasis and functions. Normal ECM dynamics are essential for maintaining tissue integrity and keep rare tumor-prone cells, together with resident fibroblasts, eosinophils, macrophages, and other stromal cells, in check by maintaining an overall healthy microenvironment. (B) With age or under pathological conditions, tissues can enter a series of tumorigenic events. One of the earlier events is the generation of activated fibroblasts or CAFs (stage 1), which contributes to abnormal ECM buildup and deregulated expression of ECM remodeling enzymes (stage 2). Abnormal ECM has profound impacts on surrounding cells, including epithelial, endothelial, and immune cells and other stromal cell types. Deregulated ECM promotes epithelial cellular transformation and hyperplasia (stage 3). (C) In late-stage tumors, immune cells are often recruited to the tumor site to promote cancer progression (stage 4). In addition, deregulated ECM affects various aspects of vascular biology and promotes tumor-associated angiogenesis (stage 5). Creation of a leaky tumor vasculature in turn facilitates tumor cell invasion and metastasis to distant sites (stage 6). (D) At distant sites, cancer cells leave the circulation and take hold of the local tissue. Together with local stromal cells, cancer cells express ECM remodeling enzymes and create a local metastatic niche. Abnormal niche ECM promotes extravasation, survival, and proliferation of cancer cells (stage 7). At later stages when cancer cells awake from dormancy, abnormal ECM turns on the angiogenic switch (stage 8), presumably using a mechanism similar to that used at the primary site (stage 5), and promotes the rapid growth of cancer cells and an expansion of micrometastasis to macrometastasis (see ref. [5]).

http://dx.doi.org/10.5772/64495

of local invasion, entry into blood and lymphatic vessels (intravasation), intravenous journey, exit from the veins (extravasation), development of micrometastases, and finally the growth of the micrometastases into macroscopic tumors [18, 19]. As it might be expected, any one of these phases may be interrupted by factors associated with the tumor or host. The series of metastatic events may also be divided into two phases, namely (1) ECM invasion and (2) intravenous dissemination of tumor cells and their homing in distant tissues/organs [20].

2.1. Characteristics, function, and invasion of ECM

As known, human tissues are composed of a series of compartments separated from each other by two types of ECMs, namely basal membranes and interstitial connective tissues. Although organized in different manners, each ECM type is composed of collagens, glycoproteins, and proteoglycans [21].

In addition to the ECM molecules, the general critical functions are important also for developmental events (**Figure 2**). Extracellular compartment comprises various ECM components

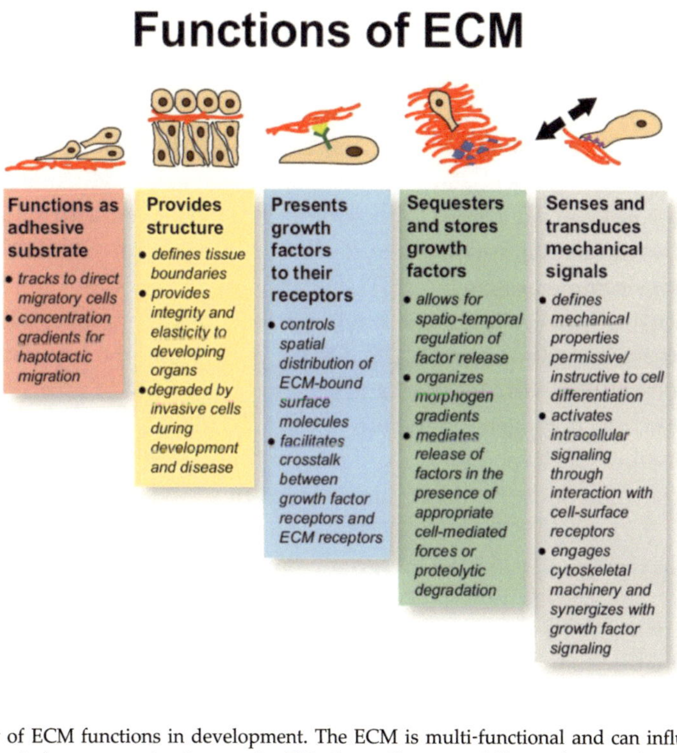

Figure 2. Summary of ECM functions in development. The ECM is multi-functional and can influence multiple biochemical and mechanical processes simultaneously. This figure illustrates different functional states of the ECM and their biological contexts. The five categories are not mutually exclusive. When interpreting ECM loss-of-function phenotypes, one should consider that multiple processes may be compromised thus specific roles of individual ECM components are difficult to glean. A couple of important properties of ECM are not illustrated in this cartoon. First, ECMs are highly dynamic and can be modified by the cells that come into contact with them creating a bi-directional mode of cell-matrix communication. Second, ECM-ECM interactions vary the chemical and mechanical composition of the extracellular microenvironment. In this review, we incorporate several examples of how the functions of ECM are utilized during embryonic development (see ref. [1]).

and this organization and composition modifies the development with the initiation of fertilization. The most prominent characteristic of cell-ECM interaction is that it is mutual. On one hand, cells are continuously formed, destroyed, or rearranged. ECM components modify one or multiple characteristics of ECM. On the other hand, as ECM arranges different cellular behaviors, this will impact adjacent cells as a result of any different cellular activity and modify its behaviors [22]. This feedback regulating mechanism between the cells and ECM enables rapid adaptation to the surrounding of cells and tissues [23].

The extracellular matrix (ECM) structure is dynamic and may be destroyed by the enzyme family known as the matrix metalloproteinases (MMPs). These enzymes are actually secreted by stromal cells or heparinase (this is an endoglycosidase enzyme which separates heparin sulfate chains expressed and secreted particularly by tumor cells). Thus, the microenvironment may contribute to tumor dormancy or metastatic growth with the impact of MMPs. The expression and secretion of MMPs by leukocytes and macrophages may lead to the release of angiostatic factors inhibiting angiogenesis and metastatic growth from ECM. These anti-angiogenesis factors comprise endostatin, restin, arrestin, three chains of collagen IV, and macrophage elastase [24]. Similarly, stromal MMPs may release cytokines and angiogenic factors affiliated with ECM such as fibroblast growth factor (FGF) and vascular endothelial growth factor (VEGF) and may initiate the angiogenic switch required for the transition from micrometastatic dormancy to metastatic growth. MMPs may also contribute to the formation of a suitable place for the transition from dormancy to metastatic growth. For instance, modifications in ECM components, such as the arrangement and production of type I collagen and fibronectin, were detected in gene expression signals associated with metastasis and poor prognosis in breast cancer [25]. Furthermore, the leukocyte secretion of MMP2 and MMP9 may activate latent transforming growth factor (TGF)-beta localized in ECM. The activation of TGF-beta may enhance the Type I collagen and lysyl oxidase expression synthesis and thus provide a suitable setting for metastatic growth [26]. On the other hand, the heparinase synthesis of tumor cells regulates the re-arrangement and destruction of ECM in association with angiogenic factors promoting angiogenesis and tumor cell migration [27]. In summary, the crosstalk between dormant tumor cells and ECM regulated by stromal and tumor cells may control the initiation or termination of the dormant status of the cell.

2.2. Dormancy of tumor cells and the metastatic process

Tumor dormancy may be defined as the long-term asymptomatic, non-detectable and latent state of disseminated tumor cells (DTCs). This period is a stage where the residual disease exists, but is not clinically visible. The cells in dormant state avail of the capacity to grow slowly, escape treatment and the immune system of the host and to renew themselves. Tumor dormancy may contribute to the progression and relapse of the tumor metastatically both in local and distant sites. Cancer cells go into a dormant stage at the beginning of the disease or following the first treatment and may remain dormant even for years or for decades after the first treatment. The mechanisms and the sleep markers regulating the transition between the dormancy and proliferation phases have not been fully designated [28]. A part of the latent period in all patients may take place as the slow accumulation of the genetic modifications leading to immortality (TP53, RB1, P16 loss, and/or telomerase gain, etc.) and the transformations during and/or following carcinogenesis (Ras-activating mutations, ERBB2 amplification, BRAF-activating mutations, etc.). Breast and prostate tumors, melanoma, B-cell lymphoma, and leukemia are malignancies displaying dormant cancer cells [29, 30].

The metastatic growth of disseminated tumor cells (DTCs) from the primary tumor constitutes the main reason of cancer-associated deaths. DTCs should survive around the circulation when they mix with blood and avoid physical damage and immune system attacks. Thus, DTCs adapt themselves to the new microenvironment of the secondary site and the reprogramming periods to the micrometastasis or quiescent state begin according to the characteristics of the microenvironment [31].

Various metastasis suppressant genes responding to microenvironmental stress may regulate the dormancy. Metastasis suppressant genes have the capacity to encourage apoptosis or the dormancy of cells and prevent the development of metastasis. KISS-1 is a tumor suppressor gene contained inside kisspeptins, and it has been demonstrated that the cells expressing kisspeptins remain dormant in many organs. Kangai 1 (Kai1/CD82) is a cell surface transmembrane protein which joins the inhibition of invasion and cancer cell migration by forming complexes with integrins. Furthermore, Kai 1 reduces the formation of distant metastasis upon binding to duffy antigen-chemokine receptor on the surface of vascular endothelial cells [32]. It was demonstrated that in melanoma, colon, breast, and lung cancer models that the metastasis is suppressed via the Nm23–1H (NME1) protein [33, 34]. Mitogen-activated protein kinase 4 (MKK4) is a specific kinase which plays a role in dormancy in the micrometastatic stage. MKK7 and MKK6 are other kinases with less metastasis suppressor effects. BRMS1, SMAD7, SSeCKS, RhoGD12, and CTGF are metastasis suppressor genes which play a potential role in dormancy. In case of more activated P38 in the cell, tumor cells may be encouraged to enter dormancy [35].

2.3. ECM's invasion and the stages of invasion

It is necessary for a carcinoma first to pass through the basal membrane beneath and then through the interstitial tissue and consequently reach the circulation upon penetrating into the basal membrane in the veins. The referred cycle is repeated also when the tumor cells embolisms extravasate from a different site. Due to these reasons, a tumor cell may metastasize only when they pass through different and high number of basal membranes and at least two interstitial matrices [36, 37]. The ECM invasion is achieved in four steps.

The first step of the series of metastatic events is the relaxation of tumor cells. E-cadherins act as intercellular adhesives and their parts within the cytoplasm bind to β-catenin. Neighboring E-cadherin molecules hold together cells, and as also explained earlier, they may send anti-proliferative signals over the β-catenin sequestration [38]. The E-cadherin function in almost all epithelial-derived cancers is lost due to the mutations achieved via the β-catenin gene activation of the E-cadherin genes or the inadequate expression of the SNAIL and TWIST transcription factors suppressing the E-cadherin expression [39, 40].

The second step in the invasion is composed of the local disintegration of the basal membrane and the interstitial connective tissue. The tumor cells themselves secrete proteolytic enzymes or stimulate stroma cells such as fibroblasts and inflammatory cells so that they secrete proteases. It was expressed indirectly that many different protease families, such as matrix metalloproteinases (MMPs), cathepsin D and urokinase plasminogen activators, play a role in the achievement of the invasive characteristic in the tumor cell. Matrix metalloproteinases regulate the tumor invasion not only by reshaping the insoluble components of the basal membrane and interstitial matrix but also by releasing the growth factors at ECM [41]. Actually, the cleavage collagens and proteoglycans also have effects which promote chemotactic, angiogenic, and growth. For instance, MMP-9 is a gelatinase which may release type IV collagen in the basal membrane of the epithelial and the veins; furthermore, it also stimulates the VEGF secretion of ECM from sequestered pools. Type IV collagenous activity, which is very rare in the benign tumors of the breast, large intestine, and stomach is at an abundant amount in the malignant tumors of the same organs. Meanwhile, indeed, an overexpression of metalloproteases and other proteases was reported for many tumors [42–44].

The third step of tumor invasion involves changes in the adhesion of tumor cells to ECM proteins. There are receptors in the normal epithelial cells, such as integrin, which belong to the basal membrane laminin polarized on the basal surfaces and to collagens, and these help the cell to maintain its undifferentiated status at rest. While the loss of adhesion initiates apoptosis in normal cells, tumor cells are resistant to the death of cells to take place via this path [36]. Furthermore, the matrix itself is changed in a manner so as to promote invasion and the occurrence of metastasis. For instance, the cleavage of basal membrane proteins (collagen IV and laminin) by MMP-2 or MMP-9 creates new sites to which the receptors in the tumor cells may bind and stimulate the migration [42, 44].

The final step of the tumor invasion is the locomotion of malignant cells. During the locomotion process, the tumor cells pass through fragmented basal membranes and proteolyzed matrix regions and translocate. The migration of cancerous cells is a multi-phased process, which impacts the cytoskeleton in the actin structure at the end and where many receptor families and the signalization protein family play a role (**Figure 3**). This last step appears to be a process which is promoted and directed by cytokines deriving from the tumor cell such as the autocrine motility factor. Furthermore, the cleavage products of the matrix proteins (such as collagen and laminin) and some growth factors (such as insulin-like growth factor I and II) have a chemotaxis effect on these cells.

Moreover, the stroma cells also produce paracrine effector factors such as HGF/SCF (hepatocyte growth factor/diffusion factor) which bind to the receptors on the tumor cells. HGF inhibition is as effective as standard chemotherapy in inhibiting local tumor growth [45]. The fact that the concentration of these factors is high in the peripheral region of glioblastoma multiform, which is a strong brain tumor with advanced invasion skills, supports the view that they play a role in motility [46].

http://dx.doi.org/10.5772/64495

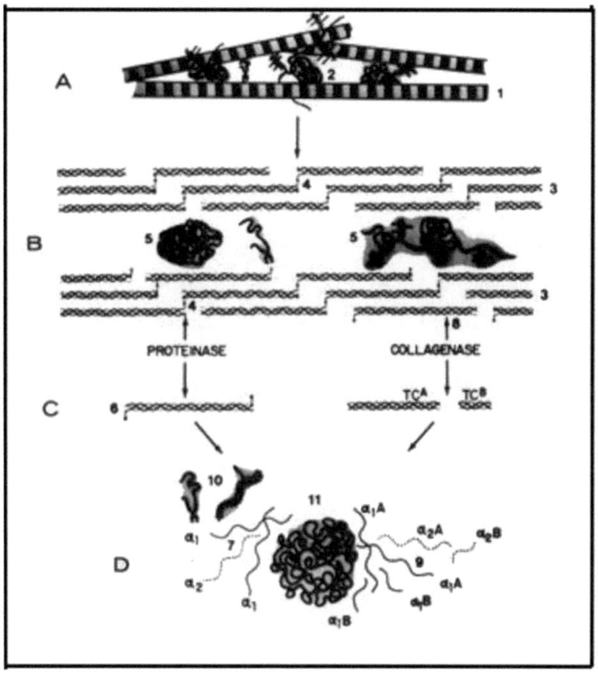

Figure 3. Schematic model of enzymatic disruption of extracellular matrix at the tumor invasion zone: (A) The tumor-surrounding extracellular matrix consists of a meshwork of collagen fibers (1) and interdispersed glycosaminoglycan-containing proteoglycans (2) that provide swelling pressure to maintain tissue volume; (B) collagen molecules (3) are aligned in staggered fashion overlapping by one quarter of their length to form a cross-striated collagen fiber (1). Covalent cross links (4) between neighboring collagen molecules are responsible for tensile strength and insolubility of the fiber meshwork. The interdispersed proteoglycans shows limited aggregation with hyaluronate (5). It is restricted from swelling by an intact collagen network; (C) collagen fibers are degraded by two enzymatic pathways: (a) proteinases (i.e., cathepsins, elastase, plasmin, thrombin) act as "cross-linkases" (4) to liberate collagen monomers from fibers (6). Collagen monomers then denature (7), solubilize, and become susceptible to many proteinases. (b) Vertebrate collagenases specifically cleave the collagen triple helix at the ¾-¼ point between the NH2- and COOH-termini (8). The resulting TCA and TCS fragments denature (9) and are further cleaved by neutral proteinases: (D) Collagen and concomitant proteoglycan degradation (10) transforms the matrix from an insoluble (solid) to a liquified (fluid) state. The remaining proteoglycans swell (11) due to breakdown of the restricting collagen network. These physical changes may allow locomotion and tumor cell penetration (see ref. [6]).

2.4. How does ECM deregulation signal cancer?

The structure of tumor-associated ECM is basically different than that of the normal tissue stroma. Relaxed, non-oriented fibrils and collagen I are significantly oriented with epithelia which are significantly linearized and attached in the breast tissue or are designed vertically to the tissue [41].

Abnormal ECM dynamics have been well documented in clinical studies as a sign of many diseases and cancer. For instance, excessive ECM production or decreased ECM destruction is evident in many organ fibroses [47]. The storage of various collagens containing collagen I, II, III, V, and IX increases during tumor formation [48]. These abnormal changes in the composition and rate of ECM may significantly modify the biochemical characteristics of ECM and potentialize the oncogenic effects of various growth factor signal pathways [49]. Increased collagen deposition or ECM stiffness may support cell survival and proliferation alone or with the upregulation of the integrin signal [50, 51].

Increased collagen cross links and ECM stiffness stimulate ERK and PI3 kinase signal as a result of LOX overproduction and facilitate oncogenic transformation [47].

2.5. May ECM prevent cancer cell invasion?

Studies have demonstrated that ECM is essential in the protection and achievement of tissue polarity and structure. Abnormal ECM dynamics may cause basal membranes to compromise as a physical barrier and facilitate tissue invasion of cancer cells by supporting epithelial mesenchymal transition [52, 53].

The changes in ECM topography may facilitate the migration of cancer cells. Thickening and linearization are observed in collagen fibers in cancer cases, and these are mostly seen in tissue invasion and vascular tumor sites, which demonstrates that they may play an active role in this cancer cell invasion [41, 54].

2.6. Tumor microenvironment and ECM

Tumor microenvironment plays a critical role in the progression of cancer and is the main factor determining the growth and survival of DTCs in prioritized metastatic sites [43, 55]. It was recently revealed that the stroma cells surrounding tumor cells constitute a variable environment which promotes or prevents tumor formation of mutual signalizations between the tumor and stroma cells and not as a static barrier that prevents the motility of tumor cells [56]. The congenital and adaptive immunity cells as well as fibroblasts are among stroma cells which interact with tumors. It was revealed in various studies that tumor-accompanying cells contain ECM molecules, proteases, protease inhibitors, and genes encoding various growth factors in modified forms [57]. Dormant tumor cells are in close contact via the extracellular matrix via the integrin signalization pathway regulating tumor cell growth, migration, differentiation, and survival. Metastasis-associated urokinase receptor (uPAR) causes tumor growth via fibronectin receptor alfa5beta1-integrin activation and interaction. This complex enables the functioning of EFGR which promotes focal adhesion kinase (FAK) and adhesion to fibronectin and transfers mitogenic signals via Ras extracellular signal-regulated kinase (ERK), respectively. In an *in vitro* study, the downregulation of uPAR and the loss of function of integrin reduced the proliferative signals from a fibronectin-rich microenvironment which led to the transition from a tumorigenic status to a dormant status in human carcinoma cells. Furthermore, the blockade of uPAR, beta1-integrinler, FAK or EGFR alone or in combination results in *in vivo* tumor suppression which is demonstrated to be associated with the induction of tumor cell dormancy [58, 59].

In vivo ERK1/2 signalization revealed that dormancy derives from an almost complete full inhibition of the Raf-MEK-ERK pathway and triggers the stopping of cell cycle in the G0-G1 phase as in the dormant cells. It was demonstrated that the mitogen-activated protein kinase (MAPK) signalization cascade activated with (P38/c-Jun N-terminal kinase (JNK) has an impact as a tumor suppressor via various tumor suppressor (TP53 and Rb-mediated) pathways and by the decrease of various oncogenic signals and become responsible for the stopping of the growth. The disruption of the UPAR complex activates the p38 MAPK signalization pathway. Proliferation in primary and secondary tumors requires a high ERK1/2/p38 MAPK, pathway activation—contrary to tumor dormancy. Thus, the molecular mechanisms of growth inhibition have become comprehensible during dormancy, which is observed both I the p38 MAPK pathway activation and ERK1/2 pathway inhibition [60].

Thus, tumor cells maintain their existence within a complex and constantly changing environment in which ECM, fibroblasts, and the immunity system cells communicate with one another. The cells which cooperate with the referred environment in order to fulfill their bad intentions and may adapt themselves to this environment can be the most successful tumor cells.

2.7. May fibroblasts play a role in tumor invasion?

When cells are transformed and the solid tumor mass formation is initiated, they lead to a modification in the phenotypes of the cells surrounding them. A transformation occurs in the extracellular matrix in addition to the modification in the cellular phenotype, and this tumor formation occurs simultaneously [57, 61]. It was recently discovered that increased matrix stiffness may also lead to the increase in the oncogenic YAP/TAZ complex increased in association with signal regulators comprising the Hippo signal pathway, enhanced cellular proliferation, decreased contact inhibition, increased cancer stem cell phenotype, and increased metastasis [62]. However, it was demonstrated in the recent publication by the authors that YAP/TAZ was not activate only at CAFs: Cancer associated fibroblasts, but that YAP/TAZ was necessary also for CAF development [63]. The authors demonstrated that CAF activation led to a matrix remodeling developing to increased stiffness with the myosin light-chain 2 (MYL9/MLC) expression which plays a vital role in the formation of ECM. Another point pinpointed by these authors was that the YAP/TAZ activation was not specific only to CAFs, but that it was also revealed in the normal tissue fibroblasts surrounding the cancerous tissue.

2.8. Role of ECM in vascular dissemination and homing of tumor cells

The growth of a tumor size requires an increase in the need for nutrients, oxygen, and waste exchange. Tumor vascularization constitutes the main path in metastases of cancer cells [36, 64].

When tumor cells reach the circulatory system, the host is likely to be destroyed by immune cells. Some tumor cells in the blood circulation aggregate and adhere on leukocytes in the circulation, particularly on thrombocytes, and cause embolism; thus, part of tumor cells in the circulation achieves a certain degree of protection against the antitumor effects of the effector cells of the host. However, the majority of tumor cells circulate alone in the circulation. During the extravasation of free tumor cells or the development of tumor embolism, the referred cells first adhere on the vascular endothelium and then enter the organ parenchyma upon passing through the basal membrane via mechanisms similar to those in the invasion process [64].

It is possible to estimate the site of extravasation of tumor cells and the distribution of the metastases in the organs by looking at the site of the primary tumor and the vascular or lymphatic drainage (**Figure 4**). Most tumors metastasize in the first organ they encounter in the capillary bed upon entering the circulation. However, natural drainage paths may not easily explain the distribution of metastases in many cases. Some tumors such as lung cancers frequently metastasize in the adrenals, while they almost never spread to the skeletal muscle [65]. This organ tropism may be associated with the following described mechanisms:

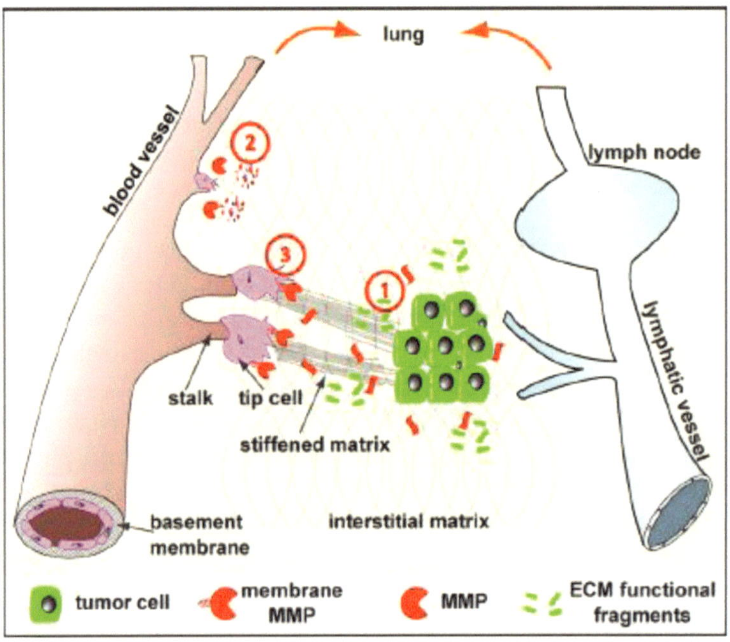

Figure 4. ECM role in tumor angiogenesis, lymphangiogenesis. Angiogenesis and lymphangiogenesis depend on the ECM. Tumor cells produce various components, including VEGF and angiogenic and antiangiogenic ECM fragments, to regulate blood vessel formation (stage 1). During branch initiation, endothelial cells secrete proteases to break down the basement membrane to grow out (stage 2). The outgrowth process of endothelial branching is propelled by at least two groups of cells: tip cells, which lead the migration toward the angiogenic chemoattractant source, and stalk cells, which depend on the ECM and its derivatives to survive and proliferate to provide building blocks for vessel formation (stage 3). Additionally, ECM components participate in cell migration and other aspects of tubulogenesis of blood vessels. Although details remain unclear, lymphangiogenesis depends on the ECM and, together with angiogenesis, provides routes for cancer cell metastasis and immune cell infiltration (see ref. [5]).

1. The expression of the ligands in the tumor cells and preferably of the adhesion molecules present in the endothelium of the target organs. 2. The expression of chemokines and their receptors. Chemokines contribute to the guided movements of leukocytes (chemotaxis), and cancer cells appear as cells which utilize similar tricks in order to settle in special tissues. Chemokine receptors named CXCR4 and CCR7 have a high expression in human breast cancer. The ligands of these receptors (CXCK12 and CCL21) are present in high amounts only in the organs where breast cancer cells have metastasized. Based on this observation, it was claimed that the blockage of chemokine receptors may limit metastases [44, 66].

http://dx.doi.org/10.5772/64495

When tumor cells reach their target, they may be colonized in that target. The factors regulating the referred colonization have not yet been fully understood. However, in order for tumor cells to proliferate after extravasation, they need a stroma that will accept them. In some cases, the target tissue may not carry a suitable environment identity for metastasis and is not the suitable soil, so to say, for the development of the tumor seeds. For instance, although the skeletal muscle is not rich in terms of vessels, it rarely becomes a stage for metastases [44].

Because, the biochemical characteristics of ECM, which play an important role in tubulogenesis during tumor angiogenesis [67, 68] in the vein lumen formation blood vessel lumen formation [69], are different in terms of displaying different branching patterns and various elasticities in these fields [70].

2.9. Details of ECM invasion

Willis et al. drew attention to the astuteness in the invasion of the devilish hidden cancer cells in the review they published [7]. Many groups reached the conclusion that cancer cells acquire an amoeboid phenotype characterized by insensitivity to proteinous inhibitors and surpass type I collagen barriers [12]. Now we know that a wide spectrum of types of cancer cells are definitely dependent on MT1-MMP when they are faced with cross-linked Type I collagen barriers [12, 71].

Still, when cancer cells encounter structural barriers, they hold the potential to adapt themselves to a protease-dependent position. Although there is limited information on the size of ECM pores, it is estimated via confocal reflection microscope that micropores range between of 40–10 μm^2 and macropores of 40–1000 μm^2 inside *in vivo* tissues [72–74]. These results increase the probability indicating that the collagen structure combined in an *in vitro* setting may not be repeated in a complex *in vivo* setting.

However, it should be noted that the defects in the migration of vascular smooth muscle cells, adipocytes differentiation, and stem cell origin displayed an *in vitro* setting duplication with the use of dense acid extracted type I collagen hydrogels in MT1-MMP-targeted mice [75–77]. Interestingly, the diameter of collagen fibers at *in vivo* neoplastic fields matched with the self-polymerized collagen hydrogels prepared in acid extractor type I collagen under standard conditions [78].

These results led to the thought that cancer cells may rapidly migrate to precleared tunnels via the proteolytic pathway through proteinaceous-independent processes similar to those in the *in vitro* setting [11, 79–81].

2.10. Role of ECM and ECM-associated proteins in metastasis

As cancer cells accumulate mutations or other molecular signals during the metastatic process, they are predisposed to become more easily malignant and lose contact with the surrounding cells and ECM in the primary tumor. These surrounding cells provide the opportunity for invasion. Thus, ECM and ECM-associated adhesion proteins play a critical role in the metastatic process [82]. Therefore, Zacharia et al. [83] published a review describing roles of the new molecules named migfilin, mitogen-inducible gene-2 (Mig-2), and Ras suppressor-1 (RSU-1) in the cell-ECM adhesion fields. The authors reached the conclusion that cell-ECM adhesion proteins are predisposed to function such as adaptor proteins in the form of multiple protein-protein interaction in the cell-ECM adhesion fields.

Even though the different effects in various types of cancer cells were discussed, they added that cell adhesion, which is crucial in terms of cell metastasis in many cases, supported cell invasion and apoptosis.

2.11. Is ECM the main constituent of niches?

Despite the "skill" they display in moving away from the site in which they were first formed, tumor cells are rather ineffective in terms of forming colonies in distant organs. Millions of cells drop off even from small tumors every single day; even though macroscopic metastases have not developed, it is possible to identify these cells in the blood circulation and in small foci in the bone marrow. The dormant state of micrometastases, which is defined as the capacity to preserve their existence for a long period without any progression, was observed in breast and prostate cancer [29, 30, 44].

In the studies demonstrating that ECM undertook a dynamic niche role in the progression of cancer in recent years [5–7], investigators indicated that the microenvironment or niche played a major role in the development of cancer. Abnormal ECM directly promotes cellular transformation and metastasis and impacted the progression of cancer [84].

A successful metastasis does not require local niche supporting only cancer cell development in the primary focus, but also necessitates the survival, colonization of the cancer cells invading the metastatic niches and their achievement of macrometastasis [85–87].

The molecular mechanisms of colonization have just begun to be enlightened in mice models, but the view claiming that tumor cells impact normal stroma cells and secrete cytokines, growth factors and proteases, which transform the site of metastasis into an environment where cancer cells may live, appears to be suitable [88, 89].

3. Concluding remarks

As metastatic mechanisms are better understood at a molecular level, it will be significantly easier for physicians to use these mechanisms as a treatment goal [90]. The identification of tissue-specific signals involved in metastatic progression will open the way to new therapeutic strategies. For this purpose, the authors [91] reviewed recent progress in the field, with particular emphasis on the mechanisms of organ-specific dissemination and colonization of breast cancer (**Figure 5**). Despite what has been described so far, it may not be possible to estimate exactly which cancer type may metastasize. But a noteworthy area of forthcoming cancer research will be to determine whether abnormal ECM could be an effective cancer therapeutic target. So we should understand how ECM composition and organization are

http://dx.doi.org/10.5772/64495

normally maintained and how they may be deregulated in cancer. Then, we may protect the ECM as a castle against to invasion of cancer.

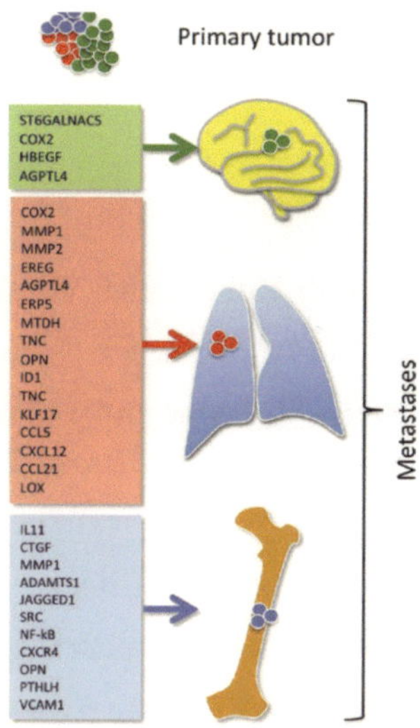

Figure 5. Gene mediating organ-specific breast cancer metastasis. Breast cancer genes promoting organ-specific metastasis to bone, lung, and brain have been identified. They include proinflammatory molecules and chemokines/receptors (e.g., COX-, CXCL12/CXCR4), matrix-degrading and modifying enzymes (e.g., MMP1/2, LOX), adhesion and extracellular matrix molecules (e.g., VCAM-1, TNC, OPN), transcription factors (e.g., ID1, KLF17), intracellular signaling proteins (e.g., SRC, NF-_B), and cell communication proteins (JAGGED1, CTGF). Some genes promote seeding (e.g., ST6GALNAC5, AGPTL4), whereas others promote colonization (e.g., OPN, CXCR4) (see ref. [91]).

Author details

Serdar Altınay

Address all correspondence to: drserdara@yahoo.com

Department of Pathology, Medical Faculty, Selcuk University , Konya, Turkey

References

[1] Rozario T, DeSimone DW. The extracellular matrix in development and morphogenesis: a dynamic view. Dev Biol. 2010;341:126–40. doi:10.1016/j.ydbio.2009.10.026. Epub 2009 Oct 23.

[2] Bissell MJ, and D. Radisky. Putting tumours in context. Nat. Rev. Cancer. 2001;1:46–54. doi:10.1038/35094059.

[3] Wiseman BS and Z Werb. Stromal effects on mammary gland development and breast cancer. Science. 2002;296:1046–1049. doi:10.1126/science.1067431.

[4] Bissell MJ and MA LaBarge. Context, tissue plasticity, and cancer:Are tumor stem cells also regulated by the microenvironment? Cancer Cell. 2005;7:17–23. doi:10.1016/j.ccr.2004.12.013.

[5] Lu P, Weaver VM, Werb Z. The extracellular matrix: a dynamic niche in cancer progression. J. Cell Biol. 2012;196:395–406. doi:10.1083/jcb.201102147.

[6] Pauli BU, Schwartz DE, Thonar EJ, Kuettner KE. Tumor invasion and host extracellular matrix. Cancer Metastasis Rev. 1983;2:129–152.

[7] Willis AL, Sabeh F, Li XY, Weiss SJ. Extracellular matrix determinants and the regulation of cancer cell invasion stratagems. J. Microsc. 2013;251:250–260. doi:10.1111/jmi.12064.

[8] Rowe RG and Weiss, SJ. Navigating ECM barriers at the invasive front: the cancer cell-stroma interface. Annu Rev Cell Dev Biol. 2009;25:567–595. doi:10.1146/annurev.cellbio.24.110707.175315.

[9] Wolf K, Mazo I, Leung H, Engelke K, von Andrian UH, Deryugina EI, Strongin AY, Bröcker EB, Friedl P. Compensation mechanism in tumor cellmigration: mesenchymal-amoeboid transition after blocking of pericellular proteolysis. J Cell Biol. 2003;160:267–277. doi:10.1083/jcb.200209006.

[10] Wolf K, Wu YI, Liu Y, Geiger J, Tam E, Overall C, Stack MS, Friedl P. Multi-step pericellular proteolysis controls the transition from individual to collective cancer cell invasion. Nat. Cell Biol. 207;9:893–904. doi:10.1038/ncb1616.

[11] Sabeh F, Ota I, Holmbeck K, Birkedal-Hansen H, Soloway P, Balbin M, Lopez-Otin C, Shapiro S, Inada M, Krane S, Allen E, Chung D, Weiss SJ. Tumor cell traffic through the extracellular matrix is controlled by the membrane-anchored collagenase MT1-MMP. J. Cell Biol. 2004;167:769–781. doi:10.1083/jcb.200408028.

[12] Sabeh F, Shimizu-Hirota R and Weiss SJ. Protease-dependent versus-independent cancer cell invasion programs: three-dimensional amoeboid movement revisited. J. Cell Biol. 2009;185:11–19. doi:10.1083/jcb.200807195.

[13] Rowe RG and Weiss SJ. Breaching the basement membrane: who, when and how? Trends Cell Biol. 2008;18:560–574. doi:10.1016/j.tcb.2008.08.007.

[14] Ehrbar M, Sala A, Lienemann P, Ranga A, Mosiewicz K, Bittermann A, Rizzi SC, Weber FE, Lutolf MP. Elucidating the role of matrix stiffness in 3D cell migration and remodeling. Biophys. J. 2011;100:284–293. doi:10.1016/j.bpj.2010.11.082.

[15] Wolf K and Friedl P. Extracellular matrix determinants of proteolytic and non-proteolytic cell migration. Trends Cell Biol. 2011;21:736–744. doi:10.1016/j.tcb.2011.09.006.

[16] Friedl P, Sahai E, Weiss S and Yamada KM. New dimensions in cell migration. Nat. Rev. Mol. Cell Biol. 2012;13:743–747. doi:10.1038/nrm3459.

[17] Petrie RJ, Gavara N, Chadwick RS and Yamada KM. Nonpolarized signaling reveals two distinct modes of 3D cell migration. J. Cell Biol. 2012;197:439–455. doi:10.1083/jcb.201201124.

[18] Sahai E: Illuminating the metastatic cascade. Nat. Rev Cancer. 2007;7:737. doi:10.1038/nrc2229.

[19] Gupta GP, Massague J. Cancer metastasis: building a framework. Cell. 2006;127:679–95. doi:10.1016/j.cell.2006.11.001.

[20] Fidler IJ. The pathogenesis of cancer metastasis: the "seed and soil" hypothesis revisited. Nat. Rev. Cancer. 2003;3:453–458. doi:10.1038/nrc1098.

[21] Radisky D, Muschler J, Bissell MJ. Order and disorder: the role of extracellular matrix in epithelial cancer. Cancer Invest. 2002;20:139–153. PMCID:PMC2933209.

[22] Butcher DT, Alliston T, and Weaver VM. A tense situation: Forcing tumour progression. Nat. Rev. Cancer. 2009;9:108–122. doi:10.1038/nrc2544.

[23] Samuel MS, Lopez JI, McGhee EJ, Croft DR, Strachan D, Timpson P, Munro J, Schröder E, Zhou J, Brunton VG, et al. Actomyosinmediated cellular tension drives increased tissue stiffness and β-catenin activation to induce epidermal hyperplasia and tumor growth. Cancer Cell. 2011;19:776–791. doi:10.1016/j.ccr.2011.05.008.

[24] Giancotti FG. Mechanisms governing metastatic dormancy and reactivation. Cell. 2013;155:750–764. doi:10.1016/j.cell.2013.10.029.

[25] Garamszegi N, Garamszegi SP, Shehadeh LA, Scully SP. Extracellular matrix-induced gene expression in human breast cancer cells. Mol. Cancer Res. 2009;7:319–329. doi:10.1158/1541-7786.MCR-08-0227.

[26] Sodek KL, Brown TJ and Ringuette MJ. Collagen I but not Matrigel matrices provide an MMP-dependent barrier to ovarian cancer cell penetration. BMC Cancer. 2008;8:223. doi:10.1186/1471-2407-8-223.

[27] Aguirre-Ghiso JA, Bragado P, Sosa MS. Metastasis awakening: targeting dormant cancer. Nat. Med. 2013;19:276–277. doi:10.1038/nm.3120.

[28] Giancotti FG. Mechanisms Governing metastatic dormancy and reactivation. Cell. 2013;155:750–764. doi:10.1016/j.cell.2013.10.029.

[29] Sih-han Wang and Shiaw-Yih Lin. Tumor dormancy: potential therapeutic target in tumor recurrence and metastasis prevention. Exp. Hematol. Oncol. 2013;2:29. doi:10.1186/2162-3619-2-29.

[30] David Paez, Melissa J. Labonte, Pierre Bohanes, Wu Zhang, Leonor Benhanim, Yan Ning, Takeru Wakatsuki, Fotios Loupakis, and Heinz-Josef Lenz. Cancer dormancy: a

model of early dissemination and late cancer recurrence. Clin. Cancer Res. 2012;18:645–653. doi:10.1158/1078-0432.CCR-11-2186.

[31] María Soledad Sosa, Paloma Bragado, Julio A. Aguirre-Ghiso. Mechanisms of disseminated cancer cell dormancy: an awakening field. Nat. Rev. Cancer. 2014;14:611–622. doi:10.1038/nrc3793.

[32] Maria Soledad Sosa, Paloma Bragado, Jayanta Debnath, Julio A. Aguirre-Ghiso. Regulation of tumor cell dormancy by tissue microenvironments and autophagy. Adv. Exp. Med. Biol. 2013;734:73–89. doi:10.1007/978-1-4614-1445-2_5.

[33] Aguirre-Ghiso JA. Models, mechanisms and clinical evidence for cancer dormancy. Nat. Rev. Cancer. 2007;7:834–846. PMCID:PMC2519109.

[34] Goss PE, Chambers AF. Does tumour dormancy offer a therapeutic target? Nat. Rev. Cancer. 2010;10:871–877. doi:10.1038/nrc2933.

[35] Kathleen P, Wilkie and Philip Hahnfeldt. Tumor-Immune dynamics regulated in the microenvironment inform the transient nature of immune-induced tumor dormancy. Cancer Res. 2013;73:3534–3544. doi:10.1158/0008-5472.CAN-12-4590.

[36] Coghlin C, Murray GI. Current and emerging concepts in tumour metastasis. J. Pathol. 2010;222:1–15. doi:10.1002/path.2727.

[37] Chaffer CL, Weinberg RA. A perspective on cancer cell metastasis. Science. 2011;331:1559–1564. doi:10.1126/science.1203543.

[38] Canel M, Serrels A, Frame MC, Brunton VG. E-cadherin-integrin crosstalk in cancer invasion and metastasis. J. Cell Sci. 2013;126(Pt 2):393–401. doi:10.1242/jcs.100115.

[39] Berx G, van Roy F. Involvement of members of the cadherin superfamily in cancer. Cold Spring Harb Perspect Biol. 2009;1:a003129. doi:10.1101/cshperspect.a003129.

[40] Barrallo-Gimeno A, Nieto MA. The Snail genes as inducers of cell movement and survival: implications in development and cancer. Development. 2005;132:3151–3161. doi:10.1242/dev.01907.

[41] Levental KR, Yu H, Kass L, Lakins JN, Egeblad M, Erler JT, et al. Matrix crosslinking forces tumor progression by enhancing integrin signaling. Cell. 2009;139:891–906. doi:10.1016/j.cell.2009.10.027.

[42] Kessenbrock K, Plaks V, Werb Z. Matrix metalloproteinases: regulators of the tumor microenvironment. Cell. 2010;141:52–67. doi:10.1016/j.cell.2010.03.015.

[43] Overall CM, Kleifeld O. Tumour microenvironment - opinion: Validating matrix metalloproteinases as drug targets and anti-targets for cancer therapy. Nat. Rev. Cancer. 2006;6:227–239. doi:10.1038/nrc1821.

[44] Kumar V, Abbas AK, Aster JC, Robbins SL. Neoplasia. In Robbins basic pathology. 9th edition. Edited by Kumar V, Abbas AK, Aster JC, Robbins SL. Philadelphia: Elsevier/ Saunders; 2013.p.162–210.

[45] Pothula SP, Xu Z, Goldstein D, Biankin AV, Pirola RC, Wilson JS, Apte MV. Hepatocyte growth factor inhibition: a novel therapeutic approach in pancreatic cancer. Br. J. Cancer. 2016;114:269–280. doi:10.1038/bjc.2015.478.

[46] Liang QL, Mo ZY, Wang P, Li X, Liu ZX, Zhou ZM. The clinical value of serum hepatocyte growth factor levels in patients undergoing primary radiotherapy for glioma: effect on progression-free survival. Med. Oncol. 2014;31:122. doi:10.1007/ s12032-014-0122-5.

[47] Frantz C, Stewart KM, and Weaver VM. The extracellular matrix at a glance. J. Cell Sci. 2010;123:4195–4200. doi:10.1242/jcs.023820.

[48] Hewitt RE, Powe DG, Morrell K, Balley E, Leach IH, Ellis IO, and Turner DR. Laminin and collagen IV subunit distribution in normal and neoplastic tissues of colorectum and breast. Br. J. Cancer. 1997;75:221–229. doi:10.1038/bjc.1997.37.

[49] Nasser NJ. Heparanase involvement in physiology and disease. Cell. Mol. Life Sci. 2008;65:1706–1715. doi:10.1007/s00018-008-7584-6.

[50] Wozniak MA, Desai R, Solski PA, Der CJ, and Keely PJ. ROCK-generated contractility regulates breast epithelial cell differentiation in response to the physical properties of a three-dimensional collagen matrix. J. Cell Biol. 2003;163:583–595. doi:10.1083/jcb. 200305010.

[51] Paszek, MJ, Zahir N, Johnson KR, Lakins JN, Rozenberg GI, Gefen A, Reinhart-King CA, et al. Tensional homeostasis and the malignant phenotype. Cancer Cell. 2005;8:241–254. doi:10.1016/j.ccr.2005.08.010.

[52] Song W, Jackson K, and McGuire PG. Degradation of type IV collagen by matrix metalloproteinases is an important step in the epithelial mesenchymal transformation of the endocardial cushions. Dev. Biol. 2000;227:606–617. doi:10.1006/dbio.2000.9919.

[53] Radisky ES and Radisky DC. Matrix metalloproteinase-induced epithelial-mesenchymal transition in breast cancer. J. Mammary Gland Biol. Neoplasia. 2010;15:201–212. doi:10.1007/s10911-010-9177-x.

[54] Condeelis J and Segall JE. Intravital imaging of cell movement in tumours. Nat. Rev. Cancer. 2003;3:921–930. doi:10.1038/nrc1231.

[55] Lorusso G, Ruegg C. The tumor microenvironment and its contribution to tumor evolution toward metastasis. Histochemistry Cell Biol. 2008;130:1091–1103. doi: 10.1007/s00418-008-0530-8.

[56] Boudreau A, van't Veer LJ, Bissell MJ. An "elite hacker": breast tumors exploit the normal microenvironment program to instruct their progression and biological diversity. Cell Adh. Migr. 2012;6:236–248. doi:10.4161/cam.20880.

[57] Kalluri R, Zeisberg M. Fibroblasts in cancer. Nat. Rev. Cancer. 2006;6:392–401. doi: 10.1038/nrc1877.

[58] Paloma Bragado, Maria Soledad Sosa, Patricia Keely, John Condeelis, Julio A. Aguirre-Ghiso. Microenvironments dictating tumor cell dormancy. Recent Results Cancer Res. 2012;195:25–39. doi:10.1007/978-3-642-28160-0_3.

[59] Klein CA. Selection and adaptation during metastatic cancer progression. Nature. 2013;501:365–372. doi:10.1038/nature12628.

[60] Sosa MS, Avivar-Valderas A, Bragado P, Wen HC, Aguirre-Ghiso JA. ERK1/2 and p38α/β signaling in tumor cell quiescence: opportunities to control dormant residual disease. Clin. Cancer Res. 2011;17:5850–5857. doi:10.1158/1078-0432.CCR-10-2574.

[61] Perentes JY, McKee TD, Ley CD, Mathiew H, Dawson M, Padera TP, Munn LL, Jain RK, Boucher Y. *In vivo* imaging of extracellular matrix remodeling by tumor-associated fibroblasts. Nat. Methods. 2009;6:143–145. doi:10.1038/nmeth.1295.

[62] Harvey KF, Zhang X and Thomas DM. The Hippo pathway and human cancer. Nat. Rev. Cancer. 2013;13:246–257. doi:10.1038/nrc3458.

[63] Calvo F, Ege N, Grande-Garcia A, Hooper S, Jenkins RP, Chaudhry SI, Harrington K, Williamson P, Moeendarbary E, Charras G, Sahai E. Mechanotransduction and YAP-dependent matrix remodelling is required for the generation and maintenance of cancer-associated fibroblasts. Nat. Cell Biol. 2013;15:637–646. doi:10.1038/ncb2756.

[64] Ahmed Z, Bicknell R. Angiogenic signalling pathways. Methods Mol. Biol. 2009;467:3–24. doi:10.1007/978-1-59745-241-0_1.

[65] Gupta GP, Nguyen DX, Chiang AC, Bos PD, Kim JY, Nadal C, et al. Mediators of vascular remodelling co-opted for sequential steps in lung metastasis. Nature. 2007;446:765–770. doi:10.1016/0959-8049(95)00353-K.

[66] Epstein RJ. The CXCL12-CXCR4 chemotactic pathway as a target of adjuvant breast cancer therapies. Nat. Rev. Cancer. 2004;4:901. doi:10.1038/nrc1473.

[67] Davis GE, and Senger DR. Endothelial extracellular matrix: biosynthesis, remodeling, and functions during vascular morphogenesis and neovessel stabilization. Circ. Res. 2005;97:1093–1107. doi:10.1161/01.RES.0000191547.64391.e3.

[68] Carmeliet P, Jain RK. Principles and mechanisms of vessel normalization for cancer and other angiogenic diseases. Nat. Rev. Drug Discov. 2011;10:417–427. doi:10.1038/nrd3455.

[69] Newman AC, Nakatsu MN, Chou W, Gershon PD, and Hughes CCW. The requirement for fibroblasts in angiogenesis: fibroblast-derived matrix proteins are essential for

endothelial cell lumen formation. Mol. Biol. Cell. 2011;22:3791–3800. doi:10.1091/mbc.E11-05-0393.

[70] Myers KA, Applegate KT, Danuser G, Fischer RS, and Waterman CM. Distinct ECM mechanosensing pathways regulate microtubule dynamics to control endothelial cell branching morphogenesis. J. Cell Biol. 2011;192:321–334. doi:10.1083/jcb.201006009.

[71] Wolf K, Te Lindert M, Krause M, Alexander S, Te Riet J, Willis AL, et al. Physical limits of cell migration: control by ECM space and nuclear deformation and tuning by proteolysis and traction force. J. Cell Biol. 2013;201:1069–1084. doi:10.1083/jcb.201210152.

[72] Conklin MW, Eickhoff JC, Riching KM, Pehlke CA, Eliceiri KW, Provenzano PP, Friedl A, Keely PJ. Aligned collagen is a prognostic signature for survival in human breast carcinoma. Am. J. Pathol. 2011;178:1221–1232. doi:10.1016/j.ajpath.2010.11.076.

[73] Wolf K, Alexander S, Schacht V, Coussens LM, von Andrian UH, van Rheenen J, Deryugina E, Friedl P. Collagen-based cell migration models *in vitro* and *in vivo*. Semin. Cell Dev. Biol. 2009;20:931–941. doi:10.1016/j.semcdb.2009.08.005.

[74] Yang YL, Motte S, Kaufman LJ. Pore size variable type I collagen gels and their interaction with glioma cells. Biomaterials 2010;31:5678–5688. doi:10.1016/j.biomaterials.2010.03.039.

[75] Filippov S, Koenig GC, Chun TH, Hotary KB, Ota I, Bugge TH, et al. MT1-matrix metalloproteinase directs arterial wall invasion and neointima formation by vascular smooth muscle cells. J. Exp. Med. 2005;202:663–671. PMCID:PMC2212885.

[76] Chun TH, Hotary KB, Sabeh F, Saltiel AR, Allen ED, Weiss SJ. A pericellular collagenase directs the 3-dimensional development of white adipose tissue. Cell. 2006;125:577–591. doi:10.1016/j.cell.2006.02.050.

[77] Tang Y, Rowe RG, Botvinick EL, Kurup A, Putnam AJ, Seiki M, et al. MT1-MMP-dependent control of skeletal stem cell commitment via a beta1-Integrin/YAP/TAZ signaling axis. Dev. Cell 2013;25:402–416. doi:10.1016/j.devcel.2013.04.011.

[78] Oldberg A, Kalamajski S, Salnikov AV, Stuhr L, Mörgelin M, Reed RK, Heldin NE, Rubin K. Collagen-binding proteoglycan fibromodulin can determine stroma matrix structure and fluid balance in experimental carcinoma. Proc. Natl. Acad. Sci. USA. 2007;104:13966–13971. PMCID:PMC1955775.

[79] Gaggioli C, Hooper S, Hidalgo-Carcedo C, Grosse R, Marshall JF, Harrington K and Sahai E. Fibroblast-led collective invasion of carcinoma cells with differing roles for RhoGTPases in leading and following cells. Nat. Cell Biol. 2007;9:1392–1400. doi:10.1038/ncb1658.

[80] Fisher KE, Sacharidou A, Stratman AN, Mayo AM, Fisher SB, Mahan RD, Davis MJ and Davis GE. MT1-MMP- and Cdc42-dependent signaling co-regulate cell invasion and

tunnel formation in 3D collagen matrices. J. Cell Sci. 2009;122:4558–4569. doi:10.1242/jcs.050724.

[81] Carey SP, Starchenko A, McGregor AL, Reinhart-King CA. Leading malignant cells initiate collective epithelial cell invasion in a three-dimensional heterotypic tumor spheroid model. Clin. Exp. Metastasis. 2013;30:615–630. doi:10.1007/s10585-013-9565-x.

[82] Hynes RO. Integrins: bidirectional, allosteric signaling machines. Cell. 2002;110:673–687. doi:10.1016/S0092-8674(02)00971-6.

[83] Zacharia LC, Gkretsi V. Cancer cell metastasis; perspectives from the focal adhesions. Adv. Mod. Oncol. Res. 2015;1:2–7. doi:10.18282/amor.v1.i1.6.

[84] Peinado H, Lavotshkin S, Lyden D. The secreted factors responsible for premetastatic niche formation: old sayings and new thoughts. Semin. Cancer Biol. 2011;21:139–146. doi:10.1016/j.semcancer.2011.01.002.

[85] Psaila B, and Lyden D. The metastatic niche: adapting the foreign soil. Nat. Rev. Cancer. 2009;9:285–293. doi:10.1038/nrc2621.

[86] Shibue T, Weinberg RA. Metastatic colonization: settlement, adaptation and propagation of tumor cells in a foreign tissue environment. Semin. Cancer Biol. 2011;21:99–106. doi:10.1016/j.semcancer.2010.12.003.

[87] Oskarsson T, Acharyya S, Zhang XH, Vanharanta S, Tavazoie SF, Morris PG, et al. Breast cancer cells produce tenascin c as a metastatic niche component to colonize the lungs. Nat. Med. 2011;17:867–874. doi:10.1038/nm.2379.

[88] Shibue T, Weinberg RA. Integrin beta1-focal adhesion kinase signaling directs the proliferation of metastatic cancer cells disseminated in the lungs. Proc. Natl. Acad. Sci. USA. 2009;106:10290–10295. doi:10.1073/pnas.0904227106.

[89] Chiang AC, Massague J. Molecular basis of metastasis. The N. Eng. J. Med. 2008;359:2814–2823. doi:10.1056/NEJMra0805239.

[90] Valastyan S, Weinberg RA. Tumor metastasis: molecular insights and evolving paradigms. Cell. 2011;147:275–292. doi:10.1016/j.cell.2011.09.024.

[91] Lorusso G, Rüegg C. New insights into the mechanisms of organ-specific breast cancer metastasis. Semin. Cancer Biol. 2012;22:226–233. doi:10.1016/j.semcancer.2012.03.007.

Chapter 3

Ovarian Cancer Metastasis: A Unique Mechanism of Dissemination

Anirban K. Mitra

Additional information is available at the end of the chapter

http://dx.doi.org/DOI:10.5772/64700

Abstract

Ovarian cancer is the most lethal of all gynecologic malignancies and has witnessed minimal improvements in patient outcomes in the past three decades. About 70% of ovarian cancer patients present with disseminated disease at the time of diagnosis. The standard of care remains a combination of debulking surgery and platinum- and taxanes-based cytotoxic chemotherapy. Even though metastasis is the leading cause of ovarian cancer related fatalities, our understanding of the process remains limited. Ovarian cancer has a unique pattern of metastasis where the hematogenous spread is less common. Ovarian cancer cells mainly metastasize within the peritoneal cavity, which involves exfoliation from the primary tumor, survival, and transport in the peritoneal fluid followed by metastatic colonization of the organs within the peritoneal cavity. A key step for successful metastasis is their attachment and productive interactions with the mesothelial cells covering the metastatic organs for the establishment of metastatic tumors. This chapter provides an overview of ovarian cancer metastasis highlighting the unique dissemination and the underlying mechanisms of regulation of the steps involved. The role of the microenvironment in the process of metastasis will also be reviewed.

Keywords: ovarian cancer, metastasis, omentum, microenvironment, ascites

1. Introduction

Ovarian cancer is the most lethal of all gynecologic malignancies. It accounts for a fifth of all cancer-related deaths among women in the United States of America. It is estimated that 22,280 women will be diagnosed with ovarian cancer and 14,240 will die of the disease in the United States in 2016 [1]. This makes it a relatively less prevalent but a very deadly form of cancer. About

90% of all ovarian cancers are epithelial in origin, which are classified into high-grade serous, low-grade serous, endometrioid, clear cell, and mucinous subtypes [2]. Of these, the high-grade serous ovarian cancer (HGSOC) is the most common subtype and is characterized by mutations in p53 and genomic instability [3]. A detailed characterization of the HGSOC tumors was done by The Cancer Genome Atlas Network, which mapped the deregulated pathways involved. In the past, these tumors were thought to originate from the ovarian surface epithelium. However, more recently researchers have started to believe that they may actually originate from the fallopian tube fimbriae based on the analysis of prophylactic salpingo-oophorectomy samples [4].

One of the reasons for the poor prognosis of ovarian cancer is the fact that most patients are diagnosed late [5]. It is a highly metastatic cancer and more than 70% of ovarian cancer patients are diagnosed with metastasis [6]. As the tumor grows within the peritoneal cavity, the symptoms produced are abdominal pain or bloating and may be confused with other bowel diseases like irritable bowel syndrome [7, 8]. Ovarian cancer is often called 'the silent cancer' or 'the disease that whispers' because of these diffuse symptoms. The presence of high levels of cancer antigen 125 (CA-125) is used as a diagnostic marker of disease progression. Pelvic ultrasound, MRI, and CT scanning is also used to determine the extent of the disease. Patients undergo a 'debulking' surgery usually conducted by a gynecologic oncologist with a goal to remove as much of the tumor masses as possible from the abdomen [9]. In addition, the tumors are also staged histopathologically as per the International Federation of Gynecology and Obstetrics (FIGO) guidelines (**Table 1**) [10]. Minimal residual disease after the surgery is considered one of the strongest prognostic factors and is highly desirable [11]. The surgery is followed by adjuvant cytotoxic chemotherapy consisting of a combination of carboplatin and paclitaxel. The response to therapy is determined by measuring the serum CA-125 levels and by imaging techniques [2]. If the disease relapses within 6 months, it is considered chemoresistant and if relapse occurs after 12 months, it is considered chemosensitive. While a majority of the patients respond well initially to chemotherapy, most eventually end up developing chemoresistance [12]. Bowel obstruction by the metastatic tumors is the predominant cause of ovarian cancer-related mortality [13]. Since many parts of the bowel get affected, it becomes extremely difficult to surgically treat this condition. In addition, extensive ascites is a cause for major discomfort. Palliative measures such as control of nausea, abdominal pain, draining ascites, and modified diet are typically resorted to [2]. Since most of the ovarian cancer patients are diagnosed with advanced disease, in effect, it is metastasis that is being treated [6]. Therefore, a greater understanding of the process and regulation of ovarian cancer metastasis is essential.

Ovarian cancer predominantly metastasizes within the peritoneal cavity and through the pelvic lymph nodes (**Figure 1**) [14, 15]. However, recent evidence suggests the possibility of hematogenous metastasis of ovarian cancer (**Figure 1**) [16]. This chapter will discuss the steps involved in the unique metastatic dissemination of ovarian cancer and will highlight what is known about the regulation of the steps involved.

Stage I: The disease limited to ovaries only

- Ia: Tumor in only one ovary or fallopian tube with intact capsule
- Ib: Tumor in both the ovaries
- Ic: Tumor on the surface of one or both ovaries/fallopian tubes with ruptured capsule and cancer cells present in peritoneal washings

Stage II: Tumors spread to the pelvis but limited to below the pelvic brim

- IIa: Tumors spread to the fallopian tubes or uterus or both
- IIb: Tumors spread to other pelvic tissues within the peritoneum

Stage III: Tumors have spread to the abdomen beyond the pelvis or has metastasized to the lymph nodes or both

- IIIa: Microscopic involvement of extra pelvic peritoneal regions
- IIIb: Tumors up to 2 cm diameter
- IIIc: Disease greater than 2 cm with or without lymph node involvement

Stage IV: Distant metastases: pleural effusions contain cancer cells and metastasis to the liver and spleen parenchyma

Table 1. International Federation of Gynecology and Obstetrics staging of ovarian cancer [10].

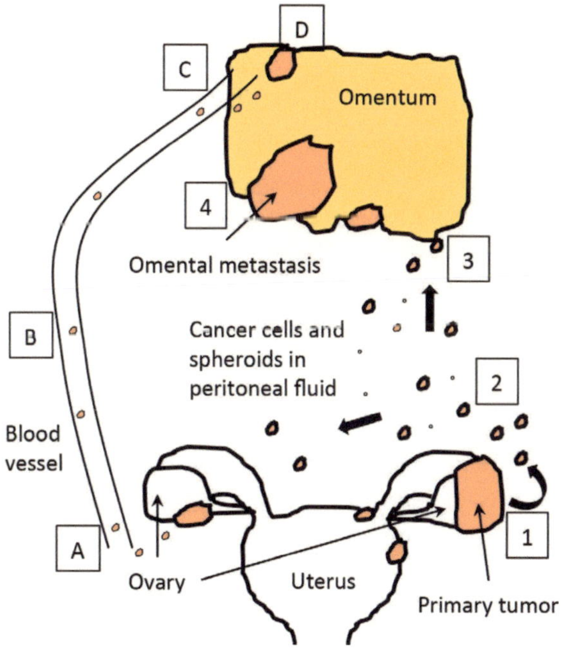

Figure 1. Mechanisms of ovarian cancer metastasis: Transcoelomic dissemination. (1) The cancer cells loose cell–cell contact and exfoliate into the peritoneal cavity. (2) They float in the peritoneal fluid and are carried all over the peritoneal cavity. (3) Attachment to the peritoneal organs like the omentum. (4) Formation of the metastatic tumor. Hematogenous metastasis. (A) Invasion and intravasation. (B) Transport of circulating cancer cells through the blood vessels. (C) Extravasation from the omental capillaries. (D) Formation of the metastatic tumor in the omentum.

2. Overview of ovarian cancer metastasis

The lack of an anatomic barrier allows the ovarian cancer cells to very conveniently spread into the peritoneal cavity. The cancer cells on the surface of the primary tumors start loosing cell–cell contact and become loosely attached to each other. As a result of this, they become prone to exfoliation into the peritoneal cavity (**Figure 1**). Exfoliation is promoted by the mechanical forces like rubbing of neighboring peritoneal organs during respiratory movements and flow of the peritoneal fluids. The cancer cells may come off as single cells or as clumps. This is a passive mode of dissemination unlike the typical invasion followed by intravasation observed in tumors undergoing hematogenous metastasis [13, 17, 18]. The peritoneal fluid naturally flows within the peritoneal cavity upward, toward the head, and then back downward, toward the feet, as a result of the diaphragm movement during respiration and gravitational pull, respectively [19]. The exfoliated ovarian cancer cells from the primary tumor are disseminated throughout the peritoneal cavity by this natural flow of the peritoneal fluid (**Figure 1**). Since normally there is only a small volume of the peritoneal fluid present, dissemination is predominantly limited to the organs in the vicinity of the primary tumor [17]. As the disease progresses, more and more ascites is produced and this enables the spread of the cancer cells to more distant sites in the abdomen. One of the predominant sites of ovarian cancer metastasis is the omentum which is a fatty double fold of the peritoneal membrane, about 8 by 8 inches in size, covering the bowels [13]. It is important to note that this mode of spreading typical of ovarian cancer is very different in terms of the hydrodynamic forces experienced by the cancer cells when they are carried rapidly in the blood vessels during hematogenous metastasis [20, 21].

Epithelial cells tend to undergo anoikis in the absence of attachment to a substratum. Therefore, the main challenge faced by the cancer cells floating in the peritoneal fluid is overcoming anoikis and surviving floatation. In addition, they have to avoid immune surveillance. The cancer cells either form aggregates or spheroids or exist as single cells (**Figure 1**) [22]. The spheroids may also contain embedded cancer-associated fibroblasts as well as activated mesothelial cells, which contribute to the development of the ascetic microenvironment [22]. The subsequent challenge for these floating cancer cells is to successfully attach to the surface of the organs in the peritoneal cavity (**Figure 1**). Debulking surgery often reveals such spheroids loosely attached to the peritoneum. The mesothelial cells covering the peritoneum and the bowels secrete mucus like substances, which help in reducing friction between surfaces as they brush against each other during the course of the organs' natural movements. The same also helps in preventing attachment of the cancer cells to some extent. However, the integrins expressed by the metastasizing cells help them to attach to the extra cellular matrix proteins (ECMs) secreted by the mesothelial cells. Thereafter, the cancer cells are able to push apart the mesothelial cells forming the protective barrier and invade into the organ [23, 24].

Having invaded through the mesothelium of the site of metastasis, the cancer cells have to now revert back to their normal self of growing attached to a substratum. However, since they are now encountering a new microenvironment with a potentially different ECM and secreted factors, they have to now adapt to these new conditions. The adaptive process involves extensive and productive reciprocal interactions between the cancer cells and the normal microenvironment of the metastatic site [6]. Those cells, which are able to successfully adapt to this new microenvironment, go on to eventually establish metastatic colonies. On the other hand, the cells that cannot productively interact and adjust to the new microenvironment eventually perish or remain dormant. The cells that are successful eventually reprogram the microenvironment to form and 'activated tumor stroma,' which include cancer-associated fibroblasts, endothelial cells, immune cells, and modified ECMs that promote tumor growth at the metastatic site. In addition to the peritoneal dissemination described above, ovarian cancer cells have been found in blood circulation and recent reports have indicated the existence of an alternative hematogenous mode of metastasis [16, 25].

The process of attaching to and developing metastatic tumors in the new organ is known as metastatic colonization (**Figure 1**). It is considered the least efficient step in the whole process of metastasis [21, 26]. This is also evidenced in mouse xenograft experiments to study ovarian cancer metastasis where many millions of cancer cells are injected intraperitoneally and result in about a hundred tumors or even less [6, 27, 28]. At the same time, the mechanism of regulation of this step and the initial cross talk between the cancer cells and the microenvironment remains a mystery for the obvious difficulty in getting access to this window. Greater understanding of the biology of this process will enable the identification of key regulators that can be targeted therapeutically to hit the metastatic disease at its most vulnerable phase.

3. Mechanism of peritoneal metastasis

The first step in the peritoneal metastasis is exfoliation of the ovarian cancer cells from the primary tumor into the peritoneal cavity. The prerequisite for this step is the loss of cell–cell contact between the cancer cells. As mentioned earlier, ovarian cancer can potentially arise from the fallopian tube epithelial cells or ovarian surface epithelium. Both express the classic epithelial marker epithelial cadherin (E-cadherin) [29]. E-cadherin plays a key role in epithelial cell behavior, tumor suppression, and tissue architecture through its function as a cell–cell adhesion molecule [30]. It is associated with the actin cytoskeleton through α, β, and γ catenins. While E-cadherin is directly involved in the formation of adherens junctions between adjacent epithelial cells, it can also regulate the formation of tight junctions and desmosomes [30, 31].

As the cancer progresses from a benign to a malignant form, the cells undergo an epithelial to mesenchymal transition (EMT). This involves molecular and morphological changes wherein they loose their epithelial characteristics and gain mesenchymal traits. This includes a loss of the compact cell-to-cell attachment, polarity, and cuboidal shape. The cells become more spindle shaped and motile. EMT also involves a change in the expression of epithelial and mesenchymal markers [32]. A very important aspect of this transition is the loss of expression of E-cadherin and a concomitant increase in the expression of neural cadherin (N-cadherin). This results in a reduction in the cell–cell interaction between cancer cells through their adherens junctions and an increase in the ability of the cancer cells to interact with the normal stromal cells present in the microenvironment. In ovarian cancer, E-cadherin expression can be regulated transcriptionally and post-transcriptionally [33]. ZEB-1, ZEB-2, Snail, and Slug are known to repress E-cadherin and can be regulated by several external cues. The signaling pathways that regulate EMT and E-cadherin expression include transforming growth factor β (TGF-β), epidermal growth factor (EGF), hepatocyte growth factor (HGF), endothelin-1 (ET-1), and bone morphogenetic protein 4 (BMP-4) [32]. Moreover, the miR-200 family of micro-RNAs can also indirectly regulate EMT by targeting ZEB-1 and ZEB-2, which results in the derepression of E-cadherin [34]. Decreased expression of miR-200 family resulted in an increase in the expression of ZEB-1 and ZEB-2, which repressed E-cadherin transcription and induced EMT in ovarian cancer.

The loss of E-cadherin expression and the resulting decrease in the cell–cell attachment promotes the dissemination of the cells into the peritoneal cavity. Interestingly, the loss in E-cadherin expression was found to lead to an induction of expression of α_5-integrin [35]. α_5-integrin forms a heterodimer with β_1-integrin that binds to fibronectin and hence is called the fibronectin receptor. The induction of α_5-integrin was not through the canonical β-catenin pathway. Instead, it was through the epithelial growth factor receptor (EGFR)/focal adhesion kinase (FAK)/mitogen-activated protein kinase (MAPK) pathway. The increase in fibronectin receptor expression was found to help the disseminated ovarian cancer cells attach to the fibronectin secreted by the mesothelial cells lining the omentum and peritoneum [35]. This is an evidence of how the loss of E-cadherin—which facilitates shedding—is coupled to preparing the cells to reattach at the distant metastatic site.

Once the cancer cells have been shed into the peritoneal fluid, it significantly affects the prognosis of the patient as evidenced by the 29% relapse rate of stage 1A ovarian cancer compared to 59% relapse rate of stage 1C [36]. However, once detached from the tumor mass, the cancer cells face several challenges in surviving in the peritoneal fluid. The peritoneal fluid is a result of continuous secretion of fluids by the peritoneal capillaries. This helps in lubricating the adjacent organs in the peritoneal cavity and allows uptake of soluble factors through the peritoneum. A majority of the peritoneal fluid is returned to the circulation through lymphatic drainage. However, in ovarian cancer patients, the increased leakiness of vasculature induced by high vascular endothelial growth factor (VEGF) levels accompanied by blocking of the lymphatic vessels by cancer cells results in ascites formation [22]. This ascites is called malignant ascites because of the presence of floating cancer cells. The malignant ascites facilitates the spread of the cancer cells throughout the peritoneal cavity.

The disseminated ovarian cancer cells floating in the ascites either as spheroids or as single cells develop resistance to anoikis and acquire cancer stem cell-like properties [37, 38]. Interestingly, the single-cell population was found to have a greater percentage of cancer stem cells [39]. The cancer stem cells enriched from ascites have highly elevated ability to form mouse xenograft tumors [40]. Just like cancer stem cells, the floating spheroids and single cells are resistant to chemotherapy. The compact nature of the spheroids serves as an additional physical barrier for the chemotherapeutic agents, preventing the inner cells from exposure to the drug [22]. Taken together, this indicates that the cancer cells floating in the ascites are stem-like and chemoresistant and have the potential to seed new metastatic tumors within the peritoneal cavity.

The spheroids have elevated levels of E-cadherin and EpCAM and concomitant diminished expression of vimentin, matrix metalloproteinases (MMPs), and CD44 [37, 39]. Therefore, the metastasizing cancer cells demonstrate plasticity in terms of their ability to switch back and forth from epithelial and mesenchymal phenotypes as per the demands of the different steps of metastasis. In addition to the cancer cells, the ascites has several normal cell types that together form the malignant ascites microenvironment and supports the floating cancer cells. The main non-cancer-cell types include cancer-associated fibroblasts (CAFs), mesothelial cells, immune cells, mesenchymal stem cells, and platelets [22]. These cells can be associated with the cancer spheroids or the single cells. They can also exist by themselves, floating in the peritoneal fluid. These supporting cells produce a milieu of factors that assist the cancer cell survival and subsequent colonization of the metastatic site. Cells like platelets also offer protection from immune surveillance by coating the cancer cells.

Having successfully survived flotation in the peritoneal fluids, the next goal of the metastasizing ovarian cancer cells is to attach to the various organs present in the peritoneal cavity. Electron micrographs of sections of normal peritoneum and omentum have revealed the architecture of the mesothelium covering them. The mesothelium consists of a monolayer of mesothelial cells that are very tightly joined end to end to form a protective barrier [24]. These mesothelial cells serve to provide a slippery surface—through the secretion of glycosaminoglycans and lubricants—facilitating normal coelomic movement as well as preventing infection and attachment of cancer cells [41]. The mesothelial cells can perform diverse functions such as secretion of ECMs, growth factors, and inflammatory cytokines for tissue repair and regeneration, proteases for fibrinolysis, and prevention of adhesions [41]. They are also actively involved in the movement of fluids and solutes across serosal cavities [42].

Early *in vitro* experiments revealed that the ovarian cancer cells force the retraction of the mesothelial cells upon attachment to the mesothelium [43]. More recently, Iwanicki et al. have demonstrated the role of the fibronectin receptor ($\alpha_5\beta_1$-integrin) expressed on the surface of the ovarian cancer cells help them attach to the fibronectin secreted on the surface of the mesothelial cells and promote the displacement of mesothelial cells through myosin-mediated traction forces [24]. Subsequent studies revealed the ovarian cancer cells with a mesenchymal phenotype had a greater propensity for mesothelial clearance [44]. The fibronectin secretion by the mesothelial cells was found to be induced by their interaction with the metastasizing ovarian cancer cells. The TGF-β secreted by the cancer cells activated a RAC1/SMAD-mediated signaling pathway in the mesothelial cells, which resulted in the transcriptional upregulation of the fibronectin gene and also induced an EMT-like phenotype in the mesothelial cells [45]. This would probably help in subsequent mesothelial clearance and also may potentially serve as a source of cancer-associated fibroblasts in the microenvironment of the metastatic tumor [46].

The increased expression of the fibronectin receptor in the ovarian cancer cells is also beneficial in coupling attachment to growth factor signaling to promote metastasis. Inhibition of the interaction of $\alpha_5\beta_1$-integrin on the cancer cells with the fibronectin on the surface of the omentum and peritoneum in mouse xenograft models of ovarian cancer metastasis resulted in a decreased metastatic burden in both prevention and intervention settings [28]. Since inhibition of $\alpha_5\beta_1$-integrin can also inhibit angiogenesis, it was further investigated whether the effects on metastasis were actually due to disruption of the human cancer cell $\alpha_5\beta_1$-integrin interaction with fibronectin or that of the mouse endothelial cell $\alpha_5\beta_1$-integrin. The effect of an anti-murine $\alpha_5\beta_1$-integrin-blocking antibody was compared to that of the anti-human $\alpha_5\beta_1$-integrin-blocking antibody. Interestingly, the murine-blocking antibody did not show any significant effect and, therefore, confirmed the key role of the interactions of the cancer cell $\alpha_5\beta_1$-integrin with the fibronectin of the microenvironment in promoting ovarian cancer metastasis [28]. Further investigation revealed that the activation of $\alpha_5\beta_1$-integrin resulted in the activation and phosphorylation of the receptor tyrosine kinase c-Met independent of its ligand—hepatocyte growth factor (HGF) [28]. This attachment induced activation of the growth factor receptor lead to increased invasiveness and growth through the subsequent activation of the FAK/Src signaling pathways in the cancer cells. The expression of a constitutively active FAK could abrogate the inhibitory effects of the $\alpha_5\beta_1$-integrin-blocking antibody on the ovarian cancer cells [28].

Another effect of adhesion of the ovarian cancer cells to the surface of the omentum is the increased secretion of the extracellular protease MMP-2. It cleaves fibronectin and vitronectin present on the surface of the mesothelium into smaller fragments, which enhances binding of the cancer cells to these ECMs through their specific integrin receptors $\alpha_5\beta_1$-integrin and $\alpha_v\beta_3$-integrin, respectively [47]. Inhibition of MMP-2 in the ovarian cancer cells as a prevention measure inhibited their adhesion to the omentum in nude mice. However, the host MMP-2 did not play a role in this process as evidenced in MMP-2 knockout mouse xenograft experiments [47].

Once the cancer cells attach to the mesothelial cells on the surface of the omentum, they embark on a process of adapting to the new microenvironment of the site of metastasis. As evidenced by the ECM-cancer cell interactions and their consequences above, more productive reciprocal interactions between the cancer cells and their new microenvironment are essential for successful establishment of the metastatic tumors. The cancer cells have to revert from surviving anoikis while floating in the peritoneal fluid to an attached growth in the presence of new ECMs and growth factors available in the microenvironment of the omentum and peritoneum. This involves significant changes in the gene expression profiles of the colonizing cancer cells and, therefore, would involve the activation/repression of transcriptional/translational regulators dependent on microenvironmental cues. One such important microenvironment regulated translational regulator was reported to be the micro-RNA miR-193b [6]. miR-193b is a tumor suppressor micro-RNA that was found to be downregulated in the metastasizing ovarian cancer upon their interaction with the mesothelial cells covering the surface of the omentum. This downregulation promoted growth and invasiveness of the cancer cells *in vitro,* colonization of human omentum *ex vivo,* and decreased metastasis in mouse xenografts [6]. Interestingly, the miR-193b downregulation was induced by the hypermethylation of its promoter as a result of the cross talk between the cancer cells and the mesothelial cells. The promoter hypermethylation was catalyzed by the increased expression of DNMT1 in the cancer cells stimulated by their interaction with the mesothelium [6]. miR-193b was found to directly target urokinase. A decrease in miR-193b expression resulted in increased expression of urokinase, which mediated the functional effects of miR-193b in driving metastatic colonization of the omentum [6].

As the cancer cells adapt to the new microenvironment of the metastatic site and start to proliferate, they also recruit resident and non-resident normal cells and convert them into the tumor-associated stroma or 'activated stroma' [48]. It is well known that the tumors consist of 10–50% of non-cancer cells or the tumor stroma [49]. The key components of this tumor stroma are the cancer-associated fibroblasts (CAFs), tumor-associated macrophages (TAMs), and other immune cells, endothelial cells, pericytes, adipocytes, extracellular matrix proteins, etc. [50]. All these stromal components are essential for successful growth and progression of the tumors as they are a critical source of growth and tropic factors, help in evasion of immune surveillance, angiogenesis, ECM remodeling, invasiveness, etc. Therefore, the eventual success of the cancer cells in colonizing the omentum will depend upon their ability to develop an active tumor stroma.

The metastasizing ovarian cancer cells were found to recruit the resident normal fibroblasts in the basement membrane of the omentum and reprogram them into CAFs. This reprogramming was driven by the decreased expression of miR-214, miR-31, and an increase in the expression of miR-155 in the normal fibroblasts induced by the cancer cells [49]. The resulting CAFs promoted ovarian cancer cell migration, invasion, and colony formation *in vitro* and tumor growth and metastasis *in vivo*. Interestingly, CAFs could be converted back into normal fibroblasts by the combined overexpression of miR-214 and miR-31 and inhibition of miR-155. The micro-RNAs mediated their effects through an array of targets, most of which were identified as chemokines and cytokines. The main mediator was found to be CCL5, which was a direct target of miR-214. Inhibition of CCL5 in nude mice injected with a mixture of ovarian cancer cells and CAFs significantly decreased the ability of the CAFs to promote tumor growth and metastasis [49].

An important and abundant cellular component of the omentum is adipocytes. Until recently, not much was known about the direct role of the omental adipocytes in promoting ovarian cancer metastasis to the omentum even though it is well established that omentum is one of the main sites of ovarian cancer metastasis and that it is a predominantly fatty tissue. Dr. Lengyel's group went on to demonstrate that the omental adipocytes secrete adipokines that promote the homing of the metastasizing ovarian cancer cells to the omentum [51]. The cancer cells, thereafter, could induce metabolic reprogramming of the adipocytes and induce lipolysis in them. The adipocytes in turn induced the expression of FABP4—a fatty acid transporter—in the cancer cells. As a result of this, the cancer cells efficiently take up the free fatty acids released by the adipocytes and utilize them as a source of energy and building blocks to drive tumor growth [51]. This explains why the omentum tumor is usually the largest one in the peritoneal cavity with sometimes the whole omentum getting converted into a solid, hard omental cake. By that time, all the adipocytes have been depleted and used for the growth of the metastatic tumor.

4. Other mechanism of dissemination

While the transcoelomic route of peritoneal dissemination is thought to be the predominant mode of ovarian cancer spread, other mechanisms do exist. The ascites produced in the peritoneal cavity is typically drained through the lymph vessels present in the diaphragm [36]. This provides the cancer cells present in the ascites, the opportunity to metastasize to the lymph nodes. Moreover, the lymphatic vessels drain into the left subclavian vein via the thoracic duct. This enables some cancer cells to enter into the blood circulation.

Although circulating ovarian cancer cells have long been reported to be present in the blood [52], it has typically been considered a mode of dissemination only in the very late stages of the disease. The prevalent reasoning being that although the ovarian cancer cells enter into the circulation, they are not yet adept at surviving in the circulation and establish metastatic tumors in a very different 'soil.' However, recent reports have suggested that hematogenous metastasis may be more commonly occurring in ovarian cancer that we had thought [16, 53]. Using a parabiosis model, Pradeep et al. have very elegantly demonstrated the haematogenous metastasis of the ovarian cancer cells from the primary tumor in one mouse to the omentum of the paired mouse [16]. The expression of $ErBB_3$ in the ovarian cancer cells entering into circulation and the omental expression of NRG1 was found to be the key players responsible for the hematogenous metastasis [16]. Interestingly, the use of mouse models of hematogenous ovarian cancer metastasis revealed a preferential homing of the cancer cells to the ovary followed by the development of ascites and subsequent peritoneal metastasis [53]. When the ovaries were removed before injecting the cancer cells, peritoneal metastasis and ascites formation were completely abolished [53]. Taken together, recent evidences point toward a more significant role of hematogenous dissemination in ovarian cancer that previously thought.

5. Conclusion

Ovarian cancer is a malignancy where most patients are treated for metastatic disease because they are usually diagnosed at an advanced stage. A better understanding of the process of metastasis and the underlying mechanisms of regulation is crucial for development of effective therapies. However, our knowledge in this field remains limited. It has become increasingly clear that there are multiple different ways in which the cancer cells disseminate, and the transcoelomic rout remains the most predominant mode. While it appears to be a relatively simpler way to metastasize, the steps involved pose their own unique challenges to the cancer cells. Moreover, the absence of the need for invasion, intravasation, and extravasation can potentially enable the cancer cells to metastasize earlier and in greater numbers than in case of hematogenous metastasis. Studying the underlying mechanisms have remained challenging but the evolution of *in vitro* organotypic 3D culture models have opened up opportunities to conduct more meaningful experiments and have lead to significant leaps in knowledge [6, 24, 45]. Use of ovarian cancer cell lines that closely resemble the mutational profile of clinical

http://dx.doi.org/DOI:10.5772/64700

HGSOC samples will also contribute toward meaningful progress in research in this field [54, 55]. The use of such models will hopefully provide greater insights into the regulation of metastatic colonization and enable therapeutic targeting of the disease at the stage in which they are most vulnerable. Moreover, considering the key roles played by the microenvironment of the site of metastasis as well as the tumor stroma, these 'normal' components can be targeted as well as the cross talk between them and the cancer cells. Since these cells are genetically stable and provide multiple different modes of support to the cancer cells, there will hopefully be reduced chances of development of drug resistance.

Acknowledgements

A Department of Defense Ovarian Cancer Academy Award supported AKM.

Author details

Anirban K. Mitra[1,2,3*]

Address all correspondence to: anmitra@indiana.edu

1 Medical Sciences Program, Indiana University School of Medicine, Bloomington, IN, USA

2 Indiana University Melvin and Bren Simon Cancer Center, Indianapolis, IN, USA

3 Department of Medical and Molecular Genetics, Indiana University School of Medicine, Indianapolis, IN, USA

References

[1] Siegel RL, Miller KD, Jemal A. Cancer statistics, 2016. CA: A Cancer Journal for Clinicians. 2016; 66(1):7–30.

[2] Jayson GC, Kohn EC, Kitchener HC, Ledermann JA. Ovarian cancer. Lancet (London, England). 2014; 384(9951):1376–1388.

[3] Integrated genomic analyses of ovarian carcinoma. Nature. 2011; 474(7353):609–615.

[4] Perets R, Drapkin R. It's totally tubular....riding the new wave of ovarian cancer research. Cancer research. 2016; 76(1):10–17.

[5] Vaughan S, Coward JI, Bast RC, Jr., Berchuck A, Berek JS, Brenton JD, Coukos G, Crum CC, Drapkin R, Etemadmoghadam D, Friedlander M, Gabra H, Kaye SB, et al. Re-

thinking ovarian cancer: recommendations for improving outcomes. Nature reviews Cancer. 2011; 11(10):719–725.

[6] Mitra AK, Chiang CY, Tiwari P, Tomar S, Watters KM, Peter ME, Lengyel E. Microenvironment-induced downregulation of miR-193b drives ovarian cancer metastasis. Oncogene. 2015; 34(48):5923–5932.

[7] Goff BA, Mandel LS, Melancon CH, Muntz HG. Frequency of symptoms of ovarian cancer in women presenting to primary care clinics. Jama. 2004; 291(22):2705–2712.

[8] Bankhead CR, Collins C, Stokes-Lampard H, Rose P, Wilson S, Clements A, Mant D, Kehoe ST, Austoker J. Identifying symptoms of ovarian cancer: a qualitative and quantitative study. BJOG: An International Journal of Obstetrics and Gynaecology. 2008; 115(8):1008–1014.

[9] Seward SM, Winer I. Primary debulking surgery and neoadjuvant chemotherapy in the treatment of advanced epithelial ovarian carcinoma. Cancer Metastasis Reviews. 2015; 34(1):5–10.

[10] Prat J. Staging classification for cancer of the ovary, fallopian tube, and peritoneum. International Journal of Gynaecology and Obstetrics: The Official Organ of the International Federation of Gynaecology and Obstetrics. 2014; 124(1):1–5.

[11] du Bois A, Reuss A, Pujade-Lauraine E, Harter P, Ray-Coquard I, Pfisterer J. Role of surgical outcome as prognostic factor in advanced epithelial ovarian cancer: a combined exploratory analysis of 3 prospectively randomized phase 3 multicenter trials: by the Arbeitsgemeinschaft Gynaekologische Onkologie Studiengruppe Ovarialkarzinom (AGO-OVAR) and the Groupe d'Investigateurs Nationaux Pour les Etudes des Cancers de l'Ovaire (GINECO). Cancer. 2009; 115(6):1234–1244.

[12] Thibault B, Castells M, Delord JP, Couderc B. Ovarian cancer microenvironment: implications for cancer dissemination and chemoresistance acquisition. Cancer Metastasis Reviews. 2014; 33(1):17–39.

[13] Lengyel E. Ovarian cancer development and metastasis. The American Journal of Pathology. 2010; 177(3):1053–1064.

[14] Amadori D, Sansoni E, Amadori A. Ovarian cancer: natural history and metastatic pattern. Frontiers in Bioscience: A Journal and Virtual Library. 1997; 2:g8–10.

[15] Tsuruchi N, Kamura T, Tsukamoto N, Akazawa K, Saito T, Kaku T, To N, Nakano H. Relationship between paraaortic lymph node involvement and intraperitoneal spread in patients with ovarian cancer--a multivariate analysis. Gynecologic Oncology. 1993; 49(1):51–55.

[16] Pradeep S, Kim SW, Wu SY, Nishimura M, Chaluvally-Raghavan P, Miyake T, Pecot CV, Kim SJ, Choi HJ, Bischoff FZ, Mayer JA, Huang L, Nick AM, et al. Hematogenous metastasis of ovarian cancer: rethinking mode of spread. Cancer Cell. 2014; 26(1):77–91.

[17] Yeung TL, Leung CS, Yip KP, Au Yeung CL, Wong ST, Mok SC. Cellular and molecular processes in ovarian cancer metastasis. A review in the theme: cell and molecular processes in cancer metastasis. American Journal of Physiology Cell Physiology. 2015; 309(7):C444–456.

[18] Naora H, Montell DJ. Ovarian cancer metastasis: integrating insights from disparate model organisms. Nature Reviews Cancer. 2005; 5(5):355–366.

[19] Carmignani CP, Sugarbaker TA, Bromley CM, Sugarbaker PH. Intraperitoneal cancer dissemination: mechanisms of the patterns of spread. Cancer Metastasis Reviews. 2003; 22(4):465–472.

[20] Valastyan S, Weinberg RA. Tumor metastasis: molecular insights and evolving paradigms. Cell. 2011; 147(2):275–292.

[21] Chambers AF, Groom AC, MacDonald IC. Dissemination and growth of cancer cells in metastatic sites. Nature Reviews Cancer. 2002; 2(8):563–572.

[22] Ahmed N, Stenvers KL. Getting to know ovarian cancer ascites: opportunities for targeted therapy-based translational research. Frontiers in Oncology. 2013; 3:256.

[23] Kenny HA, Nieman KM, Mitra AK, Lengyel E. The first line of intra-abdominal metastatic attack: breaching the mesothelial cell layer. Cancer Discovery. 2011; 1(2):100–102.

[24] Iwanicki MP, Davidowitz RA, Ng MR, Besser A, Muranen T, Merritt M, Danuser G, Ince TA, Brugge JS. Ovarian cancer spheroids use myosin-generated force to clear the mesothelium. Cancer Discovery. 2011; 1(2):144–157.

[25] Pecot CV, Bischoff FZ, Mayer JA, Wong KL, Pham T, Bottsford-Miller J, Stone RL, Lin YG, Jaladurgam P, Roh JW, Goodman BW, Merritt WM, Pircher TJ, et al. A novel platform for detection of CK+ and CK- CTCs. Cancer Discovery. 2011; 1(7):580–586.

[26] Chaffer CL, Weinberg RA. A perspective on cancer cell metastasis. Science (New York, NY). 2011; 331(6024):1559–1564.

[27] Mitra AK, Davis DA, Tomar S, Roy L, Gurler H, Xie J, Lantvit DD, Cardenas H, Fang F, Liu Y, Loughran E, Yang J, Sharon Stack M, et al. *In vivo* tumor growth of high-grade serous ovarian cancer cell lines. Gynecologic Oncology. 2015; 138(2):372–377.

[28] Mitra AK, Sawada K, Tiwari P, Mui K, Gwin K, Lengyel E. Ligand-independent activation of c-Met by fibronectin and alpha(5)beta(1)-integrin regulates ovarian cancer invasion and metastasis. Oncogene. 2011; 30(13):1566–1576.

[29] Burkhalter RJ, Westfall SD, Liu Y, Stack MS. Lysophosphatidic acid initiates epithelial to mesenchymal transition and induces beta-catenin-mediated transcription in epithelial ovarian carcinoma. The Journal of Biological Chemistry. 2015; 290(36):22143–22154.

[30] van Roy F, Berx G. The cell–cell adhesion molecule E-cadherin. Cellular and Molecular Life Sciences: CMLS. 2008; 65(23):3756–3788.

[31] van Hengel J, Gohon L, Bruyneel E, Vermeulen S, Cornelissen M, Mareel M, von Roy F. Protein kinase C activation upregulates intercellular adhesion of alpha-catenin-negative human colon cancer cell variants via induction of desmosomes. The Journal of Cell Biology. 1997; 137(5):1103–1116.

[32] Vergara D, Merlot B, Lucot JP, Collinet P, Vinatier D, Fournier I, Salzet M. Epithelial-mesenchymal transition in ovarian cancer. Cancer Letters. 2010; 291(1):59–66.

[33] Wu C, Cipollone J, Maines-Bandiera S, Tan C, Karsan A, Auersperg N, Roskelley CD. The morphogenic function of E-cadherin-mediated adherens junctions in epithelial ovarian carcinoma formation and progression. Differentiation; Research in Biological Diversity. 2008; 76(2):193–205.

[34] Park SM, Gaur AB, Lengyel E, Peter ME. The miR-200 family determines the epithelial phenotype of cancer cells by targeting the E-cadherin repressors ZEB1 and ZEB2. Genes and Development. 2008; 22(7):894–907.

[35] Sawada K, Mitra AK, Radjabi AR, Bhaskar V, Kistner EO, Tretiakova M, Jagadeeswaran S, Montag A, Becker A, Kenny HA, Peter ME, Ramakrishnan V, Yamada SD, et al. Loss of E-cadherin promotes ovarian cancer metastasis via alpha 5-integrin, which is a therapeutic target. Cancer Research. 2008; 68(7):2329–2339.

[36] Tan DS, Agarwal R, Kaye SB. Mechanisms of transcoelomic metastasis in ovarian cancer. The Lancet Oncology. 2006; 7(11):925–934.

[37] Latifi A, Luwor RB, Bilandzic M, Nazaretian S, Stenvers K, Pyman J, Zhu H, Thompson EW, Quinn MA, Findlay JK, Ahmed N. Isolation and characterization of tumor cells from the ascites of ovarian cancer patients: molecular phenotype of chemoresistant ovarian tumors. PloS One. 2012; 7(10):e46858.

[38] Ahmed N, Abubaker K, Findlay J, Quinn M. Epithelial mesenchymal transition and cancer stem cell-like phenotypes facilitate chemoresistance in recurrent ovarian cancer. Current Cancer Drug Targets. 2010; 10(3):268–278.

[39] Wintzell M, Hjerpe E, Avall Lundqvist E, Shoshan M. Protein markers of cancer-associated fibroblasts and tumor-initiating cells reveal subpopulations in freshly isolated ovarian cancer ascites. BMC Cancer. 2012; 12:359.

[40] Zhang S, Balch C, Chan MW, Lai HC, Matei D, Schilder JM, Yan PS, Huang TH, Nephew KP. Identification and characterization of ovarian cancer-initiating cells from primary human tumors. Cancer Research. 2008; 68(11):4311–4320.

[41] Mutsaers SE. Mesothelial cells: their structure, function and role in serosal repair. Respirology (Carlton, Vic). 2002; 7(3):171–191.

[42] Leak LV, Rahil K. Permeability of the diaphragmatic mesothelium: the ultrastructural basis for "stomata". The American Journal of Anatomy. 1978; 151(4):557–593.

[43] Niedbala MJ, Crickard K, Bernacki RJ. Interactions of human ovarian tumor cells with human mesothelial cells grown on extracellular matrix. An *in vitro* model system for

studying tumor cell adhesion and invasion. Experimental Cell Research. 1985; 160(2): 499–513.

[44] Davidowitz RA, Selfors LM, Iwanicki MP, Elias KM, Karst A, Piao H, Ince TA, Drage MG, Dering J, Konecny GE, Matulonis U, Mills GB, Slamon DJ, et al. Mesenchymal gene program-expressing ovarian cancer spheroids exhibit enhanced mesothelial clearance. The Journal of Clinical Investigation. 2014; 124(6):2611–2625.

[45] Kenny HA, Chiang CY, White EA, Schryver EM, Habis M, Romero IL, Ladanyi A, Penicka CV, George J, Matlin K, Montag A, Wroblewski K, Yamada SD, et al. Mesothelial cells promote early ovarian cancer metastasis through fibronectin secretion. The Journal of Clinical Investigation. 2014; 124(10):4614–4628.

[46] Rynne-Vidal A, Jimenez-Heffernan JA, Fernandez-Chacon C, Lopez-Cabrera M, Sandoval P. The mesothelial origin of carcinoma associated-fibroblasts in peritoneal metastasis. Cancers. 2015; 7(4):1994–2011.

[47] Kenny HA, Kaur S, Coussens LM, Lengyel E. The initial steps of ovarian cancer cell metastasis are mediated by MMP-2 cleavage of vitronectin and fibronectin. The Journal of Clinical Investigation. 2008; 118(4):1367–1379.

[48] Ko SY, Naora H. Adaptation of ovarian cancer cells to the peritoneal environment: Multiple mechanisms of the developmental patterning gene HOXA9. Cancer Cell and Microenvironment. 2014; 1(6):e379.

[49] Mitra AK, Zillhardt M, Hua Y, Tiwari P, Murmann AE, Peter ME, Lengyel E. MicroRNAs reprogram normal fibroblasts into cancer-associated fibroblasts in ovarian cancer. Cancer Discovery. 2012; 2(12):1100–1108.

[50] Hanahan D, Coussens LM. Accessories to the crime: functions of cells recruited to the tumor microenvironment. Cancer Cell. 2012; 21(3):309–322.

[51] Nieman KM, Kenny HA, Penicka CV, Ladanyi A, Buell-Gutbrod R, Zillhardt MR, Romero IL, Carey MS, Mills GB, Hotamisligil GS, Yamada SD, Peter ME, Gwin K, et al. Adipocytes promote ovarian cancer metastasis and provide energy for rapid tumor growth. Nature Medicine. 2011; 17(11):1498–1503.

[52] Judson PL, Geller MA, Bliss RL, Boente MP, Downs LS, Jr., Argenta PA, Carson LF. Preoperative detection of peripherally circulating cancer cells and its prognostic significance in ovarian cancer. Gynecologic Oncology. 2003; 91(2):389–394.

[53] Coffman LG, Burgos-Ojeda D, Wu R, Cho K, Bai S, Buckanovich RJ. New models of hematogenous ovarian cancer metastasis demonstrate preferential spread to the ovary and a requirement for the ovary for abdominal dissemination. Transl Res. 2016 Mar 30. pii: S1931-5244(16)00108-0. doi: 10.1016/j.trsl.2016.03.016. [Epub ahead of print] PubMed PMID: 27083386.

[54] Haley J, Tomar S, Pulliam N, Xiong S, Perkins SM, Karpf AR, Mitra S, Nephew KP, Mitra AK. Functional characterization of a panel of high-grade serous ovarian cancer cell lines as representative experimental models of the disease. Oncotarget. 2016.

[55] Domcke S, Sinha R, Levine DA, Sander C, Schultz N. Evaluating cell lines as tumour models by comparison of genomic profiles. Nature Communications. 2013; 4:2126.

Chapter 4

Role of Aquaporins in Breast Cancer Progression and Metastasis

Maitham A. Khajah and Yunus A. Luqmani

Additional information is available at the end of the chapter

http://dx.doi.org/10.5772/64446

Abstract

There are various limitations regarding the current pharmacological options for the treatment of breast cancer in terms of efficacy, target selectivity, side effect profile and survival. Endocrine-based therapy for hormone-sensitive cancers such as that of the breast is one of the most effective and well-tolerated therapeutic options but is hampered by either intrinsic or acquired resistance, resulting in a more aggressive form of the disease. It is generally agreed that this process occurs in parallel with cellular transition from epithelial to mesenchymal phenotype (EMT), with consequent enhancement of proliferative capacity, migrative ability and invasive potential. Aquaporins (AQPs) represent a large family of water channel proteins which are widely distributed in various tissues and which play a role in the physiological maintenance of the extracellular environment particularly to regulate electrolyte-water balance. Accumulating evidence shows that expression of several AQPs is modulated in cancer tissues, and this correlates with tumor grade. AQPs 1 and 3–5 are also involved in breast cancer invasion, through modulating the activity of various growth factors, signaling molecules and proteolytic enzymes. We review current data on the involvement of these proteins in processes associated with malignant progression and discuss possible applications of AQP-based therapy as an effective means of inhibiting cancer cells from metastasizing.

Keywords: breast cancer, metastasis, aquaporin, transport, ion channels

1. Introduction

Breast cancer remains the leading cause of tumor-associated mortality in women worldwide. Estrogen, acting through predominantly nuclear-located receptors (ER), has a significant detrimental impact during its pathogenesis [1]. This forms the basis for endocrine therapy, with the application of pharmacological antagonists generally termed selective estrogen receptor modulators, such as tamoxifen. These have resulted in significant improvements in quality of life as well as improved prognosis [2] in a significant proportion of patients with clinically defined ER+ve status [3]. Unfortunately, *de novo* resistance to tamoxifen occurs in about 30–40% of patients (those with very low level of ER expression, clinically designated as ER−ve) and even in about 50% of the clinically defined ER+ve patients. Furthermore, almost all initially responsive patients with late stage metastatic disease eventually relapse due to the development of *acquired* resistance to anti-estrogen therapy. These forms of endocrine resistance invariably lead to a more aggressive form of resurgent disease [4], and occur in parallel with cellular transition from epithelial to mesenchymal phenotype (EMT). There is a strong association between the EMT process and metastasis, which involves detachment of individual epithelial cells from neighboring cells, loss of polarity, scattering, acquisition of enhanced motility and invasion into the extracellular matrix (ECM) before entering blood and lymphatic vessels. Many phenotypic changes occur during this process which includes the loss of cell-cell adhesion as a result of reduced E-cadherin and catenins expression in adherens junctions, reduced claudins and occludins expression at tight junctions and reduced expression of various epithelial cytokeratins such as KRT8, 18 and 19 which presumably aids in disruption of cytoskeletal connections that maintain tissue architecture. These changes are also paralleled with up-regulation of mesenchymal markers such as vimentin, fibronectin, alpha smooth muscle actin (ACTA2), N-cadherin and various matrix metalloproteinases (MMPs) [4, 5]. Attempts to overcome endocrine resistance include the use of pure estrogen antagonists such as fulvestrant (in place of tamoxifen, which is associated with some agonist actions with prolonged administration) or agents which inhibit peripheral extragonadal synthesis of estrogen (aromatase inhibitors such as anastrazole), which delays but does not resolve this problem [6, 7]. In addition, receptor tyrosine kinase (RTK) inhibitors have been used recently in the treatment of endocrine-resistant breast cancer [8], but they have limitations in terms of target specificity and clinical outcomes. For example, the reversible inhibitor of epidermal growth factor receptor (EGFR) erlotinib also blocks ERBB2 [9, 10], AKT (the downstream target of phosphatidylinositide 3-kinases; PI3K) and mitogen-activated protein kinase (MAPK) phosphorylation in breast cancer cells [11]. Furthermore, imatinib inhibits the activity of the tyrosine kinase domain of various targets such as ABL, KIT and platelet-derived growth factor receptor (PDGFR) [12, 13]. The lack of specificity of these agents might increase the risk of side effects and therefore limits their clinical usage and utility. Since the current therapeutic options for endocrine insensitive breast cancer patients have various limitations (including severe side effect profile and resistance), there is a need to find better therapeutic targets to control this condition and improve its prognosis.

Aquaporins (AQPs) represent a family of 13–14 small hydrophobic integral transmembrane water channel proteins which are widely distributed in various tissues in the body. Their function is to transport mainly water (through passive transport), glycerol, solutes (such as urea, carbon dioxide, ammonia and nitric oxide) [14–20], as well as larger polar solutes (such as sugars and hydrogen peroxide) [21–23]. The first discovered family member of these proteins was initially called CHIP28, but it is now known as AQP 1 [24, 25]. AQPs are classified on the basis of their substrate permeability: (a) the classical water permeable AQPs 0, 1, 2, 4, 5, 6 and 8; (b) the water and small solute (e.g., glycerol and urea) permeable aquaglyceroporins AQPs 3, 7, 9, 10 and 12; (c) gas (carbon dioxide and nitric oxide) and ammonia permeable AQPs 1, 4 and 5; and (d) small ion (e.g., sodium and potassium) conducting AQP 1 [25]. Besides their main role in maintaining salt and water homeostasis, recent evidence suggests their involvement in various disease conditions including neoplasms such as breast cancer. These membrane channels have received much attention in recent years as potential novel drug targets for reducing cancer angiogenesis and metastasis. This chapter will provide evidence from recent studies regarding the involvement of various AQPs in breast cancer pathogenesis and will highlight their role in disease diagnosis, prognosis and treatment.

2. Structure of AQPs

Unlike other types of channels, AQPs do not show gating, saturation or membrane potential-dependent behavior. AQP family members share 25–60% protein sequence homology [14, 26, 27], and are assembled on the cell membrane and cytoplasmic compartments as homotetramers [28]. Each monomer is about 28–30 kDa in size and has its own water pore. Some members of this family such as AQPs 0 and 4 have unique features in that their tetramers assemble into higher order supramolecular structures described as orthogonal arrays of particles [29, 30]. The monomeric units of AQPs consist of six transmembrane α-helices (M 1, 2, 4–7 and 8), two half helices (M 3 and 7) and five connecting loops (a–e) [31]. Both the N- and carboxyterminal domains are present in the cytoplasmic compartment. Water movement occurs through a narrow pore (<0.3 nm) in which steric and electrostatic factors prevent the transport of protons and other small molecules [32]. Several studies have also indicated that the central pore allows the rapid transport of oxygen, carbon dioxide and nitric oxide (seen in AQPs 1, 4 and 5) [19, 33]. On the other hand, the aquaglyceroporins have a less constricted pore with a larger proportion of hydrophobic residues [34, 35]. **Figure 1** illustrates a schematic arrangement of an AQP channel.

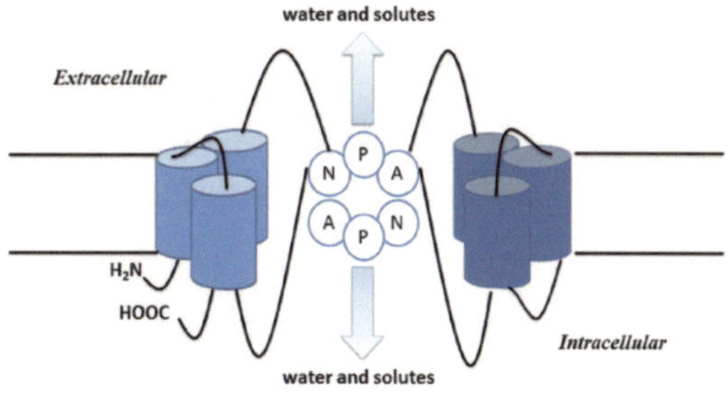

Figure 1. Schematic diagram of the aquaporin channel. The aquaporins are formed by two tandem repeats of three membrane-spanning helices. Two connecting loops, each containing a conserved sequence motif of Asn-Pro-Ala (NPA) on the loops, bend into molecules to pair with each other and form a channel in the plasma membrane through which water and solutes can pass between the cell and its environment.

3. Expression profile of AQPs

3.1. Normal tissues

These channel proteins exhibit a wide tissue distribution. Several AQPs (1–4) play a role in kidney function [36, 37]. For example, AQP 2 translocates from the intracellular vesicles to the apical plasma membrane of the collecting duct in response to vasopressin stimulation leading to water reabsorption by the kidney [37, 38]. AQP 1 allows carbon dioxide transport in the proximal tubules, for regulation of arterial pH during metabolic acidosis [39]. In the brain, AQP 4 is expressed in the perivascular astrocyte foot process region and plays a role in solute clearance from the interstitial fluid [40] and the neuro-excitatory processes [41]. In the skin, AQP 3 is expressed in the stratum corneum (SC) and plays a role in maintaining skin hydration and elasticity, and epidermal proliferation [42]. In the adipocytes, AQP 7 is involved in glycerol movement across the cell [36]. Several AQPs are expressed in various regions of the eye and play a role in ocular surface hydration, intraocular pressure regulation and visual signal transduction [43]. Other AQPs are expressed elsewhere but their physiological functions remain to be determined. For example, AQP 4 is expressed in the basolateral region of gastric parietal cells but its deletion in mice does not alter acid secretion [36, 44]. Furthermore, tissue-specific expression of AQP 4 in skeletal muscle [45], AQP 5 in sweat glands [46] and AQP 8 in various tissues [47] have not yet been linked with any specific physiological role.

3.2. Tumors

There is accumulating evidence to suggest a role for several AQPs in cancer pathogenesis through their modulated expression profile in several tumors. It is speculated that AQPs facilitate water penetration into the growing tumor leading to its expansion through edema formation [48, 49]. They also appear to be involved in angiogenesis, tumor proliferation and migration/invasion [50–53]. About twenty types of tumors have been shown to express AQPs *in vivo*. For example, the expression level of AQPs 1, 4 and 9 are increased in astrocytoma [48, 54–57], while the level of AQP 1 was shown to be either increased [58] or decreased [59] in cholangiocarcinoma. Increased levels of AQPs 1, 3 and 5 [60–62] and decreased level of AQP 8 [63, 64] have been reported in colorectal cancer. In lung cancer, AQPs 1, 3, 4 and 5 were shown to be overexpressed [65–67]. Increased levels of AQPs 1, 3 and 5 were observed in cervical cancer [68, 69]. AQP 5 was increased in chronic myelogenous leukemia [70] and esophageal cancer [71]. In liver cancer, high levels of AQPs 3 and 5 [72] and low levels of AQPs 8 and 9 were observed [73].

There is a direct correlation between the expression level of several AQPs and tumor grade. High levels of AQPs 1, 4 and 9 were observed in astrocytoma correlating with advanced disease stage [48, 54–57]. Enhanced AQP 9 expression was evident in malignant compared to benign ovarian tissues and was positively correlated with tumor grade [74]. Furthermore, enhanced expression of AQP 1 was seen in lung adenocarcinoma and its inhibition reduced cell invasion [66].

4. Physiological role of AQPs

4.1. Fluid transport and osmotic equilibrium

It has been suggested that at least eight (of the known 13) AQPs transport water, while others such as AQPs 3, 7, 9 and 10 are also able to transport glycerol (termed aquaglyceroporins) [44, 75]. Their expression in various organs such as the kidney tubules, lung and alveoli facilitate active fluid absorption and secretion by the creation of an osmotic gradient across the cell membrane and subsequent fluid movement through these channels. Genetic knockout of AQP 5 in mice resulted in impaired salivary [76, 77] and airway submucosal gland secretion [78]. In addition, tissue-specific knockout of AQP 1 in mice leads to impaired secretion of the cerebrospinal fluid [79] and ocular aqueous fluid [80], and inappropriate hypertonic fluid absorption in the proximal kidney tubules [81]. It should be noted, however, that other data suggest that knockout of various AQPs does not lead to impaired fluid absorption or secretion [82–86], suggesting that the requirement of AQPs to facilitate active fluid transport depends on the rate of such transport in each compartment. AQPs (specifically 1–4 and 7) are also involved in maintaining the osmotic equilibrium across the kidney tubules and the formation of concentrated urine. Marked polyuria and low urine osmolality was seen in AQPs 1 and 3 knockout mice, which led to severe dehydration [87, 88]. Reduced expression of AQP 2 also leads to acquired forms of nephrogenic diabetes insipidus (NDI) due to the inability of the kidneys to concentrate urine owing to the insensitivity of the distal nephron to the antidiuretic hormone arginine vasopressin [89]. AQP 4 is expressed in the glial cells of the brain and spinal cord, and plays an important role in water balance in the brain. A significant reduction in osmotic water permeability in glial cells was demonstrated in AQP-4-deficient mice which led to brain edema and swelling [90, 91]. In addition, several AQPs (0, 1, 3, 4 and 5) are expressed in various compartments of the eye and play an important role in the regulation of fluid movement and intraocular pressure [92–95].

4.2. CNS functions

AQP 4 was shown to be expressed in the glial cells in the brain particularly at astrocyte end-feet at the blood-brain barrier and the ependymal-cerebrospinal fluid barrier [96]. AQP 4 deficiency in mice resulted in reduced seizure susceptibility in response to pentylenetetrazol treatment [97], as well as in electrically-induced seizure following hippocampal stimulation [98]. Delayed potassium uptake from the brain extracellular space (ECS) [98, 99], and expanded ECS which dilutes the released potassium levels [100, 101], has been suggested to be responsible for the reduced seizure susceptibility in AQP-4-deficient mice. AQP 4 also increases water exit from the brain in vasogenic edema, as AQP-4-deficient mice show greater water accumulation in various models of brain edema [102–105]. Also, AQP 1 was shown to be expressed in the dorsal root ganglion neurons and nociceptive C-fibers, and AQP 1 deficiency in mice leads to reduced pain perception in response to thermal inflammatory pain in part through modulation of voltage gated sodium channel Nav 1.8 activity [105–107].

4.3. Glycerol transport

AQP 3 was shown to be expressed in the stratum corneum (SC) at the basal layer of the keratinocytes and plays a role in skin hydration. In AQP-3-deficient mice, SC hydration was significantly reduced due to reduced water content, decreased skin elasticity and wound healing [108]. An important factor which was also attributed to reduced skin hydration in AQP-3-deficient mice is the impaired glycerol transport from the blood to the epidermis through the basal keratinocytes, suggesting the importance of AQP 3 in glycerol transport. Dysregulated expression of AQP 3 has been found in various skin disorders associated with altered epidermal proliferation [109, 110]. In fact, topical or systemic replacement of glycerol prevented skin abnormalities (less hydration and elasticity and impaired barrier function) in the deficient mice [111].

4.4. Cell proliferation

A role for AQP 3 in cell proliferation has been suggested in various cell types. Using corneal epithelial cells, delayed restoration of full-thickness epithelia was seen in AQP-3-deficient mice after scraping. This was confirmed by reduction in proliferating BrdU-positive cells during healing [112]. Reduced keratinocyte cell proliferation was also evident in AQP-3-deficient mice or with siRNA-mediated knockout of AQP 3 in keratinocytes in part through reduction of p38 MAPK activity [113]. Furthermore, the proliferative rate of mouse colonic epithelial cells was significantly reduced in AQP-3-deficient mice, which might explain the enhanced colitis severity in these mice compared to WT mice in the dextran sulfate sodium model of colitis [114].

4.5. Cell adhesion

AQP 0 is thought to be involved in cell-cell adhesion. It has been found to be expressed in lens fiber cells in the eye and plays a role in maintaining their structure [115]. Loss-of-function mutation of AQP 0 in humans and mice resulted in congenital cataracts [34, 92]. In addition, AQP 4 was shown to mediate weak cell-cell interaction through its short helix in the extracellular loop [116]. Overexpression of AQP 4 in L-cells (which lack endogenous adhesion molecules) resulted in cell cluster formation, which supports the role of this AQP in intercellular adhesion.

4.6. Cell migration

Various AQPs have been shown to be involved in the cell migrative process. AQP 1 is expressed on the leading edge of migrating cultured endothelial cells in association with increased lamellipodia formation. AQP 1 deficiency in cultured endothelial cells results in significant reduction in their migration. Overexpression of AQP 1 or 4 enhanced cell migration along with prominent membrane ruffling at the leading edge [53]. The role of AQP 1 in cell migration was also confirmed using kidney proximal tubule cells where its deficiency reduced cell migration and its overexpression led to enhanced cell migration through the formation of lamella-like membrane protrusions at the cell leading edge [50]. Furthermore, AQP 4 was localized on the leading edge of migrating cultured astroglia cells, and its expression was increased by inducing a small extracellular osmotic gradient. AQP 4 deficiency (by siRNA treatment or cell isolation from AQP-4-deficient mice) resulted in marked reduction in their migratory potential [51, 52]. AQP 3 deficiency in mammalian corneal epithelial cells [51], keratinocytes [113] and fibroblasts [117] also reduced their migrative ability both *in vitro* and *in vivo.*

AQPs enhance cell migration through various mechanisms. They facilitate rapid changes in cell volume and shape, which allows the cells to squeeze through the narrow and irregularly shaped extracellular space; this has been referred to as amoeboidal movement [118]. Also, they increase the local hydrostatic pressure (that push apart adjacent stationary cells), and actin repolymerization, to stabilize cell membrane protrusions at the leading edge which is required for the migratory process [119]. There is some evidence regarding the role of AQP 4 in regulating a complex of intracellular molecules such as alpha-syntrophin involved in membrane protrusions [120]. Some evidence also suggests a role for AQP 3 in reducing keratinocyte cell migration through reduced p38 MAPK activity [113]; this is generally recognized as an important signaling molecule for cell migration.

5. Involvement of AQPs in the etiology of cancer

There is accumulating evidence for the involvement of several forms of AQPs in various types of cancer which also correlates with tumor stage.

With respect to tumor proliferation, AQP 5 interacts with the Ras-MAPK pathway and cyclin D1/CDK4 complexes in colon cancer [121] and with the EGFR/ERK1/2/p38 MAPK signaling cascade in lung cancer [122], resulting in enhanced proliferation, differentiation and survival. A role for AQP 3 has also been suggested for controlling proliferation of epidermal cancer cells through the facilitation of glycerol transport and increase in ATP generation [123]. In non-small-cell lung cancer cells, its effects appear to be associated with enhancement of the expression of p53, increase in the ratio of cleaved to procaspase 3 and reduction in the expression of proliferating cell nuclear antigen and B-cell lymphoma-2 (Bcl-2) [124]. AQP 4 is involved in glioblastoma cell proliferation; siRNA-mediated knockdown of AQP 4 induced cell apoptosis in part through modulation of key proteins involved in this process such as cytochrome c, Bcl-2 and Bad [125].

With regard to tumor migration/invasion and angiogenesis, AQP 3 silencing in non-small lung cancer cells resulted in significant inhibition of cell invasion through reduction of the activity of matrix metalloproteinases (MMPs) 2 and 9 and AKT phosphorylation, as well as reduction in angiogenesis through interaction with the HIF-2α-VEGF pathway [124]. Overexpression of AQP 1 in B16F10 melanoma cells and 4T1 breast cancer cells resulted in enhanced cell invasion and tumor spread when injected through the tail vein in mice [53, 126]. siRNA-mediated knockdown of AQP 1 in melanoma cells also resulted in reduced cell proliferation and invasion [127]. Overexpression of AQP 1 in colon cancer cells increased their invasive potential through actin relocalization and RhoA and Rac activation [128]. In glioma cells, AQP 1 facilitated the shunting of H^+ from the intracellular to the extracellular compartment and the release of lactate dehydrogenase (LDH) and cathepsin B, which results in the acidification of the tumor microenvironment leading to enhanced tumor angiogenesis and invasion [129]. AQP 4 also plays a role in glioblastoma cell migration and invasion through rearrangement of the actin cytoskeleton [130]. Furthermore, overexpression of AQP 5 in non-small lung cancer cells enhanced cell metastasis through c-Src activation and induction of the EMT process [122].

6. Role of AQPs in the pathogenesis of breast cancer

While AQPs have been shown to be involved in the delivery of water to the mammary glands which is critical for milk production and secretion during lactation [131], their expression in breast tumors is modified and correlates with tumor grade.

6.1. AQP 1

Immunostaining indicates a predominantly membranous localization with some presence in the cytoplasm in large tumor cells (more pronounced at the tumor invasion front), but no expression was seen in smaller tumor cells. All of the AQP 1 positive invasive carcinomas are found to be of ductal type, ER−ve and HER2/neu −ve (triple −ve form), and its expression was significantly associated with poor clinical prognosis [132, 133]. A recent report suggested that the cytoplasmic expression of AQP 1 promotes breast cancer progression and was associated with a shorter survival rate especially in luminal subtype patients [134]. Its cytoplasmic expression was positively correlated with advanced pathological features of invasive ductal carcinoma and lymph node metastasis [134]. Another study reported that AQP 1 was highly expressed in blood vessels (mainly in CD31+ve endothelial cells) of human breast and endometrial carcinoma tissues, suggesting a role in tumor angiogenesis [135]. Using human umbilical vein endothelial cells (HUVECs), Zou et al. [135] showed that estrogen treatment significantly up-regulated AQP 1 expression in a time- and dose-dependent fashion, which was mediated through a functional estrogen response element motif in the promoter region of the AQP1 gene. Estrogen treatment significantly increased HUVEC proliferation, migration, invasion and tubule formation; all of these effects were inhibited by pretreatment of cells with AQP1-specific siRNA. These data suggest an important role of AQP 1 in cell invasion in part through regulating actin stress fiber formation through colocalization with the ezrin/radixin/moesin protein complex [135]. Qin et al. [134] showed that overexpression of AQP 1 in MCF-7 and MDA-MB-231 cells significantly enhanced (by approximately 2 fold) cell proliferation and invasion. Epidermal growth factor (EGF) stimulation induced AQP 1 redistribution from the cytoplasm to the cell membrane, further supporting a role in promoting cell invasion. In the mouse mammary tumor virus-driven polyoma middle T oncogene (MMTV-PyVT) model (which spontaneously develops a well-differentiated luminal-type breast carcinoma with lung metastasis), AQP 1 deficiency significantly reduced the breast tumor mass (by 46%) and volume (by 50%), vessel density and the number of lung metastases compared to the control group [136]. This effect was in part due to decreased expression of vascular endothelial growth factor receptor-2 (VEGFR2) and increased levels of hypoxia inducible factor-1α (HIF-1α) in the AQP 1 knockout mice [136].

6.2. AQP 3

AQP 3 overexpression in early breast cancer patients was shown to be associated with worse prognosis in patients with HER2-overexpressing phenotype after curative surgery [137]. Its expression was correlated with advanced stage, large tumor size and lymphatic and vascular invasion, highlighting its role in angiogenesis and invasion. In addition, Huang et al. [138] showed higher AQP 3 protein expression in breast cancer tissues (mainly in the cell membrane and the cytoplasm) of premenopausal compared to postmenopausal patients, and was associated with higher histopathological grade and lymph node metastasis in ER+ve breast cancer patients. Estrogen stimulation significantly up-regulated AQP 3 expression in ER+ve breast cancer cells (MCF-7 and T47D) by activating the estrogen response elements (EREs) in the promoter region of the AQP 3 gene. siRNA mediated knockdown of AQP 3 in ER+ve breast cancer cells significantly reduced estrogen-induced cell migration (by 30–70%) and invasion (by 43–71%). Overexpression of AQP 3 in T47D cells significantly enhanced cell migration and invasion. The role of AQP 3 in cell invasion was suggested to be in part through mediating actin cytoskeleton rearrangement (by the formation of filopodia and stress fibers required for invasion) and EMT induction (evident by reduced expression of the epithelial marker E-cadherin, and increased levels of the mesenchymal markers N-cadherin and snail-1) [138]. Using breast cancer cell lines MDA-MB-231 and Bcap-37, Cao et al. [139] showed that fibroblast growth factor-2 (FGF-2) significantly increased AQP 3 expression, and lentivirus-mediated shRNA inhibition of AQP3 expression significantly reduced FGF-2 induced cell migration by approximately 50%. This effect was mediated through AQP-3-induced activation of Akt and ERK1/2. A recent report showed that AQP 3 expression in the triple negative breast cancer cell lines MDA-MB-231 and DU4475 (as well as in HUVEC) was required for the transport of extracellular hydrogen peroxide into the cells in response to CXCL-12 stimulation to induce directional cell migration [140]. AQP 3 silencing in these cells was associated with impaired CXCL-12 induced directional migration due to impaired F-actin polymerization, PTEN and PTP1B oxidation, Akt phosphorylation, and the accumulation of the intracellular hydrogen peroxide at the reading edge of migrating cells was needed for polarity sensing. Furthermore, the role of AQP3 in invasion was tested by the injection of fluorescently labeled breast cancer cells into severe combined immunodeficient (SCID) mice. Lung metastasis was significantly reduced in AQP-3-deficient breast cancer cells, whereas its overexpression significantly increased the number of cells migrating to the lungs [140]. In addition, the expression of AQP 3 was also increased in MCF-7 cells by treatment with the chemotherapeutic agent 5′-deoxy-5-fluorouridine (5′-DFUR) [141], which was required for the 5′-DFUR-induced cell cycle arrest (through its action on G1/S phase transition and up-regulation of p21 and FAS).

6.3. AQP 4

The role of this AQP is not well studied in breast cancer, however, one report showed that AQP 4 expression (at both mRNA and protein level) was significantly higher in normal compared to cancer tissue [133], and was mainly expressed in the cell membrane and the cytoplasmic compartments.

6.4. AQP 5

Immunohistochemical analysis shows significant overexpression of AQP 5 in breast tumors from early breast cancer patients, and was correlated with the disease prognosis particularly in patients with ER/PR+ve tumors [142]. This observation was also confirmed by another group who showed that AQP 5 was not detectable in normal breast tissues, but was expressed mainly in the cell membrane of mammary carcinoma and associated with cellular differentiation, lymph node invasion and tumor stage [133]. The 5-year survival rate was decreased from 80% in AQP 5 −ve patients to 50% in AQP5+ve patients, suggesting that its expression was associated with short overall survival [133]. In another report, AQP 5 expression was observed in the ductal epithelial cells of human breast tissues with significant overexpression in invasive compared to benign tumors [143]. It was also expressed in MCF7 and MDA-MB-231 breast cancer cell lines (at mRNA and protein level); shRNA, or hyperosmotic stress-induced reduction in AQP 5 expression significantly reduced cell proliferation and migration toward fetal bovine serum (FBS) gradient. Some reports have suggested that AQP 5 induces tumorigenesis (at least in lung epithelial cells) upon phosphorylation of the cAMP protein kinase consensus site located in its cytoplasmic loop [144, 145].

7. AQPs: cancer diagnostic markers in breast cancer

There is no clinical data so far which confirms the use of AQPs as diagnostic markers for breast cancer. However, many reports suggest a strong correlation between the expression profile of certain types of AQPs and breast cancer pathogenesis and prognosis. For example, AQP 1 expression was associated with poor clinical prognosis in ductal type, ER −ve and HER2/neu −ve breast cancer patients [132]. The cytoplasmic expression of AQP 1 was also correlated with advanced pathological features of invasive ductal carcinoma, lymph node metastasis and shorter survival [134]. Overexpression of AQP 3 in HER2-overexpressing patients [137] as well as in premenopausal ER+ve breast cancer patients [138] was associated with advanced stage. AQP 5 expression was also shown to be associated with poor clinical prognosis [133], particularly in patients with ER/PR+ve tumors [142], and in the ductal epithelial cells of human breast tissues [143].

Detection of serum AQP 4 auto-antibodies has shown promising indication as a diagnostic tool in neuromyelitis optica (NMO), an inflammatory demyelinating disease that selectively affects optic nerves and spinal cord. It is claimed to be significantly associated with a higher number of relapses and longer disease duration [146, 147]. There are also reports suggesting a role for other AQPs: AQP 2 in determining the etiology of metabolic disorders dependent on the arginine vasopressin [148], AQP 3 in eczema [149] and AQP 4 in epilepsy [150].

8. AQPs: therapeutic targets for breast cancer

There appears to be potential for the use of AQP-based therapies (such as cysteine-reactive heavy metal-based inhibitors, AQP-induced water permeation, monoclonal AQP-specific antibodies and AQP gene transfer) to treat various conditions including breast cancer. Several heavy metals have been shown to inhibit AQP 1. These include mercury II chloride (through covalent interaction with the Cys189 residue in the water pore of AQP 1) [151, 152] and silver and gold III compounds (through interaction with the cysteine residue near the conserved NPA domain) [153, 154]. Gold III compounds were also shown to inhibit AQP 3 through interaction with the Cys40 in its extracellular domain [154, 155]. Other nonmetal containing small molecule inhibitors include tetraethylammonium (TEA^+), which reversibly inhibits AQP 1 through interaction with the Tyr186 site [156, 157]. The carbonic anhydrase inhibitor acetazolamide was also shown to inhibit AQPs 1 and 4 [158, 159]. Several antiepileptics, and the loop diuretic bumetanide, are reported to inhibit AQP 4 [159–161]. The other loop diuretic furosemide was also found to inhibit AQP 1 [162]. Furthermore, AQP gene transfer therapy is also in its early phases; AQP 1 cDNA transfer into the parotid glands for treating salivary gland hypofunction after radiation therapy is currently in phase I clinical trials [163–165].

In noncancerous conditions, some AQPs (1–4 and 7) are required for the formation of concentrated urine, which suggests that AQP-inhibitors might act as a unique form of diuretics to treat various disorders such as heart failure [87, 88]. Increased expression of AQP 4 exacerbated water accumulation in the brain, suggesting that AQP 4 inhibitors might be used to treat cytotoxic edema [90, 91]. Other potential therapeutic uses of AQP-therapies include treatment of various exocrine disorders, obesity and glaucoma [166].

AQP 1 is expressed on the endothelial cells of microvessels in various tumors including the breast [167], with a clear role in mediating angiogenesis and invasion through interaction with the actin cytoskeletal machinery, EGF, VEGF and HIF-1α. It has been suggested that the carbonic anhydrase inhibitor acetozolamide, and the antiepileptic drug topiramate, suppress tumor invasion in part through inhibiting AQP 1 gene expression [168, 169]. AQP 3 was also shown to be involved in breast cancer cell invasion through interaction with the actin cytoskeleton proteins, ER, chemokines and growth factors (CXCL-12, FGF-2), downstream signaling molecules (ERK1/2, Akt, PTEN and PTP1B) and induction of the EMT process. Furthermore, AQP 5 also enhanced breast cancer invasion in part through interaction with cAMP. The chemotherapeutic drug cisplatin inhibits the expression of AQP 5 in ovarian cancer and leads to reduced lymph node metastasis [170]. Therefore [171], inhibitors of the above-mentioned AQPs may have potential applications in breast cancer therapy through their inhibitory actions on tumor angiogenesis and invasion.

9. Conclusion

There is growing evidence in several tumors (including that of the breast) to indicate that several growth factors (e.g., EGF, VEGF and FGF-2) which are known to enhance cell invasion, may do so, at least in part, through increasing expression of a number of AQPs, suggesting a prometastatic role for these channels. This is likely to be mediated by interaction with various signaling molecules involved in cell invasion such as Ras, MAPK and PI3K, leading to rearrangement of the actin cytoskeleton (through interaction with RhoA/Rac), extracellular acidification (through interaction with LDH and HIF-1α, which by itself enhances cell invasion), enhanced secretion of proteolytic enzymes needed to degrade the extracellular matrix (ECM) (e.g., MMP2/9 and cathepsin B) and induction of the EMT process. AQPs also enhance cell invasion through a 'rounding' of the cell to enable it to squeeze through the ECM (termed amoeboidal motility). **Figure 2** summarizes the putative role of AQPs in cancer pathogenesis.

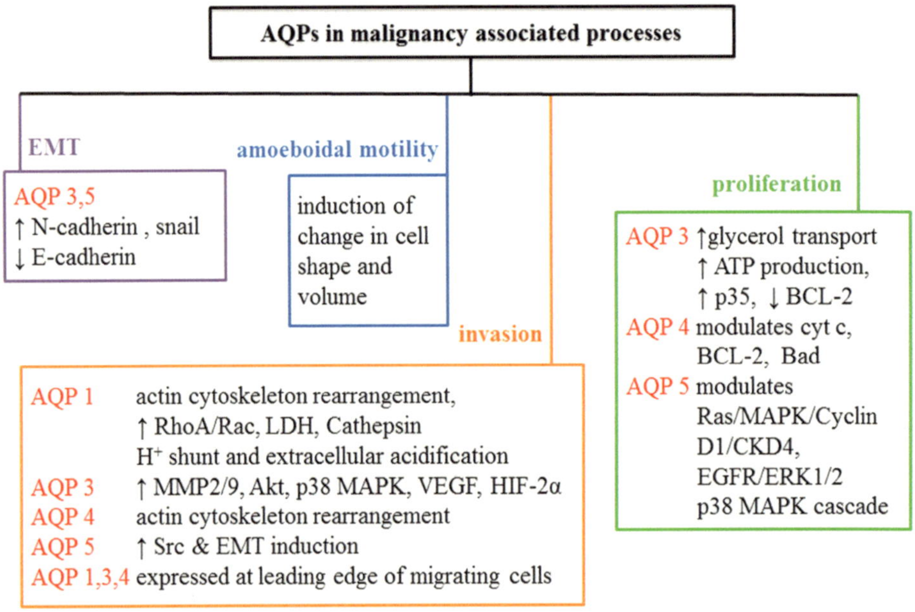

Figure 2. Role of AQPs in cancer pathogenesis. AQPs play an important role in cancer pathogenesis through enhancement of cancer cell proliferation, invasion and induction of epithelial to mesenchymal transition (EMT) as well as induction of amoeboidal motility. The mediators through which each AQP modulates these functions are elaborated in the scheme.

Author details

Maitham A. Khajah[1] and Yunus A. Luqmani[2*]

*Address all correspondence to: yunus@hsc.edu.kw

1 Department of Pharmacology and Therapeutics, Faculty of Pharmacy, Kuwait University, Safat, Kuwait

2 Department of Pharmaceutical Chemistry, Faculty of Pharmacy, Kuwait University, Safat, Kuwait

References

[1] Adamo V, Iorfida M, Montalto E, Festa V, Garipoli C, Scimone A, et al. Overview and new strategies in metastatic breast cancer (MBC) for treatment of tamoxifen-resistant patients. Ann Oncol. 2007;18(6):vi53-vi57.

[2] Berry DA, Cronin KA, Plevritis SK, Fryback DG, Clarke L, Zelen M, et al. Effect of screening and adjuvant therapy on mortality from breast cancer. N Engl J Med. 2005;353(17):1784-1792.

[3] Strasser-Weippl K, Goss PE. Advances in adjuvant hormonal therapy for postmenopausal women. J Clin Oncol. 2005;23(8):1751-1759.

[4] Al Saleh S, Sharaf LH, Luqmani YA. Signalling pathways involved in endocrine resistance in breast cancer and associations with epithelial to mesenchymal transition (Review). Int J Oncol. 2011;38(5):1197-1217.

[5] Luqmani YA, Al Azmi A, Al Bader M, Abraham G, El Zawahri M. Modification of gene expression induced by siRNA targeting of estrogen receptor alpha in MCF7 human breast cancer cells. Int J Oncol. 2009;34(1):231-242.

[6] Massarweh S, Schiff R. Unraveling the mechanisms of endocrine resistance in breast cancer: new therapeutic opportunities. Clin Cancer Res. 2007;13(7):1950-1954.

[7] Osborne CK, Schiff R. Mechanisms of endocrine resistance in breast cancer. Annu Rev Med. 2011;62:233-247.

[8] Normanno N, Morabito A, De Luca A, Piccirillo MC, Gallo M, Maiello MR, et al. Target-based therapies in breast cancer: current status and future perspectives. Endocr Relat Cancer. 2009;16(3):675-702.

[9] Normanno N, Bianco C, De Luca A, Maiello MR, Salomon DS. Target-based agents against ErbB receptors and their ligands: a novel approach to cancer treatment. Endocr Relat Cancer. 2003;10(1):1-21.

[10] Schaefer G, Shao L, Totpal K, Akita RW. Erlotinib directly inhibits HER2 kinase activation and downstream signaling events in intact cells lacking epidermal growth factor receptor expression. Cancer Res. 2007;67(3):1228-1238.

[11] Guix M, Granja Nde M, Meszoely I, Adkins TB, Wieman BM, Frierson KE, et al. Short preoperative treatment with erlotinib inhibits tumor cell proliferation in hormone receptor-positive breast cancers. J Clin Oncol. 2008;26(6):897-906.

[12] Gambacorti-Passerini C. Part I: Milestones in personalised medicine – imatinib. Lancet Oncol. 2008;9(6):600.

[13] Deininger MW, Druker BJ. Specific targeted therapy of chronic myelogenous leukemia with imatinib. Pharmacol Rev. 2003;55(3):401-423.

[14] Agre P, King LS, Yasui M, Guggino WB, Ottersen OP, Fujiyoshi Y, et al. Aquaporin water channels – from atomic structure to clinical medicine. J Physiol. 2002;542(Pt 1): 3-16.

[15] Verkman AS, Mitra AK. Structure and function of aquaporin water channels. Am J Physiol Renal Physiol. 2000;278(1):F13-F28.

[16] Wang Y, Tajkhorshid E. Nitric oxide conduction by the brain aquaporin AQP4. Proteins. 2010;78(3):661-670.

[17] Herrera M, Hong NJ, Garvin JL. Aquaporin-1 transports NO across cell membranes. Hypertension. 2006;48(1):157-164.

[18] Holm LM, Jahn TP, Moller AL, Schjoerring JK, Ferri D, Klaerke DA, et al. NH3 and NH4+ permeability in aquaporin-expressing Xenopus oocytes. Pflugers Arch. 2005;450(6):415-428.

[19] Musa-Aziz R, Chen LM, Pelletier MF, Boron WF. Relative CO2/NH3 selectivities of AQP1, AQP4, AQP5, AmtB, and RhAG. Proc Natl Acad Sci U S A. 2009;106(13): 5406-5411.

[20] Hub JS, Grubmuller H, de Groot BL. Dynamics and energetics of permeation through aquaporins. What do we learn from molecular dynamics simulations? Handb Exp Pharmacol. 2009;190:57-76.

[21] Miller EW, Dickinson BC, Chang CJ. Aquaporin-3 mediates hydrogen peroxide uptake to regulate downstream intracellular signaling. Proc Natl Acad Sci U S A. 2010;107(36): 15681-15686.

[22] Hara-Chikuma M, Chikuma S, Sugiyama Y, Kabashima K, Verkman AS, Inoue S, et al. Chemokine-dependent T cell migration requires aquaporin-3-mediated hydrogen peroxide uptake. J Exp Med. 2012;209(10):1743-1752.

[23] Tsukaguchi H, Weremowicz S, Morton CC, Hediger MA. Functional and molecular characterization of the human neutral solute channel aquaporin-9. Am J Physiol. 1999;277(5 Pt 2):F685-F696.

[24] Preston GM, Carroll TP, Guggino WB, Agre P. Appearance of water channels in Xenopus oocytes expressing red cell CHIP28 protein. Science. 1992;256(5055):385-387.

[25] Agre P, Preston GM, Smith BL, Jung JS, Raina S, Moon C, et al. Aquaporin CHIP: the archetypal molecular water channel. Am J Physiol. 1993;265(4 Pt 2):F463-F476.

[26] Fujiyoshi Y, Mitsuoka K, de Groot BL, Philippsen A, Grubmuller H, Agre P, et al. Structure and function of water channels. Curr Opin Struct Biol. 2002;12(4):509-515.

[27] Takata K, Matsuzaki T, Tajika Y. Aquaporins: water channel proteins of the cell membrane. Prog Histochem Cytochem. 2004;39(1):1-83.

[28] Walz T, Fujiyoshi Y, Engel A. The AQP structure and functional implications. Handb Exp Pharmacol. 2009;190:31-56.

[29] Crane JM, Verkman AS. Determinants of aquaporin-4 assembly in orthogonal arrays revealed by live-cell single-molecule fluorescence imaging. J Cell Sci. 2009;122(Pt 6): 813-821.

[30] Rash JE, Yasumura T, Hudson CS, Agre P, Nielsen S. Direct immunogold labeling of aquaporin-4 in square arrays of astrocyte and ependymocyte plasma membranes in rat brain and spinal cord. Proc Natl Acad Sci U S A. 1998;95(20):11981-11986.

[31] Verkman AS, Anderson MO, Papadopoulos MC. Aquaporins: important but elusive drug targets. Nat Rev Drug Discov. 2014;13(4):259-277.

[32] Hub JS, de Groot BL. Mechanism of selectivity in aquaporins and aquaglyceroporins. Proc Natl Acad Sci U S A. 2008;105(4):1198-1203.

[33] Herrera M, Garvin JL. Aquaporins as gas channels. Pflugers Arch. 2011;462(4):623-630.

[34] Chepelinsky AB. Structural function of MIP/aquaporin 0 in the eye lens; genetic defects lead to congenital inherited cataracts. Handb Exp Pharmacol. 2009;190:265-297.

[35] Yang B, Brown D, Verkman AS. The mercurial insensitive water channel (AQP-4) forms orthogonal arrays in stably transfected Chinese hamster ovary cells. J Biol Chem. 1996;271(9):4577-4580.

[36] Verkman AS. Aquaporins in clinical medicine. Annu Rev Med. 2012;63:303-316.

[37] Noda Y, Sohara E, Ohta E, Sasaki S. Aquaporins in kidney pathophysiology. Nat Rev Nephrol. 2010;6(3):168-178.

[38] Deen PM, Verdijk MA, Knoers NV, Wieringa B, Monnens LA, van Os CH, et al. Requirement of human renal water channel aquaporin-2 for vasopressin-dependent concentration of urine. Science. 1994;264(5155):92-95.

[39] Skelton LA, Boron WF, Zhou Y. Acid-base transport by the renal proximal tubule. J Nephrol 2010(23):S4-S18.

[40] Yang L, Kress BT, Weber HJ, Thiyagarajan M, Wang B, Deane R, et al. Evaluating glymphatic pathway function utilizing clinically relevant intrathecal infusion of CSF tracer. J Transl Med. 2013;11(107):1479-5876.

[41] Verkman AS, Ratelade J, Rossi A, Zhang H, Tradtrantip L. Aquaporin-4: orthogonal array assembly, CNS functions, and role in neuromyelitis optica. Acta Pharmacol Sin. 2011;32(6):702-710.

[42] Hara-Chikuma M, Verkman AS. Roles of aquaporin-3 in the epidermis. J Invest Dermatol. 2008;128(9):2145-2151.

[43] Verkman AS, Ruiz-Ederra J, Levin MH. Functions of aquaporins in the eye. Prog Retin Eye Res. 2008;27(4):420-433.

[44] Rojek A, Praetorius J, Frokiaer J, Nielsen S, Fenton RA. A current view of the mammalian aquaglyceroporins. Annu Rev Physiol. 2008;70:301-327.

[45] Yang B, Verbavatz JM, Song Y, Vetrivel L, Manley G, Kao WM, et al. Skeletal muscle function and water permeability in aquaporin-4 deficient mice. Am J Physiol Cell Physiol. 2000;278(6):C1108-C1115.

[46] Song Y, Sonawane N, Verkman AS. Localization of aquaporin-5 in sweat glands and functional analysis using knockout mice. J Physiol. 2002;541(Pt 2):561-568.

[47] Yang B, Song Y, Zhao D, Verkman AS. Phenotype analysis of aquaporin-8 null mice. Am J Physiol Cell Physiol. 2005;288(5):12.

[48] Saadoun S, Papadopoulos MC, Davies DC, Krishna S, Bell BA. Aquaporin-4 expression is increased in oedematous human brain tumours. J Neurol Neurosurg Psychiatry. 2002;72(2):262-265.

[49] Warth A, Simon P, Capper D, Goeppert B, Tabatabai G, Herzog H, et al. Expression pattern of the water channel aquaporin-4 in human gliomas is associated with blood-brain barrier disturbance but not with patient survival. J Neurosci Res. 2007;85(6): 1336-1346.

[50] Hara-Chikuma M, Verkman AS. Aquaporin-1 facilitates epithelial cell migration in kidney proximal tubule. J Am Soc Nephrol. 2006;17(1):39-45.

[51] Auguste KI, Jin S, Uchida K, Yan D, Manley GT, Papadopoulos MC, et al. Greatly impaired migration of implanted aquaporin-4-deficient astroglial cells in mouse brain toward a site of injury. Faseb J. 2007;21(1):108-116.

[52] Saadoun S, Papadopoulos MC, Watanabe H, Yan D, Manley GT, Verkman AS. Involvement of aquaporin-4 in astroglial cell migration and glial scar formation. J Cell Sci. 2005;118(Pt 24):5691-5698.

[53] Saadoun S, Papadopoulos MC, Hara-Chikuma M, Verkman AS. Impairment of angiogenesis and cell migration by targeted aquaporin-1 gene disruption. Nature. 2005;434(7034):786-792.

[54] Jelen S, Parm Ulhoi B, Larsen A, Frokiaer J, Nielsen S, Rutzler M. AQP9 expression in glioblastoma multiforme tumors is limited to a small population of astrocytic cells and CD15(+)/CalB(+) leukocytes. PLoS One. 2013;8(9):2013.

[55] Saadoun S, Papadopoulos MC, Davies DC, Bell BA, Krishna S. Increased aquaporin 1 water channel expression in human brain tumours. Br J Cancer. 2002;87(6):621-623.

[56] Zhu SJ, Wang KJ, Gan SW, Xu J, Xu SY, Sun SQ. Expression of aquaporin8 in human astrocytomas: correlation with pathologic grade. Biochem Biophys Res Commun. 2013;440(1):168-172.

[57] El Hindy N, Bankfalvi A, Herring A, Adamzik M, Lambertz N, Zhu Y, et al. Correlation of aquaporin-1 water channel protein expression with tumor angiogenesis in human astrocytoma. Anticancer Res. 2013;33(2):609-613.

[58] Mazal PR, Susani M, Wrba F, Haitel A. Diagnostic significance of aquaporin-1 in liver tumors. Hum Pathol. 2005;36(11):1226-1231.

[59] Aishima S, Kuroda Y, Nishihara Y, Taguchi K, Iguchi T, Taketomi A, et al. Down-regulation of aquaporin-1 in intrahepatic cholangiocarcinoma is related to tumor progression and mucin expression. Hum Pathol. 2007;38(12):1819-1825.

[60] Yoshida T, Hojo S, Sekine S, Sawada S, Okumura T, Nagata T, et al. Expression of aquaporin-1 is a poor prognostic factor for stage II and III colon cancer. Mol Clin Oncol. 2013;1(6):953-958.

[61] Moon C, Soria JC, Jang SJ, Lee J, Obaidul Hoque M, Sibony M, et al. Involvement of aquaporins in colorectal carcinogenesis. Oncogene. 2003;22(43):6699-6703.

[62] Shi X, Wu S, Yang Y, Tang L, Wang Y, Dong J, et al. AQP5 silencing suppresses p38 MAPK signaling and improves drug resistance in colon cancer cells. Tumour Biol. 2014;35(7):7035-7045.

[63] Wang W, Li Q, Yang T, Bai G, Li D, Sun H. Expression of AQP5 and AQP8 in human colorectal carcinoma and their clinical significance. World J Surg Oncol. 2012;10(242): 1477-7819.

[64] Fischer H, Stenling R, Rubio C, Lindblom A. Differential expression of aquaporin 8 in human colonic epithelial cells and colorectal tumors. BMC Physiol. 2001;1(1):23.

[65] Machida Y, Ueda Y, Shimasaki M, Sato K, Sagawa M, Katsuda S, et al. Relationship of aquaporin 1, 3, and 5 expression in lung cancer cells to cellular differentiation, invasive growth, and metastasis potential. Hum Pathol. 2011;42(5):669-678.

[66] Hoque MO, Soria JC, Woo J, Lee T, Lee J, Jang SJ, et al. Aquaporin 1 is overexpressed in lung cancer and stimulates NIH-3T3 cell proliferation and anchorage-independent growth. Am J Pathol. 2006;168(4):1345-1353.

[67] Xie Y, Wen X, Jiang Z, Fu HQ, Han H, Dai L. Aquaporin 1 and aquaporin 4 are involved in invasion of lung cancer cells. Clin Lab. 2012;58(1-2):75-80.

[68] Chen R, Shi Y, Amiduo R, Tuokan T, Suzuk L. Expression and prognostic value of aquaporin 1, 3 in cervical carcinoma in women of Uygur ethnicity from Xinjiang, China. PLoS One. 2014;9(2):2014.

[69] Zhang T, Zhao C, Chen D, Zhou Z. Overexpression of AQP5 in cervical cancer: correlation with clinicopathological features and prognosis. Med Oncol. 2012;29(3): 1998-2004.

[70] Chae YK, Kang SK, Kim MS, Woo J, Lee J, Chang S, et al. Human AQP5 plays a role in the progression of chronic myelogenous leukemia (CML). PLoS One. 2008;3(7):0002594.

[71] Liu S, Zhang S, Jiang H, Yang Y, Jiang Y. Co-expression of AQP3 and AQP5 in esophageal squamous cell carcinoma correlates with aggressive tumor progression and poor prognosis. Med Oncol. 2013;30(3):013-0636.

[72] Guo X, Sun T, Yang M, Li Z, Gao Y. Prognostic value of combined aquaporin 3 and aquaporin 5 overexpression in hepatocellular carcinoma. Biomed Res Int. 2013;2013(206525):9.

[73] Jablonski EM, Mattocks MA, Sokolov E, Koniaris LG, Hughes FM, Jr., Fausto N, et al. Decreased aquaporin expression leads to increased resistance to apoptosis in hepatocellular carcinoma. Cancer Lett. 2007;250(1):36-46.

[74] Yang JH, Yan CX, Chen XJ, Zhu YS. Expression of aquaglyceroporins in epithelial ovarian tumours and their clinical significance. Int Med Res.2011; 39(3):702-711.

[75] Verkman AS. More than just water channels: unexpected cellular roles of aquaporins. J Cell Sci. 2005;118(Pt 15):3225-3232.

[76] Ma T, Song Y, Gillespie A, Carlson EJ, Epstein CJ, Verkman AS. Defective secretion of saliva in transgenic mice lacking aquaporin-5 water channels. J Biol Chem. 1999;274(29): 20071-20074.

[77] Krane CM, Melvin JE, Nguyen HV, Richardson L, Towne JE, Doetschman T, et al. Salivary acinar cells from aquaporin 5-deficient mice have decreased membrane water permeability and altered cell volume regulation. J Biol Chem. 2001;276(26):23413-23420.

[78] Song Y, Verkman AS. Aquaporin-5 dependent fluid secretion in airway submucosal glands. J Biol Chem. 2001;276(44):41288-41292.

[79] Oshio K, Watanabe H, Song Y, Verkman AS, Manley GT. Reduced cerebrospinal fluid production and intracranial pressure in mice lacking choroid plexus water channel Aquaporin-1. Faseb J. 2005;19(1):76-78.

[80] Zhang D, Vetrivel L, Verkman AS. Aquaporin deletion in mice reduces intraocular pressure and aqueous fluid production. J Gen Physiol. 2002;119(6):561-569.

[81] Schnermann J, Chou CL, Ma T, Traynor T, Knepper MA, Verkman AS. Defective proximal tubular fluid reabsorption in transgenic aquaporin-1 null mice. Proc Natl Acad Sci U S A. 1998;95(16):9660-9664.

[82] Bai C, Fukuda N, Song Y, Ma T, Matthay MA, Verkman AS. Lung fluid transport in aquaporin-1 and aquaporin-4 knockout mice. J Clin Invest. 1999;103(4):555-561.

[83] Ma T, Fukuda N, Song Y, Matthay MA, Verkman AS. Lung fluid transport in aquaporin-5 knockout mice. J Clin Invest. 2000;105(1):93-100.

[84] Song Y, Fukuda N, Bai C, Ma T, Matthay MA, Verkman AS. Role of aquaporins in alveolar fluid clearance in neonatal and adult lung, and in oedema formation following acute lung injury: studies in transgenic aquaporin null mice. J Physiol. 2000;3:771-779.

[85] Song Y, Jayaraman S, Yang B, Matthay MA, Verkman AS. Role of aquaporin water channels in airway fluid transport, humidification, and surface liquid hydration. J Gen Physiol. 2001;117(6):573-582.

[86] Yang B, Folkesson HG, Yang J, Matthay MA, Ma T, Verkman AS. Reduced osmotic water permeability of the peritoneal barrier in aquaporin-1 knockout mice. Am J Physiol. 1999;276(1 Pt 1):C76-C81.

[87] Ma T, Yang B, Gillespie A, Carlson EJ, Epstein CJ, Verkman AS. Severely impaired urinary concentrating ability in transgenic mice lacking aquaporin-1 water channels. J Biol Chem. 1998;273(8):4296-4299.

[88] Ma T, Song Y, Yang B, Gillespie A, Carlson EJ, Epstein CJ, et al. Nephrogenic diabetes insipidus in mice lacking aquaporin-3 water channels. Proc Natl Acad Sci U S A. 2000;97(8):4386-4391.

[89] Khanna A. Acquired nephrogenic diabetes insipidus. Semin Nephrol. 2006;26(3): 244-248.

[90] Thiagarajah JR, Papadopoulos MC, Verkman AS. Noninvasive early detection of brain edema in mice by near-infrared light scattering. J Neurosci Res. 2005;80(2):293-299.

[91] Papadopoulos MC, Verkman AS. Aquaporin-4 gene disruption in mice reduces brain swelling and mortality in pneumococcal meningitis. J Biol Chem. 2005;280(14): 13906-13912.

[92] Berry V, Francis P, Kaushal S, Moore A, Bhattacharya S. Missense mutations in MIP underlie autosomal dominant 'polymorphic' and lamellar cataracts linked to 12q. Nat Genet. 2000;25(1):15-17.

[93] Thiagarajah JR, Verkman AS. Aquaporin deletion in mice reduces corneal water permeability and delays restoration of transparency after swelling. J Biol Chem. 2002;277(21):19139-19144.

[94] Li J, Patil RV, Verkman AS. Mildly abnormal retinal function in transgenic mice without Muller cell aquaporin-4 water channels. Invest Ophthalmol Vis Sci. 2002;43(2):573-579.

[95] Levin MH, Verkman AS. Aquaporin-dependent water permeation at the mouse ocular surface: in vivo microfluorimetric measurements in cornea and conjunctiva. Invest Ophthalmol Vis Sci. 2004;45(12):4423-4432.

[96] Nielsen S, Nagelhus EA, Amiry-Moghaddam M, Bourque C, Agre P, Ottersen OP. Specialized membrane domains for water transport in glial cells: high-resolution immunogold cytochemistry of aquaporin-4 in rat brain. J Neurosci. 1997;17(1):171-180.

[97] Binder DK, Oshio K, Ma T, Verkman AS, Manley GT. Increased seizure threshold in mice lacking aquaporin-4 water channels. Neuroreport. 2004;15(2):259-262.

[98] Binder DK, Yao X, Zador Z, Sick TJ, Verkman AS, Manley GT. Increased seizure duration and slowed potassium kinetics in mice lacking aquaporin-4 water channels. Glia. 2006;53(6):631-636.

[99] Padmawar P, Yao X, Bloch O, Manley GT, Verkman AS. K+ waves in brain cortex visualized using a long-wavelength K+-sensing fluorescent indicator. Nat Methods. 2005;2(11):825-827.

[100] Binder DK, Papadopoulos MC, Haggie PM, Verkman AS. In vivo measurement of brain extracellular space diffusion by cortical surface photobleaching. J Neurosci. 2004;24(37): 8049-8056.

[101] Zador Z, Magzoub M, Jin S, Manley GT, Papadopoulos MC, Verkman AS. Microfiber-optic fluorescence photobleaching reveals size-dependent macromolecule diffusion in extracellular space deep in brain. Faseb J. 2008;22(3):870-879.

[102] Papadopoulos MC, Manley GT, Krishna S, Verkman AS. Aquaporin-4 facilitates reabsorption of excess fluid in vasogenic brain edema. Faseb J. 2004;18(11):1291-1293.

[103] Bloch O, Papadopoulos MC, Manley GT, Verkman AS. Aquaporin-4 gene deletion in mice increases focal edema associated with staphylococcal brain abscess. J Neurochem. 2005;95(1):254-262.

[104] Tait MJ, Saadoun S, Bell BA, Verkman AS, Papadopoulos MC. Increased brain edema in aqp4-null mice in an experimental model of subarachnoid hemorrhage. Neuroscience. 2010;167(1):60-67.

[105] Bloch O, Auguste KI, Manley GT, Verkman AS. Accelerated progression of kaolin-induced hydrocephalus in aquaporin-4-deficient mice. J Cereb Blood Flow Metab. 2006;26(12):1527-1537.

[106] Saadoun S, Bell BA, Verkman AS, Papadopoulos MC. Greatly improved neurological outcome after spinal cord compression injury in AQP4-deficient mice. Brain. 2008;131(Pt 4):1087-1098.

[107] Kimura A, Hsu M, Seldin M, Verkman AS, Scharfman HE, Binder DK. Protective role of aquaporin-4 water channels after contusion spinal cord injury. Ann Neurol. 2010;67(6):794-801.

[108] Ma T, Hara M, Sougrat R, Verbavatz JM, Verkman AS. Impaired stratum corneum hydration in mice lacking epidermal water channel aquaporin-3. J Biol Chem. 2002;277(19):17147-17153.

[109] Kim NH, Lee AY. Reduced aquaporin3 expression and survival of keratinocytes in the depigmented epidermis of vitiligo. J Invest Dermatol. 2010;130(9):2231-2239.

[110] Nakahigashi K, Kabashima K, Ikoma A, Verkman AS, Miyachi Y, Hara-Chikuma M. Upregulation of aquaporin-3 is involved in keratinocyte proliferation and epidermal hyperplasia. J Invest Dermatol. 2011;131(4):865-873.

[111] Hara M, Verkman AS. Glycerol replacement corrects defective skin hydration, elasticity, and barrier function in aquaporin-3-deficient mice. Proc Natl Acad Sci U S A. 2003;100(12):7360-7365.

[112] Levin MH, Verkman AS. Aquaporin-3-dependent cell migration and proliferation during corneal re-epithelialization. Invest Ophthalmol Vis Sci. 2006;47(10):4365-4372.

[113] Hara-Chikuma M, Verkman AS. Aquaporin-3 facilitates epidermal cell migration and proliferation during wound healing. J Mol Med. 2008;86(2):221-231.

[114] Thiagarajah JR, Zhao D, Verkman AS. Impaired enterocyte proliferation in aquaporin-3 deficiency in mouse models of colitis. Gut. 2007;56(11):1529-1535.

[115] Sindhu Kumari S, Gupta N, Shiels A, FitzGerald PG, Menon AG, Mathias RT, et al. Role of Aquaporin 0 in lens biomechanics. Biochem Biophys Res Commun. 2015;462(4): 339-345.

[116] Hiroaki Y, Tani K, Kamegawa A, Gyobu N, Nishikawa K, Suzuki H, et al. Implications of the aquaporin-4 structure on array formation and cell adhesion. J Mol Biol. 2006;355(4):628-639.

[117] Cao C, Sun Y, Healey S, Bi Z, Hu G, Wan S, et al. EGFR-mediated expression of aquaporin-3 is involved in human skin fibroblast migration. Biochem J. 2006;400(2): 225-234.

[118] Sahai E, Marshall CJ. Differing modes of tumour cell invasion have distinct requirements for Rho/ROCK signalling and extracellular proteolysis. Nat Cell Biol. 2003;5(8): 711-719.

[119] Condeelis J. Life at the leading edge: the formation of cell protrusions. Annu Rev Cell Biol. 1993;9:411-444.

[120] Neely JD, Amiry-Moghaddam M, Ottersen OP, Froehner SC, Agre P, Adams ME. Syntrophin-dependent expression and localization of Aquaporin-4 water channel protein. Proc Natl Acad Sci U S A. 2001;98(24):14108-14113.

[121] Kang SK, Chae YK, Woo J, Kim MS, Park JC, Lee J, et al. Role of human aquaporin 5 in colorectal carcinogenesis. Am J Pathol. 2008;173(2):518-525.

[122] Zhang Z, Chen Z, Song Y, Zhang P, Hu J, Bai C. Expression of aquaporin 5 increases proliferation and metastasis potential of lung cancer. J Pathol. 2010;221(2):210-220.

[123] Hara-Chikuma M, Verkman AS. Prevention of skin tumorigenesis and impairment of epidermal cell proliferation by targeted aquaporin-3 gene disruption. Mol Cell Biol. 2008;28(1):326-332.

[124] Xia H, Ma YF, Yu CH, Li YJ, Tang J, Li JB, et al. Aquaporin 3 knockdown suppresses tumour growth and angiogenesis in experimental non-small cell lung cancer. Exp Physiol. 2014;99(7):974-984.

[125] Ding T, Zhou Y, Sun K, Jiang W, Li W, Liu X, et al. Knockdown a water channel protein, aquaporin-4, induced glioblastoma cell apoptosis. PLoS One. 2013;8(8):2013.

[126] Hu J, Verkman AS. Increased migration and metastatic potential of tumor cells expressing aquaporin water channels. Faseb J. 2006;20(11):1892-1894.

[127] Nicchia GP, Stigliano C, Sparaneo A, Rossi A, Frigeri A, Svelto M. Inhibition of aquaporin-1 dependent angiogenesis impairs tumour growth in a mouse model of melanoma. J Mol Med. 2013;91(5):613-623.

[128] Jiang Y. Aquaporin-1 activity of plasma membrane affects HT20 colon cancer cell migration. IUBMB Life. 2009;61(10):1001-1009.

[129] Hayashi Y, Edwards NA, Proescholdt MA, Oldfield EH, Merrill MJ. Regulation and function of aquaporin-1 in glioma cells. Neoplasia. 2007;9(9):777-787.

[130] Ding T, Gu F, Fu L, Ma YJ. Aquaporin-4 in glioma invasion and an analysis of molecular mechanisms. J Clin Neurosci. 2010;17(11):1359-1361.

[131] Mobasheri A, Barrett-Jolley R. Aquaporin water channels in the mammary gland: from physiology to pathophysiology and neoplasia. J Mammary Gland Biol Neoplasia. 2014;19(1):91-102.

[132] Otterbach F, Callies R, Adamzik M, Kimmig R, Siffert W, Schmid KW, et al. Aquaporin 1 (AQP1) expression is a novel characteristic feature of a particularly aggressive subgroup of basal-like breast carcinomas. Breast Cancer Res Treat. 2010;120(1):67-76.

[133] Shi Z, Zhang T, Luo L, Zhao H, Cheng J, Xiang J, et al. Aquaporins in human breast cancer: identification and involvement in carcinogenesis of breast cancer. J Surg Oncol. 2012;106(3):267-272.

[134] Qin F, Zhang H, Shao Y, Liu X, Yang L, Huang Y, et al. Expression of aquaporin1, a water channel protein, in cytoplasm is negatively correlated with prognosis of breast cancer patients. Oncotarget. 2016; 7(7):8143-8154.

[135] Zou LB, Shi S, Zhang RJ, Wang TT, Tan YJ, Zhang D, et al. Aquaporin-1 plays a crucial role in estrogen-induced tubulogenesis of vascular endothelial cells. J Clin Endocrinol Metab. 2013;98(4):2012-4081.

[136] Esteva-Font C, Jin BJ, Verkman AS. Aquaporin-1 gene deletion reduces breast tumor growth and lung metastasis in tumor-producing MMTV-PyVT mice. Faseb J. 2014;28(3):1446-1453.

[137] Kang S, Chae YS, Lee SJ, Kang BW, Kim JG, Kim WW, et al. Aquaporin 3 Expression Predicts Survival in Patients with HER2-positive Early Breast Cancer. Anticancer Res. 2015;35(5):2775-2782.

[138] Huang YT, Zhou J, Shi S, Xu HY, Qu F, Zhang D, et al. Identification of estrogen response element in aquaporin-3 gene that mediates estrogen-induced cell migration and invasion in estrogen receptor-positive breast cancer. Sci Rep. 2015;5:12484.

[139] Cao XC, Zhang WR, Cao WF, Liu BW, Zhang F, Zhao HM, et al. Aquaporin3 is required for FGF-2-induced migration of human breast cancers. PLoS One. 2013;8(2):28.

[140] Satooka H, Hara-Chikuma M. Aquaporin-3 controls breast cancer cell migration by regulating hydrogen peroxide transport and its downstream cell signaling. Mol Cell Biol. 2016;36(7):1206-1218.

[141] Trigueros-Motos L, Perez-Torras S, Casado FJ, Molina-Arcas M, Pastor-Anglada M. Aquaporin 3 (AQP3) participates in the cytotoxic response to nucleoside-derived drugs. BMC Cancer. 2012;12(434):1471-2407.

[142] Lee SJ, Chae YS, Kim JG, Kim WW, Jung JH, Park HY, et al. AQP5 expression predicts survival in patients with early breast cancer. Ann Surg Oncol. 2014;21(2):375-383.

[143] Jung HJ, Park JY, Jeon HS, Kwon TH. Aquaporin-5: a marker protein for proliferation and migration of human breast cancer cells. PLoS One. 2011;6(12):1.

[144] Woo J, Lee J, Chae YK, Kim MS, Baek JH, Park JC, et al. Overexpression of AQP5, a putative oncogene, promotes cell growth and transformation. Cancer Lett. 2008;264(1): 54-62.

[145] Sidhaye V, Hoffert JD, King LS. cAMP has distinct acute and chronic effects on aquaporin-5 in lung epithelial cells. J Biol Chem. 2005;280(5):3590-3596.

[146] Lennon VA, Kryzer TJ, Pittock SJ, Verkman AS, Hinson SR. IgG marker of optic-spinal multiple sclerosis binds to the aquaporin-4 water channel. J Exp Med. 2005;202(4): 473-477.

[147] Mader S, Lutterotti A, Di Pauli F, Kuenz B, Schanda K, Aboul-Enein F, et al. Patterns of antibody binding to aquaporin-4 isoforms in neuromyelitis optica. PLoS One. 2010;5(5):0010455.

[148] Ishikawa S. Urinary excretion of aquaporin-2 in pathological states of water metabolism. Ann Med. 2000;32(2):90-93.

[149] Olsson M, Broberg A, Jernas M, Carlsson L, Rudemo M, Suurkula M, et al. Increased expression of aquaporin 3 in atopic eczema. Allergy. 2006;61(9):1132-1137.

[150] Lee TS, Eid T, Mane S, Kim JH, Spencer DD, Ottersen OP, et al. Aquaporin-4 is increased in the sclerotic hippocampus in human temporal lobe epilepsy. Acta Neuropathol. 2004;108(6):493-502.

[151] Zhang R, van Hoek AN, Biwersi J, Verkman AS. A point mutation at cysteine 189 blocks the water permeability of rat kidney water channel CHIP28k. Biochemistry. 1993;32(12):2938-2941.

[152] Preston GM, Jung JS, Guggino WB, Agre P. The mercury-sensitive residue at cysteine 189 in the CHIP28 water channel. J Biol Chem. 1993;268(1):17-20.

[153] Niemietz CM, Tyerman SD. New potent inhibitors of aquaporins: silver and gold compounds inhibit aquaporins of plant and human origin. FEBS Lett. 2002;531(3): 443-447.

[154] Martins AP, Ciancetta A, de Almeida A, Marrone A, Re N, Soveral G, et al. Aquaporin inhibition by gold(III) compounds: new insights. ChemMedChem. 2013;8(7):1086-1092.

[155] Martins AP, Marrone A, Ciancetta A, Galan Cobo A, Echevarria M, Moura TF, et al. Targeting aquaporin function: potent inhibition of aquaglyceroporin-3 by a gold-based compound. PLoS One. 2012;7(5):18.

[156] Brooks HL, Regan JW, Yool AJ. Inhibition of aquaporin-1 water permeability by tetraethylammonium: involvement of the loop E pore region. Mol Pharmacol. 2000;57(5):1021-1026.

[157] Detmers FJ, de Groot BL, Muller EM, Hinton A, Konings IB, Sze M, et al. Quaternary ammonium compounds as water channel blockers. Specificity, potency, and site of action. J Biol Chem. 2006;281(20):14207-14214.

[158] Ma B, Xiang Y, Mu SM, Li T, Yu HM, Li XJ. Effects of acetazolamide and anordiol on osmotic water permeability in AQP1-cRNA injected Xenopus oocyte. Acta Pharmacol Sin. 2004;25(1):90-97.

[159] Gao J, Wang X, Chang Y, Zhang J, Song Q, Yu H, et al. Acetazolamide inhibits osmotic water permeability by interaction with aquaporin-1. Anal Biochem. 2006;350(2): 165-170.

[160] Huber VJ, Tsujita M, Yamazaki M, Sakimura K, Nakada T. Identification of arylsulfonamides as Aquaporin 4 inhibitors. Bioorg Med Chem Lett. 2007;17(5):1270-1273.

[161] Huber VJ, Tsujita M, Kwee IL, Nakada T. Inhibition of aquaporin 4 by antiepileptic drugs. Bioorg Med Chem. 2009;17(1):418-424.

[162] Ozu M, Dorr RA, Teresa Politi M, Parisi M, Toriano R. Water flux through human aquaporin 1: inhibition by intracellular furosemide and maximal response with high osmotic gradients. Eur Biophys J. 2011;40(6):737-746.

[163] Baum BJ, Zheng C, Cotrim AP, Goldsmith CM, Atkinson JC, Brahim JS, et al. Transfer of the AQP1 cDNA for the correction of radiation-induced salivary hypofunction. Biochim Biophys Acta. 2006;8(7):5.

[164] Gao R, Yan X, Zheng C, Goldsmith CM, Afione S, Hai B, et al. AAV2-mediated transfer of the human aquaporin-1 cDNA restores fluid secretion from irradiated miniature pig parotid glands. Gene Ther. 2011;18(1):38-42.

[165] Baum BJ, Alevizos I, Zheng C, Cotrim AP, Liu S, McCullagh L, et al. Early responses to adenoviral-mediated transfer of the aquaporin-1 cDNA for radiation-induced salivary hypofunction. Proc Natl Acad Sci U S A. 2012;109(47):19403-19407.

[166] Wang F, Feng XC, Li YM, Yang H, Ma TH. Aquaporins as potential drug targets. Acta Pharmacol Sin. 2006;27(4):395-401.

[167] Endo M, Jain RK, Witwer B, Brown D. Water channel (aquaporin 1) expression and distribution in mammary carcinomas and glioblastomas. Microvasc Res. 1999;58(2): 89-98.

[168] Pedersen SF, Hoffmann EK, Mills JW. The cytoskeleton and cell volume regulation. Comp Biochem Physiol A Mol Integr Physiol. 2001;130(3):385-399.

[169] Ma B, Xiang Y, Li T, Yu HM, Li XJ. Inhibitory effect of topiramate on Lewis lung carcinoma metastasis and its relation with AQP1 water channel. Acta Pharmacol Sin. 2004;25(1):54-60.

[170] Yang J, Yan C, Zheng W, Chen X. Proliferation inhibition of cisplatin and aquaporin 5 expression in human ovarian cancer cell CAOV3. Arch Gynecol Obstet. 2012;285(1): 239-245.

[171] Khajah MA, Mathew PM, Alam-Eldin NS, Luqmani YA. Bleb formation is induced by alkaline but not acidic pH in estrogen receptor silenced breast cancer cells. Int J Oncol. 2015;46(4):1685-1698.

Chapter 5

Extracellular Vesicles: A Mechanism to Reverse Metastatic Behaviour as a New Approach to Cancer Therapy

Monerah Al Soraj, Salma Bargal and
Yunus A. Luqmani

Additional information is available at the end of the chapter

http://dx.doi.org/10.5772/64391

Abstract

Extracellular vesicles (EVs) are membrane-bound particles shed from nearly all cell types into the extracellular environment. This collective term includes vesicles ranging in size from 30 nm to 5 μm in diameter. Various isolation techniques are used in different studies to separate EVs with no consensus protocol. EVs are released from cells under normal physiological conditions as well as in stressful and pathological conditions. In malignancies, they have been shown to be useful circulating markers for risk assessment, early diagnosis, monitoring of therapeutic effectiveness and prognosis. In addition, they appear to influence cell death and growth, angiogenesis, immune surveillance, extracellular matrix degradation and metastasis. In this respect, EVs have generated considerable interest for their potential use in cancer therapeutics. Since they appear to be responsible for transference of cellular components between cells and thereby transfer of functional characteristics of the donor to the recipient, two strategies for their role in cancer therapeutics may be envisaged. The first would be to prevent formation and/or shedding of EVs to prevent communication to or from cancer cells. The second would be to utilize them as carriers to deliver inhibitory/toxic components into cancer cells to destroy or neutralize them. In this review, we discuss the current state of research on characterization of EVs and highlight possible strategies for their use in cancer therapy.

Keywords: cancer, microvesicles, EVs, exosomes, drug delivery

1. Introduction

Extracellular vesicles (EVs) are membrane-bound particles shed into the extracellular environment by many types of cell under different circumstances ranging from normal physiological conditions to pathological conditions like cancer. There are several ways of classifying EVs, including size and mode of biogenesis. Some authors use the designation EVs interchangeably with other terms like exosomes and microvesicles (MVs). This has led to some confusion and inconsistency as to the particles actually being studied. Therefore, we have included a section on the various isolation procedures to emphasise the importance of standardization. Indeed, in many studies, there is no or unconvincing characterization of preparations. In this chapter, we will use EVs as a broad term to encompass three categories: exosomes, microvesicles and apoptotic bodies [1]. Exosomes (30–100 nm diameter) are formed in multi-vesicular bodies (MVB) [2] and released upon MVB exocytosis [3]. They carry several kinds of cargo, depending on the surrounding physiological conditions prevailing at the time of their formation and this will determine their effect upon recipient cells. MVs (100 nm–1 μm) are produced by the outward blebbing and fission of the plasma membrane and appear to have possibly more selectively sorted cargo. MVs express surface receptors that differ depending on the membrane composition of the donor cell [2]. Apoptotic bodies (1–5 μm) are usually released by tumour cells undergoing apoptosis, are packaged indiscriminately and are often fragmented nuclei and cytoplasmic organelles [3, 4] **Figure 1**.

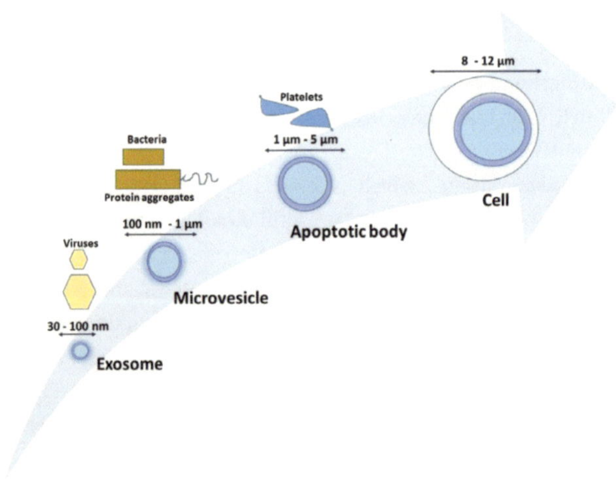

Figure 1. Schematic illustrating the relative sizes of the different classes of EVs (Adapted with permission from Ref. [3]).

When first discovered, the release of EVs from cells was thought to be a mechanism for removal of waste and harmful substances from the cell. Nowadays, they are viewed as mediators of intercellular communication through the transfer of biologically active molecules from donor to recipient cells where they can modulate the phenotype and function of those recipient cells [1]. EVs can interact through their surface proteins with receptors on the target cell, triggering

http://dx.doi.org/10.5772/64391

intracellular pathways, or by direct membrane fusion or endocytosis thereby releasing their cargo into the recipient cell [5]. Furthermore, EVs could transfer paracrine oncogenic features locally between different cells and endocrine signals to distal cells of any type through body fluids, usually blood [6].

The importance of exosomes may include antigen presentation and immune-stimulatory and inhibitory functions. Several key roles of MVs have been suggested to include contribution to the proinvasive character of tumours, induction of oncogenic cellular transformation, procoa gulant activity and fetomaternal communication [3].

2. Techniques used for collection, measurement of concentration and preservation of EVs

Because of the heterogenicity of EVs, a method of collecting a specific population of EVs of interest must be established. Moreover, the methods of efficient collection of EVs have been investigated in different studies. Previous reports have used two main methods: the ultracentrifugation method [7, 8] and FACS methods [9] for collecting EVs. Many studies have compared the efficiency of these collection methods and evaluated the effect of *in vivo* biodistribution of EVs [10, 11]. These observations suggested that bulk EVs are heterogeneous populations and that there is a need to collect a specific population of interest. In the following section, we will compare different methods for isolating EVs and different techniques used for collection and preservation of EVs.

2.1. Isolation techniques

In general, the isolation of EVs from biological fluids and cell cultures requires a series of standard differential centrifugation steps [22]. These sequentially remove dead cells and large cellular debris and then larger intracellular organelles, prior to obtaining a pellet from the cleared cell supernatant. Several modifications/elaborations of the basic procedure have been introduced to purify EVs as well as fractionate them further into discrete size groups; these are illustrated in **Figure 2**.

Heat shock proteins (HSPs), usually associated with cytoprotective functions or as receptor chaperones, are often associated with the cell surface of cancer cells. This feature has been exploited for the separation of EVs from biological fluids and conditioned cell culture growth media. Synthetic peptides called venceremin (Vn), with specific affinity to HSPs, have been used to precipitate out EVs expressing these proteins, in a procedure [16] that has advantages of speed and simplicity over those methods using standard ultracentrifugation. Further refinement of such a strategy, utilizing targets with an exclusively cell surface localization, could be used to distinguish the intracellularly generated exosomes from particles that are formed from the plasma membrane. Other techniques for separating EVs include a salting out process using sodium acetate, and the exoquick technique marketed as a kit by several companies. The latter is also based on selective precipitation of EVs but uses a commercial agglutinating agent as well as two centrifugation steps. Exoquick has been claimed to produce the highest concentration of EVs when compared to differential centrifugation or salting out methods [14].

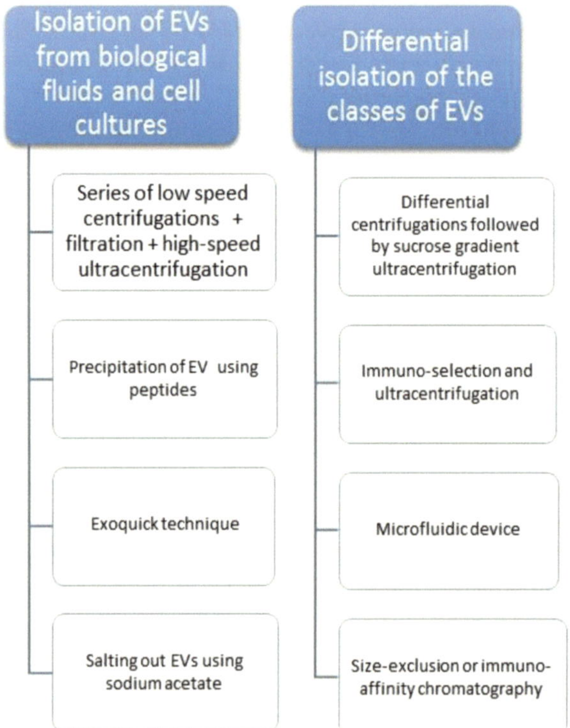

Figure 2. Summary of procedures for isolation of EVs from biological fluids or cell cultures.

Currently, there is no standard isolation protocol for clearly discriminating the different classes of EVs whether by size, density, morphology of the particles or molecular markers [2]. Various procedures have been described in an attempt to separate them. Among the different groups of EVs, the isolation of exosomes is the one most frequently reported in the literature [13]. Separation of exosomes from MVs usually involves a combination of low-speed differential centrifugation steps followed by sucrose gradient ultracentrifugation [21]. Apoptotic bodies can be collected at low-speed centrifugation of approximately 2,000 g. Microvesicles need a higher speed ranging from 10,000 to 20,000 g. Exosomes are pelleted by ultracentrifugation above 100,000 g for 1 hour or more [12]. Alternatively, immune selection of MVs can be performed instead of the differential centrifugation step. This involves the adherence of MVs to magnetic beads bearing antibodies against tumour-associated markers found on the surface of MVs. Ultracentrifugation would still be needed following this immunoselection in order to recover the exosomes in the eluate from the magnetic beads. Apoptotic bodies, on the other hand, can be separated from exosomes by flotation on a continuous sucrose gradient. Separation of exosomes from biological fluids and other EVs through the steps mentioned above takes approximately 4–6 hours.

Another procedure devised to shorten the time for preparation is based on the use of a microfluidic device, which is said to allow extraction and purification of exosomal RNA from 100 to 400 μl serum samples in an hour. This device relies on immunoaffinity isolation of exosomes from cell-free supernatant or serum samples. The sample is allowed to flow inside a microchannel coated with IgG against CD63 (which is highly expressed in exosomes from all cell origins). Specificity was demonstrated by showing that fluorescence intensity was higher in the microchannel coated with anti-CD63 antibodies compared to that coated with (control) anti-CD4 antibodies. As opposed to magnetic bead-based systems, the microfluidic device extracts exosomes directly from the serum in a single step. It does not require incubation, washing or centrifugation. This technique is not only faster compared to other methods of separation but is also cheaper, requires smaller volumes of samples, and fewer reagents [22].

Another method commonly used for isolation is size exclusion chromatography, which relies on size differences to separate EVs. Immunoaffinity chromatography is also an option for capturing exosomes with antibodies that recognize a marker on the surface of exosomes [13].

3. EVs in health and disease

3.1. Biological roles of EVs

EVs that are derived from healthy cells transfer signals to other cells, which are needed to maintain their physiological homeostasis and biological functions such as growth, differentiation and apoptotic death. They exert their effects through multiple pathways, directly activating cell surface receptors through bioactive lipid ligands and proteins, integrating their membrane contents into the recipient cell plasma membrane and delivering effectors, such as transcription factors, oncogenes, small and large non-coding regulatory RNAs, mRNAs and infectious particles into recipient cells. Consequently, EVs contribute to the maintenance of normal physiology [12].

The following are some examples of the role of EVs in maintaining a wide range of cellular and biological functions:

I. Regulation of immune responses.

EVs might trigger adaptive immune responses or suppress inflammation in a tolerogenic manner [13]. They have been shown to implement immune suppression by several mechanisms, such as enhancing the function of regulatory T cells, suppressing natural killer (NK cells, and inhibiting monocyte differentiation [12].

II. The nervous system.

The secretion of EVs can contribute to a range of neurobiological functions. For example, increased release of EVs containing neurotransmitter receptors from cortical neurons following enhanced glutamatergic activity [14].

III. Embryonic development.

EVs are likely to be involved in the regulation of embryonic development, including maintenance of morphogen gradients, collective cell migration and tissue polarity. However, this still remains an emerging field with many unanswered questions, which need further investigation [15].

IV. Tissue repair.

EVs derived from human adult mesenchymal stem cells (MSCs) have been found to prevent ischaemia-reperfusion kidney injury and improve survival in a model of lethal acute kidney injury [16]. MSC-derived EVs are reported to modify the expression of miR29c and miR150 and upregulate the expression of SDF-1, CXCR4, CXCR7, CCL2 and ANGPTL4, which are known to play essential roles in acute and chronic wounding [17].

V. Liver homeostasis.

A comprehensive study of hepatocyte-derived EVs showed the presence of several members of cytochrome P450, uridinediphosphate-glucuronosyl-transferase (UGTs) and glutathione S-transferase (GST) protein families, supporting a role of these vesicles in the metabolism of endogenous and xenobiotic compounds [18]. Recently, it has been shown that EVs from hepatocytes were able to activate stellate cells to mediate a response to liver damage [19] and many studies support an important role of these vesicles in maintaining liver homeostasis.

3.2. Pathological actions of EVs

Given their essential role in regulating biological processes, it is not surprising that EVs have a significant influence in disease pathogenesis. This has been most extensively studied in tumour biology. Several reports have indicated that EVs may be an important means of driving the formation of a pre-metastatic tumour [12, 20]. EVs can promote proliferation of their target cells, stimulate angiogenesis, induce metastasis and promote immune escape by modulating T-cell activity [21–24].

Prior to the discovery of EVs, it was known that the vesicles secreted by tumour cells retained procoagulant activity, linking cancer progression with EV-induced thrombosis [25–27]. In addition, a direct link between EVs and tumour invasion of healthy tissues was reported in 2008 [28]. It was shown that the mRNA expression of an activated mutated epidermal growth factor receptor (EGFRvII) in glioma cells can enhance vesiculation significantly and intercellular transfer of this oncoprotein to adjacent tumour cells, leading to the production of angiogenic mediators such as vascular endothelial growth factor (VEGF) [28].

Similar results were reported in another study by Skog et al. [22] showing that various miRNAs that stimulate tumour growth and angiogenesis in addition to EGFR can be transferred by human primary glioblastoma cell-derived EVs. Moreover, EVs derived from tumour cells were shown to transfer activated EGFR to endothelial cells, inducing VEGF expression and resulting in VEGF receptor activation to stimulate angiogenesis [29]. Many of the previously mentioned studies suggested that EVs can trigger tumour growth by stimulating the proliferation of cancer cells and by stimulating angiogenesis in the adjacent normal endothelial cells.

Additional data also support the association of tumour-secreted EVs in the promotion of metastasis and tumour invasion; for example, transfer of the EMMPRIN transmembrane glycoprotein, which stimulates matrix metalloproteinase (MMP) expression in fibroblasts and remodelling of the ECM [30]. Recently, it was shown that EVs derived from melanoma cells directed bone marrow cells towards a prometastatic phenotype, mediating the communication between tumour cells and normal cells [31, 32].

Furthermore, tumour-associated macrophages can secrete EVs, which contain certain miRNAs that can promote breast cancer cell invasion [33]. In addition to their role in cancer, EVs have been associated with various pathogens, including HIV-1, Epstein-Barr virus (EBV) and prions [34–36].

4. Involvement of EVs in cancer

Tumour EVs (oncosomes) are associated with many types of cancers [37–39], with elevated concentration in the plasma of cancer patients compared to healthy controls [40]; this can be up to 10-fold more than the approximately 10^{11} MVs per ml of serum measured in healthy individuals [41, 42]. Tumour EVs contain lipids and proteins as well as RNAs, genomic DNA and cellular metabolites, which can be transferred between cells [43], thus regulating the bioactivities of recipient cells. Production of EVs seems to be highly regulated. Several studies have characterised tumour EV components to identify useful cancer biomarkers [44]. For example, in two breast cancer cell lines, MCF-7 and MDA-MB 231, the cell-derived EVs show different profiles; 59 proteins were identified in MCF-7-derived EVs and 88 in EVs from MDA-MB 231, with 27 proteins common between the two exosome-like vesicle types [45]. Among all of these molecules that can be transferred from one cell to another through EVs, miRNAs have attracted most attention because of their newly recognised regulatory role in modulating gene expression. As some profiling studies have shown, miRNAs are not randomly incorporated into exosomes. According to previous studies, there exists a class of miRNAs that are preferentially sorted into exosomes, such as miR-320 and miR-150. Members of the miR-320 family are widely distributed in exosomes derived from both normal tissue and tumours [22, 46, 47] Moreover, some reports have shown that exosomal miRNA expression levels are altered under different physiological conditions. Exosomal miR-105 released from the breast cancer cell line MDA-MB-231 reduced *ZO-1* gene expression in endothelial cells and enhanced metastases to the lung and brain [48]. Exosomal miR-214, derived from the human microvascular endothelial cell line HMEC-1, stimulated migration and angiogenesis in neighbouring HMEC-1 cells [49]. Thus, it is attractive to speculate that EVs may 'export' the ability of the producer cells to metastasise, to other cells.

Stressful stimuli, such as hypoxia, acidosis, oxidative stress, radiation and cytotoxic drugs, activate signalling pathways that can trigger exosome production and secretion [50]. The p-53-regulated gene product, TSAP6 [51], as well as ceramide [52] have been documented as

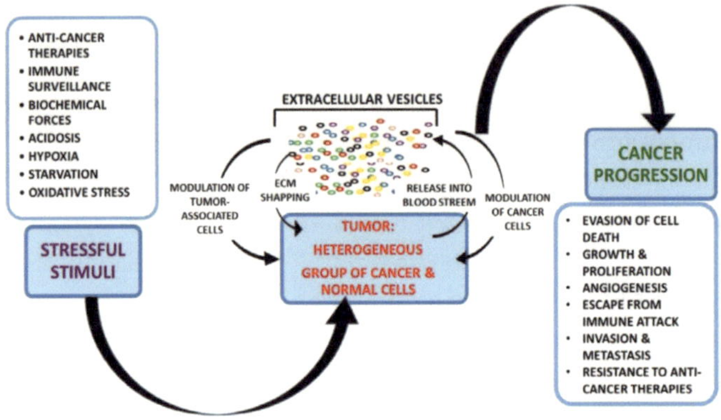

Figure 3. Extracellular vesicles (EVs) are potential carriers of stress-mediated tumour progression (Adapted with permission from Ref. [50]).

triggers. Stressful conditions can change both the molecular content and function of EVs, allowing for cancer progression through any of the processes displayed in **Figure 3**. For example, thermal and oxidative stress on leukemia/lymphoma T and B cells has been shown to induce the release of exosomes rich in Natural Killer Group 2 and member D (NKGD2) ligands that confer immunosuppressive properties to the exosomes. In addition, aggressive B-cell lymphoma cells that have been exposed to rituximab, which is an anti-CD20 chimeric antibody, started secreting CD20-poitive exosomes that protected the lymphoma cells from antibody and complement-dependent cytolysis. It is known that the phenotype of metastatic cells is a result of an accumulation of stress conditions on tumour cells. It has also been reported that while EVs derived from primary tumour cells can contain cell-adhesive proteins, those from metastatic cells are loaded with proteins that are responsible for cancer progression, invasion, metastasis and multidrug resistance. Thus, EVs can act as conveyors of stress-mediated tumour progression. Like cancer cells, stromal cells could release EVs with modulated function upon exposure to stress. As an example, mesenchymal stem cells exposed to hypoxic conditions released microvesicles with angiogenic effects [50]. The horizontal transfer of bioactive molecules by EVs can influence the different aspects of tumour progression, which include angiogenesis, decrease of immune surveillance, ECM degradation, metastasis and chemoresistance. The following sections discuss the influence of EVS on the processes that are vital for tumour progression, through horizontal transfer of bioactive molecules.

I. Neoangiogenesis.

Fibrin, the end product of the coagulation process, plays an important role in tumour growth as tumour cells can be coated with fibrin to escape immune surveillance; at the same time, the fibrin matrix enhances the outgrowth of new blood vessels. In several studies, it has been shown that EVs support coagulation through various mechanisms. They expose negatively charged phospholipids, which enable binding of coagulation factors and hence formation of prothrombinase complexes [53, 54]. In cancer, tissue factor vesicles are present in the peripheral blood [27, 55]. A part of these MVs originates from cancer cells and usually participate in thrombus formation equally to leukocyte-derived vesicles. Those MV-exposed tissue factors can promote coagulation by adhering at the site of vascular damage [56, 57].

In addition, tissue factor also plays a more direct role in angiogenesis, which is induced through cytoplasmic domain phosphorylation of the tissue factor and subsequent downstream signalling events. Consequently, thrombin will be generated through the activation of coagulation by tissue factor, which cleaves several protease-activated receptors (PARs), in order to initiate angiogenesis [58].

Besides, platelet-derived vesicles stimulate mRNA expression of angiogenic factors in cancer cells and then cancer cell-derived vesicles will contain mRNA for growth factors, such as VEGF and hepatocyte growth factor [59]. It has been showed that such vesicles fuse with monocytes, conveying their nucleic acids content and altering their biologic activity [60]. It is believed that cancer cell-derived MVs transfer mRNA to other cancer cells, enhancing their malignant potential, and it has been reported, as mentioned previously, that intercellular transfer of oncogenic growth factor receptor by cancer cell-derived EVs modify the phenotype of these cells [28].

II. Escape from immune surveillance.

Collective data suggest a relationship between stressful conditions due to the tumour environment and immunological tolerance of tumours [50]. There are many mechanisms, either direct or indirect, that have been suggested which can facilitate escape from immune surveillance. For example, cancer cells may employ vesiculation as a means to efficiently deceive the immune system and survive [13]. Another study also showed that under the pressure of oxidative stress, tumour cells release NKG2DL-expressing tumour exosomes, which facilitate tumour escape from cytotoxic immune attack [61]. Further, exosomes from various cancer cells were shown to expose Fas ligand (FasL, CD95L) of the death receptor Fas (CD95), to trigger T-cell death and to diminish the function of adaptive immune cells [62].

Tumour-associated EVs may also enhance the function of regulatory T (T_{Reg}) cells, weaken natural cytotoxic responses mediated by natural killer cells, downregulate dendritic cell differentiation from monocytes and turn these cells into immunosuppressive cells [24, 63, 64]. In addition, cancer cells can integrate with EVs derived from non-cancer cells, for example, platelets, by this means receiving lipids and transmembrane proteins, which would protect them from immune surveillance [59]. Additionally, cancer cells may hide from the immune system by mimicking the host environment.

III. Environmental degradation.

It has been shown that degradation of the ECM is needed for tumour growth [65]. EVs expose and contain several proteases, including matrix metalloproteinase (MMP)-2 and MMP-9 and urokinase-type plasminogen activator (uPA). uPA catalyzes the conversion of plasminogen into plasmin, whereas MMPs degrade basement membrane collagens. Plasmin, which is a serine protease, degrades numerous components of the ECM, including fibrin, and activates various MMP zymogens [66].

When Ginestra et al. [67] analyzed vesicle content in ascites fluids from 33 women with different gynaecologic pathologies, they found that malignant tumour fluids contained higher amounts of vesicles compared to benign proliferative cells. Moreover, they showed that the EVs from benign serous cysts had only minimal lytic activity, whereas those from cancer ascites contained active metalloproteases [67]. Furthermore, a link was found between the malignant potential of tumours and the MV-associated MMP-2 activity [68]. Another study reported an increase in numbers of vesicles in late stage ovarian cancer ascites and showed that MMP-2, MMP-9 and uPA activities were mainly concentrated within the MVs. Further, the MMP-2, MMP-9 or uPA inhibition using antibodies almost eliminated the ability of these MVs to enhance tumour invasion capacity, which highlights the significance of this pathway [69].

IV. Metastasis.

Metastasis necessitates an increase in cellular survival and invasiveness, which are both enhanced by MVs. Some evidence suggests that MVs may favour lymphogenous and haematological spread as the expression of Fas ligand by cancer cell-derived MVs plays a role in lymph node infiltration [70]. Furthermore, as mentioned above, activation of platelets by tissue factor-derived vesicles supports the haematological spread of cancer cells. Since the cancer cells will be surrounded by platelets, this would afford them some protection from immune surveillance and enhance their attachment to the vessel wall [59]. In addition, the procoagulant properties of cancer cell-derived MVs further support intravascular fibrin formation, which in turn facilitates adherence of cancer cells to the vessel wall [27].

4.1. EVs in cancer therapeutics

Since MVs appear to contribute significantly to cancer development, it is not surprising that much effort is being focused on trying to find ways of utilizing them in therapy as well. There are at least four strategies that could potentially be used to oppose EV-driven disease by inhibiting various aspects of EV function; these are summarised in **Figure 4**. The most obvious approach is to get rid of them and this can be achieved by blocking their biogenesis, by interfering with their release from the cell, removing them from the circulation or inhibiting their uptake by recipient cells [1].

4.1.1. Inhibition of EVs

I. Inhibiting EV formation.

Various cellular components are known to be vital for EV formation but until now no clear inhibition strategy has been forthcoming although many are under investigation. However, some studies showed that inhibition of ceramide formation (which is essential for endosomal sorting and exosome biogenesis) using small molecule inhibitors of neutral sphingomyelinase or through treatment with the blood pressure-lowering drug amiloride (which decreases endocytic vesicle recycling) can reduce EV formation [52, 71]. Another interesting study emphasised the importance of syndecan proteoglycans and their cytoplasmic adaptor syntenin, in regulating exosome formation and release, directly interfering with this interaction either by RNA interference (RNAi) or using small molecule inhibitors [72].

http://dx.doi.org/10.5772/64391

II. Inhibiting EV release.

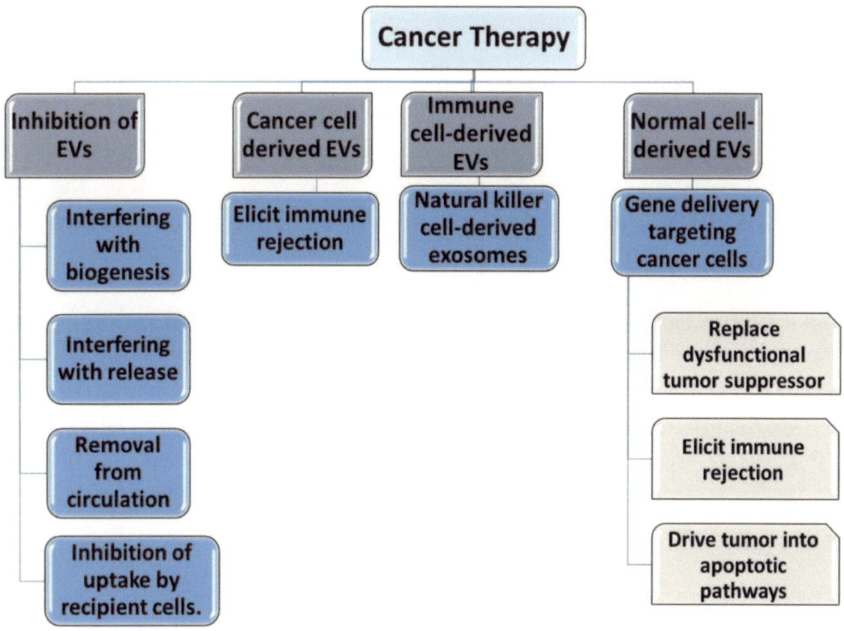

Figure 4. Flowchart showing the variety of roles of EVs in cancer therapeutics.

Many proteins have been shown to be associated with the secretion of EVs, but again the exact mechanism of regulated EV release remains unclear and probably varies between different cells. However, it has been shown that some small GTPases in some tumour cells, such as RAB27A73, can be a promising therapeutic target (by RNAi) for reducing tumour exosome-mediated signalling to inhibit neutrophils that support tumour growth [73, 74]. This approach was used in two independent studies and it showed a significant reduction in the growth rate of primary metastatic carcinoma and in metastasis progression [73, 75]. Other GTPases such as RAB11 and RAB35 might serve as alternative targets for inhibiting the release of exosomes by weakening and loosening the docking and/or fusion of multi-vesicular bodies with the plasma membrane [74].

III. Inhibiting EV uptake.

Several uptake mechanisms have been suggested for EVs, but there is insufficient information about the fundamental phases in EV trafficking and target specification. However, some studies showed that the uptake of EVs released from tumour cells can be reduced by diannexin, which can block phosphatidylserine, an important cell adhesion protein [76]. On the other hand, this concept can also be used in diseases other than cancer. For example, diffusion of HIV-1 to T cells could be reduced by targeting intercellular adhesion molecule 1 (ICAM1), which is exposed on EV-encapsulated viruses, thus preventing binding specifically to β2 integrin [77]. Moreover, another suggested mechanism of HIV-1 diffusion to non-haematopoietic cells is by the horizontal transfer of chemokine receptors through EVs, which makes these vesicles valued targets for investigation [34].

IV. Blocking specific EV components.

Blocking specific signalling components of EVs was shown to have therapeutic significance. It was demonstrated that FASL-specific monoclonal antibodies targeting FASL1 displayed on EVs reduced tumour growth in a melanoma model [78]. However, this method may lack specificity and has negative impact on immune function. In the same way, the targeting of MET oncoprotein by RNAi to inhibit its active involvement into EVs was shown to be useful in reducing metastasis in late-stage melanoma [31].

All the above approaches highlight promising targets to develop small molecule therapeutics. Nevertheless, it is important to note that interfering with EV biogenesis could result in unwanted off-target effects, given that EVs are important for the regulation of normal core cellular processes and of course such approaches will need to be translated into a drug delivery system (DDS) that is capable of targeting specific EVs.

4.1.2. Cancer cell-derived EVs

Since it is known that EVs released from normal cells trigger positive effects and those released from cells under pathological conditions usually trigger undesirable effects, it might initially seem surprising that cancer cell-derived EVs could play a therapeutic role. Cancer cell-derived MVs carrying tumour antigens could actually help in initiating immune attacks by providing these antigens to antigen-presenting cells. These cells would then activate a T cell-dependent immune response against the tumour; their antigen content theoretically makes them ideal cancer vaccines. This has been reported in a number of studies of animal models of cancer [79, 80].

4.1.3. Normal cell-derived EVs

Normal cell-derived EVs can be used as drug delivery systems that transfer therapeutic nucleic acids or proteins. Unlike synthetic liposomes and viral vectors, EVs would be immunologically protected as 'self'. In addition to being sufficiently stable with a long tissue half-life, the small size of cell-derived EVs is suitable to allow them to penetrate through the target tissues [81] and cross biological barriers [2] and at the same time be large enough to carry sufficient payload. Moreover, MVs are capable of carrying a wide range of bioactive components, including mRNA, miRNA, DNA and proteins. In this regard, most studies have focused on the delivery of genes to cancerous cells to either replace dysfunctional tumour suppressor genes or to activate immune rejection or trigger cells into apoptotic pathways. Another potential advantage of EVs that makes them competitive in the pool of delivery vehicles is the suggestion that specific peptides could be introduced into EVs to provide them with targeting abilities toward a certain tissue.

http://dx.doi.org/10.5772/64391

4.1.4. Immune cell-derived EVs

EVs that are produced by immune cells have been shown to have an important role in the regulation of immunity. They can mediate immune stimulation or suppression and they can drive inflammatory, autoimmune and infectious disease pathology. Therefore, EVs have the potential to be used as therapeutic agents to modulate the immune system. It has been found that EVs released by B cell lines carry MHC class II, co-stimulatory and adhesion molecules indicating that such vesicles could directly stimulate CD4+ T cell clones [82]. This idea was further supported by the observation that the vaccination of mice with exosomes derived from tumour peptide-pulsed dendritic cells (DCs), enhanced tumour-specific cytotoxic T lymphocytes (CTLs) and inhibited tumour growth in a T cell-dependent manner [83]. Numerous studies have shown the direct effects of EVs in T cell activation. It has been demonstrated that immature DC-derived EVs express a low ratio of co-stimulatory molecules to co-regulatory molecules on their surface and therefore act as immunosuppressives [84].

5. EVs as drug delivery tool in cancer

Effective therapeutic agents have been extensively studied and tried for many decayed to be developed in order to deliver an effective therapeutic agent to its target specifically with minimal side effects. It is well known that non-targeted drugs are inefficient and have side effects when they are delivered systemically. The purpose of a drug delivery system (DDS) is to deliver a drug efficiently, improve the effect of the drug and minimise its side effects [85, 86]. Many useful drug delivery tools and cargos have been developed, such as PEG, liposome, nanoparticles and cell penetrating peptides (CPPs) [87–89]. However, despite the persistent efforts of researchers, the delivery to specific organ and the side effect of DDS remain unsolved completely. DDSs are desirable for use in cancer therapy, and EVs have been recently proposed as promising natural drug delivery tool to serve different diseases [90, 91]. It has been noticed that EVs have a tropism to some organs or cells, and because of their biological significance, they have gain a potential benefit in drug delivery field to target organs or cells. Furthermore, EV-based DDSs are expected to have huge impact and revolution in drug delivery industry field because of their minimal side effects, as they are naturally occurring in the body, in addition to their ability to mediate tumour-selective drug delivery or to mediate organ-specific drug delivery.

5.1. Drug delivery techniques

5.1.1. Encapsulation of drugs to EVs

Drugs should be conjugated or encapsulated in EVs in order to be used as DDSs cargo or vehicle. Several methods have been utilized for encapsulating existing drugs in EVs using methods, such as sonication, extrusion and electroporation [92]. One study investigated four different methods for incorporating catalase into EVs from a Raw 264.7 macrophage cell line, where incubation at room temperature, freeze-thaw cycles, sonication and extrusion were applied [93]. Interestingly, it has been reported that melanoma cells treated with the anticancer drug cisplatin eliminated the cisplatin through EVs [94]. When human pancreatic adenocarcinoma CFPAC-1 cells were treated with EVs containing paclitaxel, this produced an anti-tumour effect [95].

5.1.2. Organ tropism of EVs

Another promising therapeutic application of EVs is through the delivery of molecules to certain organs or cells using a phenomenon known as EV tropism. There have been various attempts to use this pathway for treatment of brain disorders and cancer. For example, Alvarez-Erviti et al. [7] used EVs as part of a neuronal-specific delivery system to effect an siRNA-mediated knockdown of the β-site amyloid precursor protein cleaving enzyme 1 (BACE1), an initiating enzyme required for β-amyloid peptide synthesis. A significant reduction (60%) of the BAAlzCE1, at both mRNA and protein level, was achieved in the brain cortical tissue by this delivery system, indicating its utility for the treatment of Alzheimer's disease. Zhao et al. [96] showed that systemic administration of glial cell line-derived neurotrophic factor to a Parkinson's disease (PD) mouse model, significantly ameloriated both neurodegradation and neuroinflammation through the specific transmission of the neurotrophic factor by the released EVs into the target neurons. Also Zhuang et al. [97] showed that intranasal delivery of EVs containing curcumin or the STAT3 inhibitor JS1-124 to microglial cells in mice significantly reduced Lipopolysaccharide (LPS)-induced brain inflammation and delayed tumour growth in the GL26 tumour model. Furthermore, Pascucci et al. [95] showed a strong anti-proliferative activity of EVs delivered from mesenchymal stromal cells (MSCs) incorporated with paclitaxel, against the human pancreatic CFPAC-1 cell-line. These data suggest a more potent and specific cell target delivery system aiming to increase the anti-tumour efficiency of chemotherapeutic drugs. Skog et al. [22] demonstrated a future possibility to use EVs as a diagnostic tool for certain tumours, such as glioblastoma. These tumour cells are able to release their own EVs, which contain mRNA/miRNA and proteins into the blood stream. Various mRNA/miRNA characteristics of glioblastoma cells were detected in the blood in about one-third of the tested glioblastoma patients, suggesting its utility in diagnosis and for design of optimal treatment plans for each patient.

6. Future perspectives

EVs are endogenous carriers that facilitate intercellular communication. Although their existence has been known for a long time, they have attracted recent renewed interest because of their possible participation in the spread of particularly cancer initiating or metastasis promoting agents from tumour cells, which appear to produce them in excessive amounts. By the same token, EVs from normal cells may be able to reverse the malignant characteristics of cancer cells by transfer of tumour suppressors or pro-apoptotic molecules, providing more 'natural' therapy. In the drug delivery field, they are causing much excitement as potential therapeutics because of their efficient transfer of proteins, mRNA and miRNA, as well as existing drugs, into selective targets. They have obvious advantages over artificial liposomes or other nanoparticles. However, this requires more knowledge of EV content and how they are released, their stability and how they target cells. There is also a need for clearer quantitative and qualitative analysis of EVs in terms of their classification and production from normal and cancerous cells.

Author details

Monerah Al Soraj[1], Salma Bargal[2] and Yunus A. Luqmani[2*]

*Address all correspondence to: yluqmani@yahoo.com

1 Department of Pharmaceutics, Faculty of Pharmacy, Kuwait University, Safat, Kuwait

2 Department of Pharmaceutical Chemistry, Faculty of Pharmacy, Kuwait University, Safat, Kuwait

References

[1] Vader P, Breakefield XO, Wood MJ. Extracellular vesicles: emerging targets for cancer therapy. Trends Mol Med. 2014;20(7):385-93.

[2] Camussi G, Quesenberry PJ. Perspectives on the potential therapeutic uses of vesicles.Exosomes Microvesicles. 2013;1(6): 10.5772/57393.

[3] Gyorgy B, Szabo TG, Pasztoi M, Pal Z, Misjak P, Aradi B, et al. Membrane vesicles, current state-of-the-art: emerging role of extracellular vesicles. Cell Mol Life Sci. 2011;68(16):2667-88.

[4] D'Souza-Schorey C, Clancy JW. Tumor-derived microvesicles: shedding light on novel microenvironment modulators and prospective cancer biomarkers. Genes Dev. 2012;26(12):1287-99.

[5] Sato-Kuwabara Y, Melo SA, Soares FA, Calin GA. The fusion of two worlds: non-coding RNAs and extracellular vesicles – diagnostic and therapeutic implications (Review). Int J Oncol. 2015;46(1):17-27.

[6] Zhang HG, Grizzle WE. Exosomes: a novel pathway of local and distant intercellular communication that facilitates the growth and metastasis of neoplastic lesions. Am J Pathol. 2014;184(1):28-41.

[7] Alvarez-Erviti L, Seow Y, Yin H, Betts C, Lakhal S, Wood MJ. Delivery of siRNA to the mouse brain by systemic injection of targeted exosomes. Nat Biotechnol. 2011;29(4): 341-5.

[8] Tian Y, Li S, Song J, Ji T, Zhu M, Anderson GJ, et al. A doxorubicin delivery platform using engineered natural membrane vesicle exosomes for targeted tumor therapy. Biomaterials. 2014;35(7):2383-90.

[9] Koga K, Matsumoto K, Akiyoshi T, Kubo M, Yamanaka N, Tasaki A, et al. Purification, characterization and biological significance of tumor-derived exosomes. Anticancer Res. 2005;25(6A):3703-7.

[10] Nordin JZ, Lee Y, Vader P, Mager I, Johansson HJ, Heusermann W, et al. Ultrafiltration with size-exclusion liquid chromatography for high yield isolation of extracellular vesicles preserving intact biophysical and functional properties. Nanomedicine. 2015;11(4):879-83.

[11] Smalley DM, Sheman NE, Nelson K, Theodorescu D. Isolation and identification of potential urinary microparticle biomarkers of bladder cancer. J Proteome Res. 2008;7(5): 2088-96.

[12] Ela S, Mager I, Breakefield XO, Wood MJ. Extracellular vesicles: biology and emerging therapeutic opportunities. Nat Rev Drug Discov. 2013;12(5):347-57.

[13] Théry C, Ostrowski M, Segura E. Membrane vesicles as conveyors of immune responses. Nat Rev Immunol. 2009;9(8):581-93.

[14] Chivet M, Hemming F, Pernet-Gallay K, Fraboulet S, Sadoul R. Emerging role of neuronal exosomes in the central nervous system. Front Physiol. 2012;3:145.

[15] Yanez-Mo M, Siljander PR, Andreu Z, Zavec AB, Borras FE, Buzas EI, et al. Biological properties of extracellular vesicles and their physiological functions. J Extracell Vesicles. 2015;4:27066.

[16] Bruno S, Grange C, Collino F, Deregibus MC, Cantaluppi V, Biancone L, et al. Microvesicles derived from mesenchymal stem cells enhance survival in a lethal model of acute kidney injury. PLoS One. 2012;7(3):e33115.

[17] Trinh NT, Yamashita T, Tu TC, Kato T, Ohneda K, Sato F, et al. Microvesicles enhance the mobility of human diabetic adipose tissue-derived mesenchymal stem cells in vitro and improve wound healing in vivo. Biochem Biophys Res Commun. 2016;473(4): 1111-8.

[18] Conde-Vancells J, Gonzalez E, Lu SC, Mato JM, Falcon-Perez JM. Overview of extracellular microvesicles in drug metabolism. Expert Opin Drug Metab Toxicol. 2010;6(5): 543-54.

[19] Royo F, Schlangen K, Palomo L, Gonzalez E, Conde-Vancells J, Berisa A, et al. Transcriptome of extracellular vesicles released by hepatocytes. PLoS One. 2013;8(7):e68693.

[20] Rak J, Guha A. Extracellular vesicles--vehicles that spread cancer genes. Bioessays. 2012;34(6):489-97.

[21] Wieckowski EU, Visus C, Szajnik M, Szczepanski MJ, Storkus WJ, Whiteside TL. Tumor-derived microvesicles promote regulatory T cell expansion and induce apoptosis in tumor-reactive activated CD8+ T lymphocytes. J Immunol. 2009;183(6):3720-30.

[22] Skog J, Würdinger T, van Rijn S, Meijer DH, Gainche L, Sena-Esteves M, et al. Glioblastoma microvesicles transport RNA and proteins that promote tumour growth and provide diagnostic biomarkers. Nat Cell Biol. 2008;10(12):1470-6.

[23] Sadovska L, Eglītis J, Linē A. Extracellular vesicles as biomarkers and therapeutic targets in breast cancer. Anticancer Res. 2015;35(12):6379-90.

[24] Szajnik M, Czystowska M, Szczepanski MJ, Mandapathil M, Whiteside TL. Tumor-derived microvesicles induce, expand and up-regulate biological activities of human regulatory T cells (Treg). PLoS One. 2010;5(7):e11469.

[25] Tesselaar ME, Romijn FP, Van Der Linden IK, Prins FA, Bertina RM, Osanto S. Microparticle-associated tissue factor activity: a link between cancer and thrombosis? J Thromb Haemost. 2007;5(3):520-7.

[26] Tesselaar ME, Osanto S. Risk of venous thromboembolism in lung cancer. Curr Opin Pulm Med. 2007;13(5):362-7.

[27] Del Conde I, Shrimpton CN, Thiagarajan P, López JA. Tissue-factor-bearing microvesicles arise from lipid rafts and fuse with activated platelets to initiate coagulation. Blood. 2005;106(5):1604-11.

[28] Al-Nedawi K, Meehan B, Micallef J, Lhotak V, May L, Guha A, et al. Intercellular transfer of the oncogenic receptor EGFRvIII by microvesicles derived from tumour cells. Nat Cell Biol. 2008;10(5):619-24.

[29] Al-Nedawi K, Meehan B, Kerbel RS, Allison AC, Rak J. Endothelial expression of autocrine VEGF upon the uptake of tumor-derived microvesicles containing oncogenic EGFR. Proc Natl Acad Sci U S A. 2009;106(10):3794-9.

[30] Sidhu SS, Mengistab AT, Tauscher AN, LaVail J, Basbaum C. The microvesicle as a vehicle for EMMPRIN in tumor-stromal interactions. Oncogene. 2004;23(4):956-63.

[31] Peinado H, Alečković M, Lavotshkin S, Matei I, Costa-Silva B, Moreno-Bueno G, et al. Melanoma exosomes educate bone marrow progenitor cells toward a pro-metastatic phenotype through MET. Nat Med. 2012;18(6):883-91.

[32] Lesnik J, Antes T, Kim J, Griner E, Pedro L, Biology RPC, et al. Registered report: Melanoma exosomes educate bone marrow progenitor cells toward a pro-metastatic phenotype through MET. Elife. 2016;5:e07383.

[33] Yang M, Chen J, Su F, Yu B, Lin L, Liu Y, et al. Microvesicles secreted by macrophages shuttle invasion-potentiating microRNAs into breast cancer cells. Mol Cancer. 2011;10:117.

[34] Mack M, Kleinschmidt A, Bruhl H, Klier C, Nelson PJ, Cihak J, et al. Transfer of the chemokine receptor CCR5 between cells by membrane-derived microparticles: a

mechanism for cellular human immunodeficiency virus 1 infection. Nat Med. 2000;6(7): 769-75.

[35] Vella LJ, Sharples RA, Lawson VA, Masters CL, Cappai R, Hill AF. Packaging of prions into exosomes is associated with a novel pathway of PrP processing. J Pathol. 2007;211(5):582-90.

[36] Pegtel DM, Cosmopoulos K, Thorley-Lawson DA, van Eijndhoven MA, Hopmans ES, Lindenberg JL, et al. Functional delivery of viral miRNAs via exosomes. Proc Natl Acad Sci U S A. 2010;107(14):6328-33.

[37] Kharaziha P, Ceder S, Li Q, Panaretakis T. Tumor cell-derived exosomes: a message in a bottle. Biochim Biophys Acta. 2012;1826(1):103-11.

[38] Wendler F, Bota-Rabassedas N, Franch-Marro X. Cancer becomes wasteful: emerging roles of exosomes in cell-fate determination. J Extracell Vesicles. 2013; 2:10.3402/ jev.v2i0.22390.

[39] Zocco D, Ferruzzi P, Cappello F, Kuo WP, Fais S. Extracellular vesicles as shuttles of tumor biomarkers and anti-tumor drugs. Front Oncol. 2014;4:267.

[40] Henderson MC, Azorsa DO. The genomic and proteomic content of cancer cell-derived exosomes. Front Oncol. 2012;2:38.

[41] Lázaro-Ibáñez E, Sanz-Garcia A, Visakorpi T, Escobedo-Lucea C, Siljander P, Ayuso-Sacido A, et al. Different gDNA content in the subpopulations of prostate cancer extracellular vesicles: apoptotic bodies, microvesicles, and exosomes. Prostate. 2014;74(14):1379-90.

[42] Silva J, Garcia V, Rodriguez M, Compte M, Cisneros E, Veguillas P, et al. Analysis of exosome release and its prognostic value in human colorectal cancer. Genes Chromosomes Cancer. 2012;51(4):409-18.

[43] Howcroft TK, Zhang HG, Dhodapkar M, Mohla S. Vesicle transfer and cell fusion: Emerging concepts of cell-cell communication in the tumor microenvironment. Cancer Biol Ther. 2011;12(3):159-64.

[44] Rak J. Extracellular vesicles – biomarkers and effectors of the cellular interactome in cancer. Front Pharmacol. 2013;4:21.

[45] Kruger S, Abd Elmageed ZY, Hawke DH, Wörner PM, Jansen DA, Abdel-Mageed AB, et al. Molecular characterization of exosome-like vesicles from breast cancer cells. BMC Cancer. 2014;14:44.

[46] Guduric-Fuchs J, O'Connor A, Camp B, O'Neill CL, Medina RJ, Simpson DA. Selective extracellular vesicle-mediated export of an overlapping set of microRNAs from multiple cell types. BMC Genomics. 2012;13:357.

[47] Squadrito ML, Baer C, Burdet F, Maderna C, Gilfillan GD, Lyle R, et al. Endogenous RNAs modulate microRNA sorting to exosomes and transfer to acceptor cells. Cell Rep. 2014;8(5):1432-46.

[48] Zhou W, Fong MY, Min Y, Somlo G, Liu L, Palomares MR, et al. Cancer-secreted miR-105 destroys vascular endothelial barriers to promote metastasis. Cancer Cell. 2014;25(4):501-15.

[49] van Balkom BW, de Jong OG, Smits M, Brummelman J, den Ouden K, de Bree PM, et al. Endothelial cells require miR-214 to secrete exosomes that suppress senescence and induce angiogenesis in human and mouse endothelial cells. Blood. 2013;121(19): 3997-4006, S1-15.

[50] Kucharzewska P, Belting M. Emerging roles of extracellular vesicles in the adaptive response of tumour cells to microenvironmental stress. J Extracell Vesicles. 2013; 2:20304.

[51] Yu X, Harris SL, Levine AJ. The regulation of exosome secretion: a novel function of the p53 protein. Cancer Res. 2006;66(9):4795–801.

[52] Trajkovic K, Hsu C, Chiantia S, Rajendran L, Wenzel D, Wieland F, et al. Ceramide triggers budding of exosome vesicles into multivesicular endosomes. Science. 2008;319(5867):1244–7.

[53] Berckmans RJ, Nieuwland R, Boing AN, Romijn FP, Hack CE, Sturk A. Cell-derived microparticles circulate in healthy humans and support low grade thrombin generation. Thromb Haemost. 2001;85(4):639–46.

[54] Helley D, Banu E, Bouziane A, Banu A, Scotte F, Fischer AM, et al. Platelet microparticles: a potential predictive factor of survival in hormone-refractory prostate cancer patients treated with docetaxel-based chemotherapy. Eur Urol. 2009;56(3):479–84.

[55] Rauch U, Antoniak S. Tissue factor-positive microparticles in blood associated with coagulopathy in cancer. Thromb Haemost. 2007;97(1):9–10.

[56] Satta N, Toti F, Feugeas O, Bohbot A, Dachary-Prigent J, Eschwege V, et al. Monocyte vesiculation is a possible mechanism for dissemination of membrane-associated procoagulant activities and adhesion molecules after stimulation by lipopolysaccharide. J Immunol. 1994;153(7):3245–55.

[57] Nieuwland R, Berckmans RJ, McGregor S, Boing AN, Romijn FP, Westendorp RG, et al. Cellular origin and procoagulant properties of microparticles in meningococcal sepsis. Blood. 2000;95(3):930–5.

[58] Rickles FR, Patierno S, Fernandez PM. Tissue factor, thrombin, and cancer. Chest. 2003;124(3 Suppl):58S-68S.

[59] Janowska-Wieczorek A, Wysoczynski M, Kijowski J, Marquez-Curtis L, Machalinski B, Ratajczak J, et al. Microvesicles derived from activated platelets induce metastasis and angiogenesis in lung cancer. Int J Cancer. 2005;113(5):752–60.

[60] Baj-Krzyworzeka M, Szatanek R, Weglarczyk K, Baran J, Zembala M. Tumour-derived microvesicles modulate biological activity of human monocytes. Immunol Lett. 2007;113(2):76–82.

[61] Hedlund M, Nagaeva O, Kargl D, Baranov V, Mincheva-Nilsson L. Thermal- and oxidative stress causes enhanced release of NKG2D ligand-bearing immunosuppressive exosomes in leukemia/lymphoma T and B cells. PLoS One. 2011;6(2):e16899.

[62] Abusamra AJ, Zhong Z, Zheng X, Li M, Ichim TE, Chin JL, et al. Tumor exosomes expressing Fas ligand mediate CD8+ T-cell apoptosis. Blood Cells Mol Dis. 2005;35(2): 169–73.

[63] Clayton A, Tabi Z. Exosomes and the MICA-NKG2D system in cancer. Blood Cells Mol Dis. 2005;34(3):206–13.

[64] Valenti R, Huber V, Filipazzi P, Pilla L, Sovena G, Villa A, et al. Human tumor-released microvesicles promote the differentiation of myeloid cells with transforming growth factor-beta-mediated suppressive activity on T lymphocytes. Cancer Res. 2006;66(18): 9290–8.

[65] Hotary KB, Allen ED, Brooks PC, Datta NS, Long MW, Weiss SJ. Membrane type I matrix metalloproteinase usurps tumor growth control imposed by the three-dimensional extracellular matrix. Cell. 2003;114(1):33–45.

[66] Muralidharan-Chari V, Clancy JW, Sedgwick A, D'Souza-Schorey C. Microvesicles: mediators of extracellular communication during cancer progression. J Cell Sci. 2010;123(Pt 10):1603–11.

[67] Ginestra A, Miceli D, Dolo V, Romano FM, Vittorelli ML. Membrane vesicles in ovarian cancer fluids: a new potential marker. Anticancer Res. 1999;19(4C):3439–45.

[68] Ginestra A, La Placa MD, Saladino F, Cassara D, Nagase H, Vittorelli ML. The amount and proteolytic content of vesicles shed by human cancer cell lines correlates with their in vitro invasiveness. Anticancer Res. 1998;18(5A):3433–7.

[69] Graves LE, Ariztia EV, Navari JR, Matzel HJ, Stack MS, Fishman DA. Proinvasive properties of ovarian cancer ascites-derived membrane vesicles. Cancer Res. 2004;64(19):7045–9.

[70] Kim JW, Wieckowski E, Taylor DD, Reichert TE, Watkins S, Whiteside TL. Fas ligand-positive membranous vesicles isolated from sera of patients with oral cancer induce apoptosis of activated T lymphocytes. Clin Cancer Res. 2005;11(3):1010–20.

[71] Chalmin F, Ladoire S, Mignot G, Vincent J, Bruchard M, Remy-Martin JP, et al. Membrane-associated Hsp72 from tumor-derived exosomes mediates STAT3-depend-

ent immunosuppressive function of mouse and human myeloid-derived suppressor cells. J Clin Invest. 2010;120(2):457–71.

[72] Baietti MF, Zhang Z, Mortier E, Melchior A, Degeest G, Geeraerts A, et al. Syndecan-syntenin-ALIX regulates the biogenesis of exosomes. Nat Cell Biol. 2012;14(7):677–85.

[73] Bobrie A, Krumeich S, Reyal F, Recchi C, Moita LF, Seabra MC, et al. Rab27a supports exosome-dependent and -independent mechanisms that modify the tumor microenvironment and can promote tumor progression. Cancer Res. 2012;72(19):4920–30.

[74] Hsu C, Morohashi Y, Yoshimura S, Manrique-Hoyos N, Jung S, Lauterbach MA, et al. Regulation of exosome secretion by Rab35 and its GTPase-activating proteins TBC1D10A-C. J Cell Biol. 2010;189(2):223–32.

[75] Ostrowski M, Carmo NB, Krumeich S, Fanget I, Raposo G, Savina A, et al. Rab27a and Rab27b control different steps of the exosome secretion pathway. Nat Cell Biol. 2010;12(1):19–30; sup pp 1–13.

[76] Lima LG, Chammas R, Monteiro RQ, Moreira ME, Barcinski MA. Tumor-derived microvesicles modulate the establishment of metastatic melanoma in a phosphatidylserine-dependent manner. Cancer Lett. 2009;283(2):168–75.

[77] Chaput N, Thery C. Exosomes: immune properties and potential clinical implementations. Semin Immunopathol. 2011;33(5):419–40.

[78] Cai Z, Yang F, Yu L, Yu Z, Jiang L, Wang Q, et al. Activated T cell exosomes promote tumor invasion via Fas signaling pathway. J Immunol. 2012;188(12):5954–61.

[79] Altieri SL, Khan AN, Tomasi TB. Exosomes from plasmacytoma cells as a tumor vaccine. J Immunother. 2004;27(4):282–8.

[80] Dai S, Wei D, Wu Z, Zhou X, Wei X, Huang H, et al. Phase I clinical trial of autologous ascites-derived exosomes combined with GM-CSF for colorectal cancer. Mol Ther. 2008;16(4):782–90.

[81] Mizrak A, Bolukbasi MF, Ozdener GB, Brenner GJ, Madlener S, Erkan EP, et al. Genetically engineered microvesicles carrying suicide mRNA/protein inhibit schwannoma tumor growth. Mol Ther. 2013;21(1):101–8.

[82] Raposo G, Nijman HW, Stoorvogel W, Liejendekker R, Harding CV, Melief CJ, et al. B lymphocytes secrete antigen-presenting vesicles. J Exp Med. 1996;183(3):1161–72.

[83] Zitvogel L, Regnault A, Lozier A, Wolfers J, Flament C, Tenza D, et al. Eradication of established murine tumors using a novel cell-free vaccine: dendritic cell-derived exosomes. Nat Med. 1998;4(5):594–600.

[84] Robbins PD, Morelli AE. Regulation of immune responses by extracellular vesicles. Nat Rev Immunol. 2014;14(3):195–208.

[85] Brannon-Peppas L, Blanchette JO. Nanoparticle and targeted systems for cancer therapy. Adv Drug Deliv Rev. 2004;56(11):1649–59.

[86] Fujita Y, Kuwano K, Ochiya T. Development of small RNA delivery systems for lung cancer therapy. Int J Mol Sci. 2015;16(3):5254–70.

[87] Veronese FM, Pasut G. PEGylation, successful approach to drug delivery. Drug Discov Today. 2005;10(21):1451–8.

[88] Farokhzad OC, Langer R. Impact of nanotechnology on drug delivery. ACS Nano. 2009;3(1):16–20.

[89] Lin W, Xie X, Deng J, Liu H, Chen Y, Fu X, et al. Cell-penetrating peptide-doxorubicin conjugate loaded NGR-modified nanobubbles for ultrasound triggered drug delivery. J Drug Target. 2016;24(2):134–46.

[90] Kooijmans SA, Vader P, van Dommelen SM, van Solinge WW, Schiffelers RM. Exosome mimetics: a novel class of drug delivery systems. Int J Nanomedicine. 2012;7:1525–41.

[91] Tominaga N, Yoshioka Y, Ochiya T. A novel platform for cancer therapy using extracellular vesicles. Adv Drug Deliv Rev. 2015;95:50–5.

[92] Akao Y, Iio A, Itoh T, Noguchi S, Itoh Y, Ohtsuki Y, et al. Microvesicle-mediated RNA molecule delivery system using monocytes/macrophages. Mol Ther. 2011;19(2):395–9.

[93] Haney MJ, Klyachko NL, Zhao Y, Gupta R, Plotnikova EG, He Z, et al. Exosomes as drug delivery vehicles for Parkinson's disease therapy. J Control Release. 2015;207:18–30.

[94] Federici C, Petrucci F, Caimi S, Cesolini A, Logozzi M, Borghi M, et al. Exosome release and low pH belong to a framework of resistance of human melanoma cells to cisplatin. PLoS One. 2014;9(2):e88193.

[95] Pascucci L, Cocce V, Bonomi A, Ami D, Ceccarelli P, Ciusani E, et al. Paclitaxel is incorporated by mesenchymal stromal cells and released in exosomes that inhibit in vitro tumor growth: a new approach for drug delivery. J Control Release. 2014;192:262–70.

[96] Zhao Y, Haney MJ, Gupta R, Bohnsack JP, He Z, Kabanov AV, et al. GDNF-transfected macrophages produce potent neuroprotective effects in Parkinson's disease mouse model. PLoS One. 2014;9(9):e106867.

[97] Zhuang X, Xiang X, Grizzle W, Sun D, Zhang S, Axtell RC, et al. Treatment of brain inflammatory diseases by delivering exosome encapsulated anti-inflammatory drugs from the nasal region to the brain. Mol Ther. 2011;19(10):1769–79.

Chapter 6

Modulation of Gene Expression During Stages of Liver Colonization by Pancreatic Cancer in a Rat Model

Khamael M.K. Al-Taee, Hassan Adwan and
Martin R. Berger

Additional information is available at the end of the chapter

http://dx.doi.org/10.5772/64335

Abstract

Pancreatic ductal adenocarcinoma (PDAC) is known for its early spreading of tumor cells into the liver. The aim of this study was to investigate the modulated gene expression of PDAC cells during liver colonization. To that purpose, ASML rat pancreatic cancer cells marked with enhanced green fluorescent protein were inoculated into the portal vein of isogenic BDX rats and reisolated from livers by fluorescence-activated cell sorting sorting at early (1, 3 days), intermediate (9 days), advanced (15 days), and terminal (21 days) stages of liver colonization. Reisolated ASML cells were used for total RNA isolation and subsequently their gene expression was investigated by Illumina chip array for mRNA and miRNA species, followed by Ingenuity Pathway Analysis (IPA). Following reisolation, 7–20% of genes and 10% of miRNA species were modulated significantly in expression during the early stage of liver colonization and continuously thereafter. These overall changes led to distinguish certain categories and processes participating in cancer progression. The knowledge of these alterations in gene expression will suggest targets, which could be used for new diagnostic procedures as well as for combating liver metastasis successfully.

Keywords: pancreatic cancer, liver metastasis, ASML cells, isogenic rat model, modulation of gene expression, stages of liver colonization

1. Introduction

Pancreatic ductal adenocarcinoma (PDAC) is an extremely aggressive cancer [1, 2], as derived from the respective 5-year survival rate of about 6% [3, 4]. This poor prognosis results, at least in part, from a delayed diagnosis of the disease. All therapeutic efforts during the past 50 years, such as surgery, radiation therapy, chemotherapy, or combinations thereof, have shown little impact on the course of this aggressive neoplastic disease. It is hoped, however, that a full understanding of the molecular biology of pancreatic cancer will help in diagnosing, preventing, and treating this cancer.

A most recent study on pancreatic cancer patients describes genetic details, which have been detected through full genome sequencing and copy number analyses in 100 PDACs. Genetic drivers known for pancreatic cancer, such as K-ras, TP53, SMAD4, and mutations in CDKN2A, were confirmed, whereas newly identified mutations, such as in the KDM6A gene, highlighted the role of chromatin modifications [5]. Based on familial clustering studies, it was estimated that 10% of PDAC cases are linked to an inherited predisposition [4, 6, 7]. Germ line mutations were especially found in tumor suppressor genes, such as INK4A, BRCA2, and LKB1, the mismatch repair gene MLH1, and the cationic trypsinogen gene PRSS1 [8, 9]. These germ line mutations are responsible for onset and penetrance of PDAC, but they likely contribute more to the malignant progression of precursor lesions than to cancer initiation [10, 11]. Of course, exogenous factors, such as cigarette smoking, constitute a measurable risk, as well [12].

In the early stage of PDAC, the genetic mutations of oncogenes like K-ras and suppressor genes like TP53—or both—lead to constitutive activation of transcription factors, but in the late stage stress factors such as acidosis and hypoxia, which are frequently encountered in the tumor microenvironment, further deregulate the expression of metastasis-related proteins. PDAC metastasis is a progressive, debilitating disease that is characterized by pain, asthenia, anorexia, and cachexia. The formation of metastasis is a complex and progressive process, including four basic steps: dissociation of cells from the primary tumor, existence and survival in the circulatory system, break down and degrading of endothelium and basement membranes in target organs, and (d) establishment of a colony of metastatic cells [13].

Currently, it is hoped that new findings related to K-ras, the tumor's unique metabolic needs, and how the stroma and immune system affect the PDAC, will change the overall situation for the better [14].

In order to better understand the PDAC metastatic process, a liver metastasis model was developed by our group [15]. This model focused on the final steps of metastasis, which are related to organ colonization. To that purpose, ASML rat PDAC cells, which had been marked by luciferase ($ASML^{luc}$ [15]) were implanted intraportally into isogenic BDX rats for mimicking the final phase of liver metastasis. This process of liver colonization was related to the size of the liver and the remaining life span of a given animal. Thus, for reisolation of tumor cells from rat liver, four periods were selected and classified as early (days 1, 3), intermediate (day 6), advanced (day 15), and terminal (day 21) stages. Also, tumor cells were recultivated in vitro after their reisolation at 21 days for three additional periods (3, 6, and 9 days) to define the microenvironment effect on gene expression after residing 21 days in rat liver. Reisolated ASML tumor cells were used for total RNA isolation and then investigated by Illumina chip array for genes and miRNAs, which show modulation of their expression during liver colonization. These modulations were evaluated by Ingenuity Pathway Analysis (IPA) as described in the study of Al-Taee et al. [16].

http://dx.doi.org/10.5772/64335

The aim of this study was to establish a rat model for identifying and understanding pathophysiological processes during metastatic liver colonization, as well as for finding new and specific tumor markers as tools for diagnostic and therapeutic approaches. Here, we report on the modulation of gene expression during stages of liver colonization by ASML pancreatic cancer cells in rat liver.

2. Gene expression modulation in ASML rat PDAC cells during liver colonization

2.1. Reisolation of tumor cells from liver tissue

ASML cells, which had been implanted to BDX rats, were reisolated after various periods. The purity of these cells was based on a procedure, which involved gradient centrifugation as first step followed by FACS sorting of eGFP-labeled tumor cells. Pending on the number of tumor cells, the final grade of purity varied from 90% (day 1) to 99% (day 15) based on 1.6 to 52% of tumor cells present in the cell suspension after gradient centrifugation.

2.2. mRNA modulation of ASML cells colonizing rat liver

2.2.1. Fold changes in mRNA expression

In order to analyze the mRNA modulation, which occurs in ASML pancreatic cancer cells colonizing the rat liver, the gene expression profiles of ASML cells were determined by microarray in five batches of tumor cells that had been reisolated from rat liver after 1, 3, 6, 15, and 21 days post injection into the portal vein. For each of the five batches, representing different stages of liver colonization, 23,400 genes were analyzed in total. In an attempt to categorize the observed changes in gene expression, two parameters were chosen initially: the fold change in mRNA expression over that of respective genes in control ASML cells growing in vitro, and the time until reisolation of tumor cells from rat liver. The gene expression profile from cells isolated after days 1 and 3 was classified as reflecting early colonization, as no tumor burden was visible with naked eye. On day 6, the ASML cells showed signs of infiltrative growth in the rat liver, visible as white spots of 1–2 mm in diameter and were discernible macroscopically. The corresponding gene profile was classified as intermediate colonization. At 15 days post injection, the ASML cells colonized about 40% of the rat liver and the tumor spot size increased to ~5 mm in diameter. The respective gene expression profile was considered as advanced colonization. At 21 days post injection, ASML cells almost completely infiltrated the rat liver and the corresponding gene expression profile was classified as terminal stage. An overview for the two categories, the fold changes in mRNA expression and the respective stage of liver colonization, is shown in **Figure 1**.

The observed modulation ranged from more than 2-fold to more than 20-fold, with a similar distribution pattern regarding decreased and increased levels, thus resulting in a curve resembling a normal (Gaussian) distribution. This distribution was similarly bell shaped over all stages, thus indicating little overall variation between early and late colonization stages. There was one exception, however, regarding mRNAs with more than 20-fold increased or decreased levels: the former were distinctly more prevalent than the latter at the early stage, thus indicating a possible need for the strong activation of genes initially after tumor cell implantation.

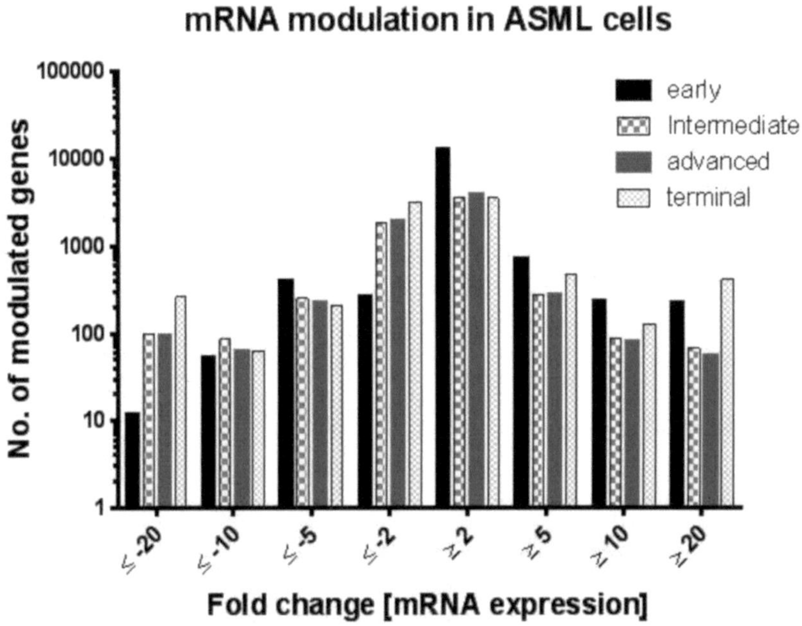

Figure 1. mRNA modulation in rat pancreatic cancer cells colonizing rat liver: Given is the fold change of mRNA expression of reisolated ASML cells during early, intermediate, advanced, and terminal stages of liver colonization relative to control cells growing in vitro.

2.2.2. *Types of mRNA modulation*

On a single gene level, several types of modulation were found during the different stages of colonization. Some examples are shown in **Figure 2**.

These included a steady increase in expression of certain genes, as seen for matrix metalloproteinase-2 (MMP-2) and ephrin type-A receptor 8 (Epha8), as well as a steady decrease, as observed for cadherin 11 (Cdh11) and 5-hydroxytryptamine (serotonin) receptor 5B (Htr5b) (see **Figure 2A**).

Another type, typical of an immediate increase or decrease in gene expression followed by a persistent plateau was observed as well. This type of modulation was seen for the expression levels of claudin-1 (Cldn1) and insulin-like growth factor 2 (IGF2), which showed a sustained increase, whereas transforming growth factor alpha (TGF-α) and MDM2 proto-oncogene/E3 ubiquitin protein ligase (Mdm2) showed a sustained decrease (see **Figure 2B**).

A third type of altered gene expression was classified as early type responsive gene (e.g. insulin-like growth factor binding protein 2 (Igfbp2) and keratin, type I cytoskeletal 42 (Krt42)) or late type responsive gene (e.g. lipolysis-stimulated lipoprotein receptor (Lsr) and family with sequence similarity 132, member A (Fam132a)), which was either activated greatly in the early stages of colonization and later showed a somewhat reduced expression or they started with a mildly increased expression level and showed intensely increased expression only at the end of the colonization period (see **Figure 2C**).

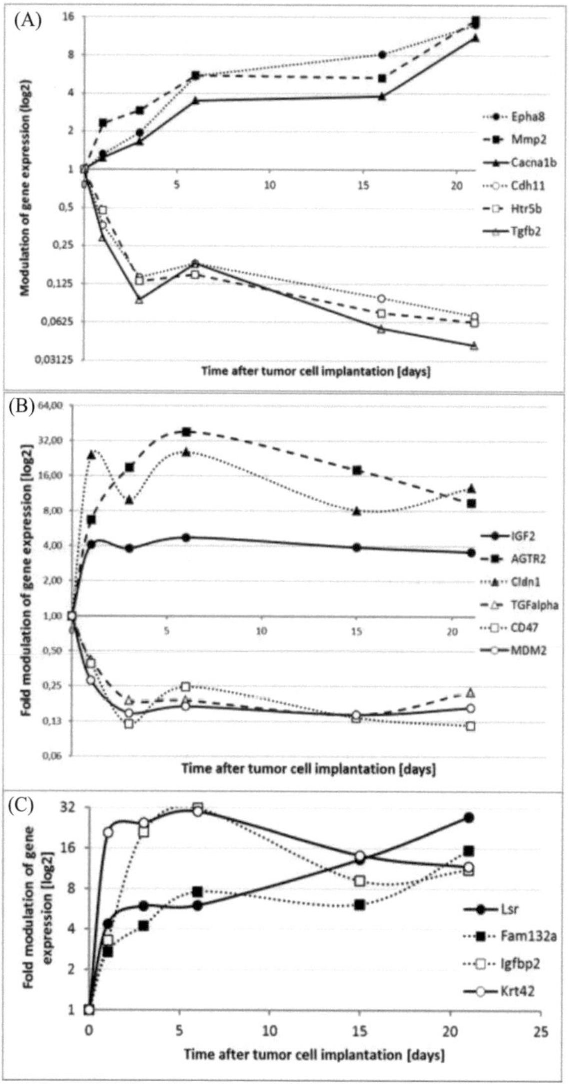

Figure 2. Types of gene expression modulation found during the different stages of liver colonization: given are examples of steady increases in expression (**A**), immediate increases or decreases in gene expression followed by a persistent plateau (**B**), and early or late type responsive genes (**C**).

Categories	Cellular movement, Hematological system, Development & function, Immune cell trafficking, Inflammatory response		Cellular development, Growth & proliferation, Connective tissue / Nervous system develop-ment & function, Tissue development		Tissue development	Lipid metabolism, Small molecule biochemistry
Diseases or Functions Annotation	movement of mononuclear leukocytes	migration of phagocytes	proliferation of fibroblasts	proliferation of neuronal cells	growth of connective tissue	fatty acid metabolism
No of genes	121	80	93	77	158	158
Early stage	Increased	Increased	Increased	Increased	Increased	Increased
p-Value	4,96E-23	6,82E-20	7,67E-19	1,30E-08	1,09E-24	1,65E-25
Activation z-score	2,812	2,563	2,436	2.461	3,143	2,751
Intermediate stage	-	not significant	not significant	Decreased	decreased	not significant
p-Value				6,24E-13	8,00E-14	
Activation z-score				-2.949	-2,034	
Advanced stage	not significant	not significant	not significant	not significant	Decreased	-
p-Value				5,47E-14	5,93E-16	
Activation z-score				-1,098	-2,159	
Final stage	Increased	Increased	Increased	-	Increased	Increased
p-Value	5,40E-30	3,21E-23	1,69E-14		1,26E-20	2,63E-05
Activation z-score	3,614	3,623	2,319		2,623	2.733

Categories	Cell cycle	Hematological system develop-ment & function, Tissue morphology	Inflammatory response	Cell-to-cell interaction, Cellular function , Inflammatory response	Cancer, organismal injury & abnormalities, Tumor morphology
Diseases or Functions Annotation	M phase of tumor cell lines	quantity of myeloid cells	immune response of cells	phagocytosis of cells	invasion of tumor
No of genes	26	78	107	56	51
Early stage	Increased	Increased	Decreased	not significant	Decreased
p-Value	5,68E-10	2,34E-16	3,56E-13	8,14E-13	2,04E-14
Activation z-score	2,123	2,498	-2,231	-2,583	-2,156
Intermediate stage	Increased	Increased	Decreased	Decreased	not significant
p-Value	1,07E-12	2,34E-16		2,83E-16	
Activation z-score	2.486	2,498		-2.574	
Advanced stage	-	Increased	Decreased	Decreased	Decreased
p-Value		3,57E-15	1,74E-14	4,25E-15	1,52E-10
Activation z-score		2,084	-3,068	-2.406	-2.301
Final stage	-		not significant	not significant	not significant
p-Value					
Activation z-score					

Table 1. Some categories and related diseases or functions annotations.

2.2.3. Categories of the tumor cell genome showing modulation

By Ingenuity Pathway Analysis (IPA), a more comprehensive way of categorizing altered gene expression was realized. In this analysis, several possibilities of grouping or ordering genes were followed. Initially, some general cellular categories were chosen, which encompass a limited number of more specific disease or function annotations. These, in turn, are characterized by a distinct number of genes participating in the disease or function. The overall status of these genes (i.e. increased in expression or decreased in expression) is used to coin an activation z-score, which is considered significant if higher than 2 (i.e. activated) or lower than −2 (decreased). In addition, a p value indicates the significance of the alteration of the respective process (**Table 1**).

Based on this analysis, the category "cellular movement" with the two function annotations "cell movement of mononuclear leukocytes" and "migration of phagocytes" with 121 and 80 genes, respectively, was significantly increased at early and terminal stages, but not significantly altered at intermediate and advanced stages. This is surprising, as it shows that movement or migration of cells is not equally important over the whole colonization period. Although this category of genes is increased initially, soon thereafter it is deactivated and reactivated only for the terminal stage (**Table 1**, top part, column 1).

Another example is the category of genes related to proliferation. As could be expected, genes belonging to this category were augmented in expression initially, as derived from the significantly increased activation z-score (2.44), but failed to show activation at intermediate and advanced stages. At these stages, genes related to neuronal cell proliferation were even decreased in expression or showed no activation. At the terminal stage, there was activation of genes related to the proliferation of fibroblasts, but not of genes related to proliferation of neuronal cells (**Table 1**, top part, column 2).

Genes related to the growth of connective tissue, fatty acid metabolism, M-phase of tumor cell lines, and quantity of myeloid cells were mainly upregulated but not throughout the whole liver colonization process. In addition, genes related to the immune response, phagocytosis, and invasion were decreased in activation (**Table 1**, top and bottom parts, columns 3–9).

2.2.4. Modulation of acute phase signaling chain genes

Subsequently, Ingenuity Pathway Analysis (IPA) was used for overlaying the findings of this study onto scaffolds of known genetic relationships. This included a scaffold for the genes of the acute phase signaling chain, which was overlaid with gene expression levels obtained at intermediate (day 6 after tumor cell implantation, **Figure 3A**) and terminal (day 21 after tumor cell implantation, **Figure 3B**) stages.

These figures show a differentiation of genes according to cellular compartments as well as to colors as indicator of expression levels. Symbols, which have been placed to the specific cellular or extracellular sites of the respective proteins, are used to report on a specific gene expression. A colored border line of the respective symbol indicates that data from the present analysis were available to describe the status of the gene. The colors used for filling the symbol denote differences in expression: red color indicates increased expression and green color indicates decreased expression, with less intense colors hinting to less pronounced increased or decreased expression.

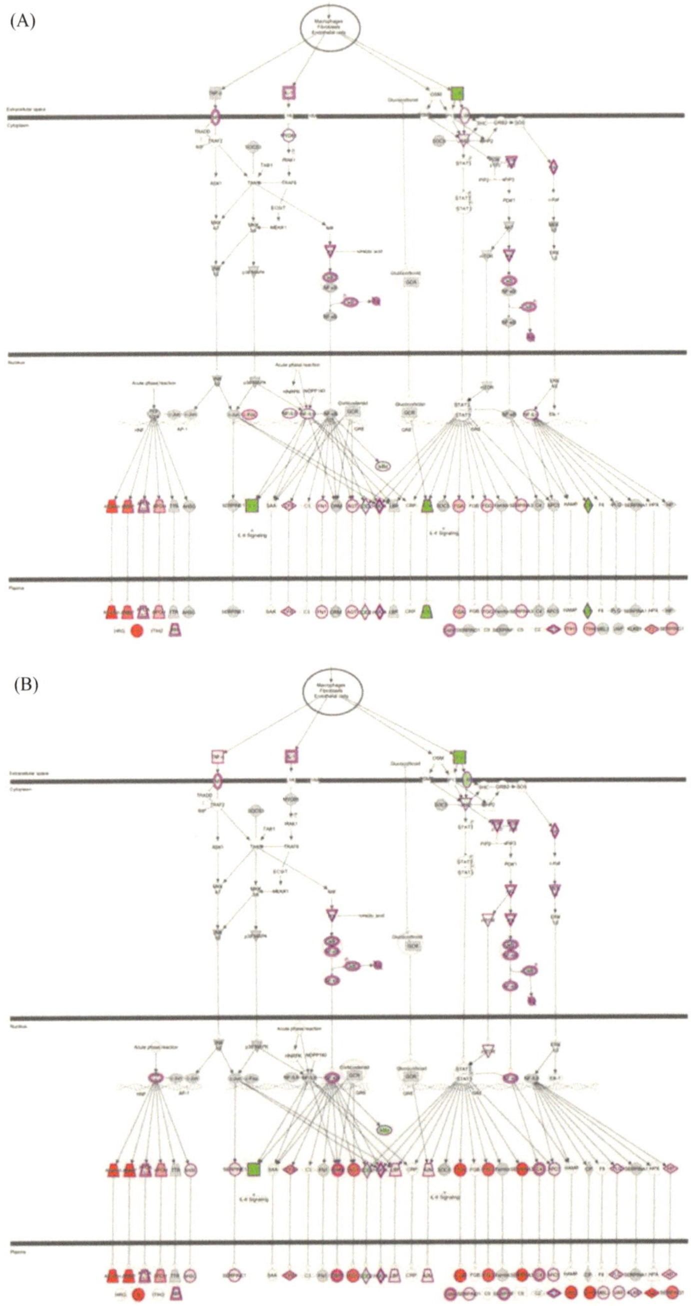

Figure 3. A) Overlay of ASML cell gene expression (day 6) on acute phase signaling chain. **B**) Overlay of ASML cell gene expression (day 21) on acute phase signaling chain.

On day 6 after tumor cell implantation, two genes (albumin and transferrin) of the acute phase signaling chain are highlighted in intense red color and three genes (interleukin 6, α-2-macroglobulin, and ceruloplasmin) in intense green color. Fifteen more genes are shown by red colors of lower intensity, indicating submaximally increased expression levels. In addition, 14 genes are highlighted in a green color of reduced intensity, indicating less than maximally decreased expression (see **Figure 3A**).

At the terminal stage, eight genes (albumin, transferrin, α-1-microglobulin, fibrinogen alpha chain, serpin family A member 3, inter-alpha-trypsin inhibitor heavy chain H3, inter-alpha-trypsin inhibitor heavy chain H4, and coagulation factor II (thrombin)) were highlighted in the most intense red color and 21 more genes in less intense red colors. Concomitantly, only 1 gene (interleukin 6) was highlighted in intense green color and 15 in less intense green colors (see **Figure 3B**), indicating a shift from reduced expression of acute phase signaling genes at the intermediate stage to increased expression at the terminal stage of liver colonization.

2.2.5. *Modulation of metastasis associated genes*

In addition to using genes of the acute phase signaling as scaffold, another overlay of was done by IPA analysis at the terminal stage of liver colonization for the three signaling cascade scaffolds known as "metastatic solid tumor," "metastasis," and "metastatic gastrointestinal tract cancer" (**Figure 4**). Because of the large overlap between the corresponding genes, all three scaffolds were combined in one scheme, resulting in a picture, in which the three scaffold designations are connected with their respective genes by straight lines. For clarity, the gene symbols are arranged according to their cellular site, i.e. extracellularly, in the plasma membrane, in the cytoplasm, or in the nucleus. In addition to the red/green color scheme known from **Figure 3A** and **B**, the straight lines are colored by yellow and blue colors, which indicate activation or inhibition of the respective gene products activity. Thus, very often a gene highlighted in a reddish color, which indicates increased expression over control, will be connected with its scaffold designation by a yellow line, indicating activation of the respective group of genes as given for the scaffold designation "metastatic solid tumor" and the gene expression of collagen, type IV, alpha 2 (Col4a2), or of coagulation factor II, thrombin (F2). This means that the increased expression of Col4a2 or F2 predicts activation of a significant share of related genes. Conversely, a gene highlighted in green color, which indicates decreased expression versus control, is sometimes connected with its scaffold designation by a straight blue line, indicating inhibition of the respective group of genes, as given for the scaffold designation "metastatic solid tumor" and the gene expression of colony stimulating factor 1 (Csf1) or interleukin 6 (IL-6). This means that the decreased expression of Csf1 or Il6 predicts inhibition of a significant share of related genes.

In addition, a gene symbol colored reddish can be connected to the scaffold designation by a yellow line, indicating that its increased expression is related to inhibition of the corresponding gene group, as for the genes apolipoprotein A1 (Apoa1) and serpin family E member 1

(Serpine1). This means that the increased expression of APOA1 or Serpine1 predicts inhibition of a significant share of related genes. Finally, a gene symbol colored greenish can be connected to the scaffold designation by an orange line, as for the genes superoxide dismutase 3 (Sod3) and TIMP metallopeptidase inhibitor 1 (Timp1). This implies that the decreased expression of Sod3 or Timp1 predicts activation of a significant share of related genes (**Figure 4A**).

As **Figure 4A** gives an overview on a multitude of genes being connected to the three signaling cascade scaffolds known as "metastatic solid tumor," "metastasis," and "metastatic gastrointestinal tract cancer," which allowed to show less details, a more complete description of a selection of metastasis genes is given in **Figure 4B**. This figure shows the respective fold changes in mRNA levels versus control as positive or negative numbers below the corresponding gene symbols.

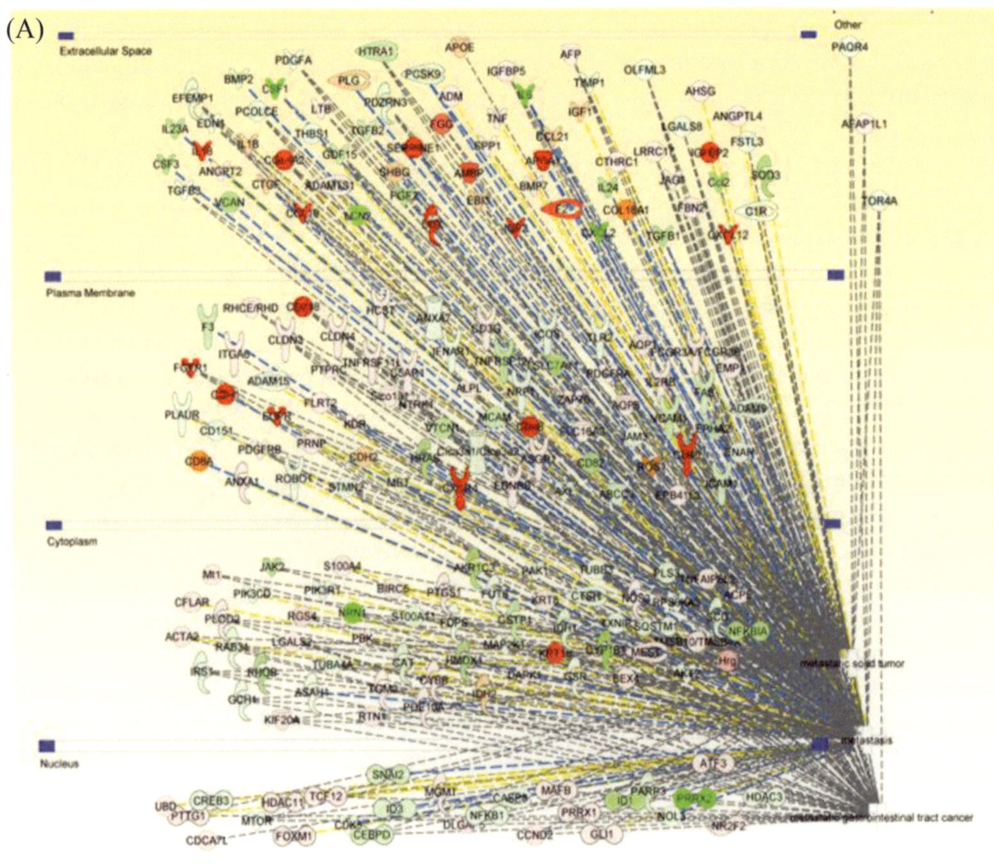

http://dx.doi.org/10.5772/64335

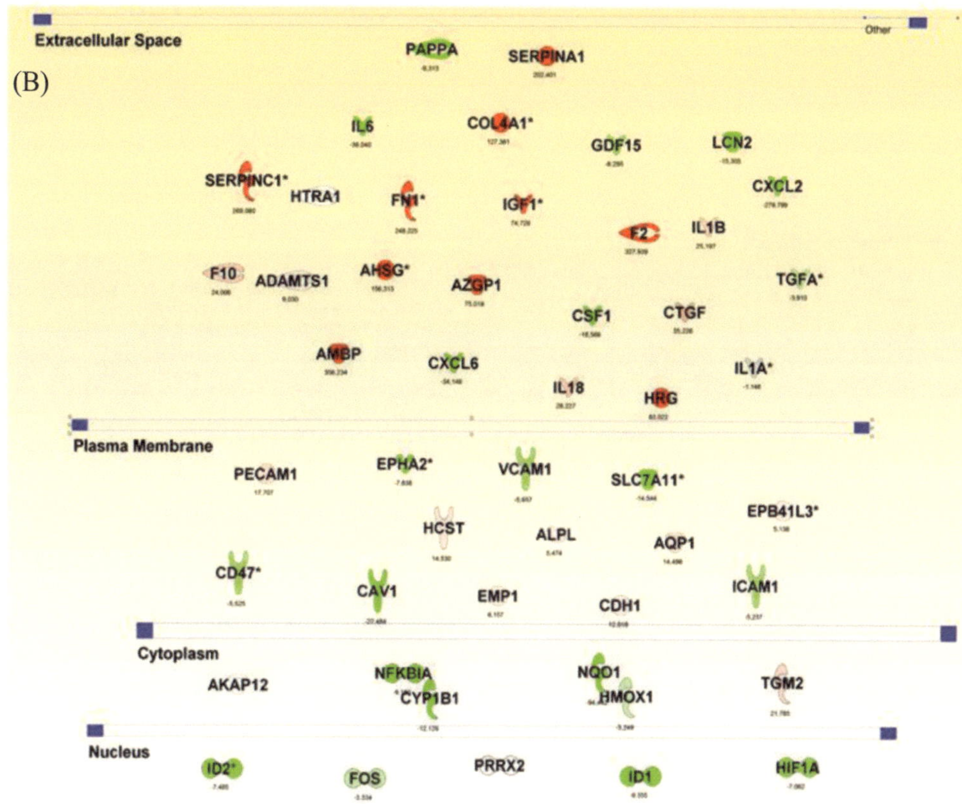

Figure 4. A) Overlay of ASML cell gene expression (day 21) on the three signaling cascade scaffolds termed "metastatic solid tumor," "metastasis," and "metastatic gastrointestinal tract cancer." The three scaffold designations are connected with their respective genes by straight lines. For clarity, the gene symbols are arranged according to their cellular site, i.e. extracellularly, in the plasma membrane, in the cytoplasm, or in the nucleus. In addition to the red/green color scheme known from **Figure 3A** and **B**, the straight lines are colored by yellow and blue colors, which indicate activation or inhibition of the respective related genes. **B**) More detailed description of a selection of metastasis genes. The respective fold changes in mRNA levels versus control are given as positive or negative numbers below the corresponding gene symbols.

2.2.6. Role of upstream regulators

The third IPA analysis concentrated on upstream regulators, which showed a significant modulation in expression and therefore altered the activation state of a whole series of downstream proteins.

From the early stage of liver colonization, six genes were selected for detailed analysis. These included member RAS oncogene family-like 6 (Rabl6), which was increased in expression and caused significant activation of downstream target genes, as well as Ras association domain family member 1 (Rassf1), nuclear protein, transcriptional regulator, 1 (Nupr1), and jun proto-oncogene (Jun), which also showed increased expression but caused inhibition of the corresponding downstream molecules (**Table 2**). Finally, the genes interleukin 1 alpha (Il1a) and inhibitor of kappa light polypeptide gene enhancer in B-cells, kinase gamma (Ikbkg) showed decreased expression and caused inhibition of their respective downstream molecules (see **Table 2**).

Upstream regulator (early stage)	Exp. fold change	Molecule type	Predicted activation state	Activation z-score / p-value of overlap	Target molecules in Ingenuity Pathway Analysis dataset
Rabl6	1,97	other	Activated	4,899 / 5,42E-14	AURKB,BUB1B,CCNA2,CCNB1,CCNE2,CENPF,CKS1B,CX3CL1,DUT,H2AFX,HMMR,HMOX1, KIF23, MAD2L1, MCM7,MELK, NDC80, PARP2, PBK,PLK1, POLD1, POLE2, PRC1,RFC3
Rassf1	2,78	other	Inhibited	-2,002 / 4,10E-08	APOE,CAV1,CCNA2,CCND2,CPE,EFEMP1,EMP1,FGF2,FOS,GDF15,LITAF,MDK,MGMT,MYL9, PAK1, SAMD5, SEPP1,SPP1, SRPX, TGM2
Nupr1	4,05	Trans-cription regulator	Inhibited	-3,543 / 5,06E-11	ARHGAP11A,ASPM,ATF3,ATP6V0A1,BUB1B,CAMK2N1,CASC5,CCDC77,CCNA2,CCNF,CDCA2, CDCA3, CDCA8, CEBPB,CENPI,CKAP2L,COL3A1,CXCL3, DHCR24,EME1, ERCC6L, ESPL1, FANCD2, FCHSD2, FHL2, FUCA1, FZD8, GBP2,GCH1,GDF15, GINS1, GMEB1, IL13RA1, IL6R, KIF11, KIF18A, KIF20A, KIF23, KIF2C, KIFC1, MAFG, MAN2B2, MKI67, MYD88, NAAA, NAPEPLD, NEIL3, NUPR1, PIK3R1, PLK1, PM20D2, POLE2, PRNP,RAB20, RAB32,SAMD4A, SERF1A/SERF1B, SGK223, SHCBP1, SHPK, SHROOM3, SKP2, SLC6A6, SPAG5, SPC25,TRIB3, TRIM16,UNC5B
Jun	3,35	Trans-cription regulator	Inhibited	-3,047 / 4,20E-20	A2M,Abcb1b,ALAS1,ANXA2,APOE,ATF3,BCL3,BIRC3,CAMP,CAV1,Ccl2,CCNA2,CCND2,CDC20,CDK1,CGA,CMTM5,CSF1,CTGF,CX3CL1,CXCL16,CXCL3, DIO2, EHD4, F3, FBLN5,FGF2,FLNC,FN1, FOS, FOSL1, FTH1, GCLC, GJA1, GSTA5, GSTP1, HES1, HMOX1, HPGD, ICAM1, IGFBP2, IL6,ITGB4,JUN, LGALS3, MDM2, MYLPF, NCAM1, NEFH, NFKBIA,NFKBIZ, Nppb, NQO1, NR0B2, PADI4, PLA2G4A, PLAUR, Prl2c2, PTX3,RGN, S100A10, SGK1, SLC6A6, SMAD7, SOD2, SPP1, STAR, STMN1, SULF2, TGFB1, TIMP1, TK1, TNC, UGT2B15, VCAM1, WNT4
Il1a	-1,82	cytokine	Inhibited	-4,061 / 1,46E-11	ADORA2A,BCL3,BIRC3,Ccl2,CCL20,CD83,CSF1,CXCL2,CXCL3,CXCL6,CYP1A1,CYP3A4,FGF2,FOS,FTH1,GCH1, HMOX1,HSD11B2,ICAM1,IGFBP5,IL11, IL18,IL6, JUN, MCAM, NFKB1, NFKBIA, NFKBIZ, NPY, NR3C1, P2RY6, PLA2G4A, PTX3, SERPINA3, SOD2, SPP1, TGFB1, TK1, TLR2, VCAM1,VEGFC
IKBKG	-1,31	kinase	Inhibited	-2,414 / 1,32E-12	AMPD3,Ccl2,CEBPB,CEBPD,CP,CSF1,CTSB,CX3CL1,CXCL2,CXCL3,CXCL6,CYP7B1,ENPP2,FOS, GBP2,GCH1, ICAM1, IGFBP6,IKBKE,IL11,IL6,Mt1,NFKB2, Nppb, Prl2c2, PTX3, RGS16, SEMA3C, SGK1, SOD3, TMEM176B

Rabl6, member RAS oncogene family-like 6; Rassf1, Ras association domain family member 1; Nupr1, nuclear protein, transcriptional regulator, 1; Jun, jun proto-oncogene; Il1a, interleukin 1 alpha; and Ikbkg, inhibitor of kappa light polypeptide gene enhancer in B-cells, kinase gamma.

Table 2. Shortlist of significantly modulated upstream regulators during the early stage of ASML cell rat liver colonization.

From the intermediate stage of liver colonization, also six genes were selected for detailed analysis. These genes included colony stimulating factor 2 (Csf2) and NK2 homeobox 3 (Nkx2-3), which showed decreased expression, but activated their respective downstream molecules. The transcription regulator forkhead box M1 (Foxm1) was increased in expression and activated the corresponding downstream genes. The genes cytochrome P450, family 2, subfamily e, polypeptide 1 (Cyp2e1), angiotensinogen (Agt), and secreted phosphoprotein 1 (Spp1) showed increased expression but inhibited their corresponding downstream genes (see **Table 3**).

Upstream regulator (intermediate stage)	Exp. fold change	Molecule type	Predicted activation state	Activation z-score / p-value of overlap	Target molecules in Ingenuity Pathway Analysis dataset
Csf2	-2,94	cytokine	Activated	3,114 / 7,97E-35	ABCA1,ANLN,ANXA1,ARG1,AURKA,BCL3,BIRC3,BIRC5,BUB1B,CASP1,Ccl2,CCL3L3,CCNA2, CCNB1, CCNF, CD14, CD74, CDC20,CDCA2,CDCA3, CDCA5, CDCA8, CDK1, CDKN2C, CHAF1A, CHAF1B, CKS1B, COL8A1, CSF1, CSF3, CXCL2, CXCR4, DSCC1,E2F8, EDN1,ERCC6L, F3, FANCA,FAS, FBXO5, FCGR2B, FOS,FOSL1,FOXM1,GCH1,GDF15,HDC,HLA-DQB1, ICAM1, ID3, IER3, IGF1, IL1B, IL3RA,IL6, INHBA, IRAK3, JAK2, KIF11,KNTC1, LAMP2, LY96,MCM5, MDM2, MKI67, MNS1, MYC, NCAPD2, NFE2, NFKBIA,NOX1, NR4A1,NUSAP1, PIM3, PLK1, POLD1, POLE,PRC1, PRNP,PTK2B, RACGAP1, REC8, RECQL4,SGK1,SKA1,SLC11A2, SLC1A5, SOD2,SPAG5, SPC25, SPP1, SQSTM1, STMN1, TGFB1, TGM2, TLR2, TNFRSF1A, TNFRSF1B, TNFRSF9,TRIP13,UHRF1,UPP1,VTCN1
Nkx2-3	-1,27	Transcription regulator	Activated	2,351 / 5,76E-09	ADM,ALPL,ANGPTL4,ANKRD37,ANLN,ARHGDIB,BMP2,CASP1,CEP55,CSRNP1,CX3CL1, CXCL16,EDN1,FAM198B, FGF2, FLRT2, GBP2,GCH1, GDF15, GIMAP7, GNG12, HIST2H2AA3 / HIST2H2AA4, HIST2H2AC,MFNG,MYD88,NR2F1, NT5DC2, PAPSS2, PIM3,PLA1A, PSAT1, PTPRE, RTP4, SHMT2, SRPX, VCAM1
Foxm1	2,91	Transcription regulator	Activated	3,840 / 2,40E-17	ANXA1,AURKB,BIRC5,BRIP1,BUB1B,CCNA2,CCNB1,CCND2,CCNF,CDC20,CDC25B,CDK1, CENPA,CENPF,CKS1B, FOXM1, FZD1, HSD11B2, IGF1, IL6, KDR, KIF20A, MCM8, MYC, PECAM1, PLAUR, PLK1, PLK4,PRC1,PTCH1,SKP2,STMN1, VCAN, VIM
Cyp2e1	3,93	enzyme	Inhibited	-2,762/ 7,73E-06	CAT,Ccl2,CD14,Cyp4a14,GCLC,HMOX1,IL6, MGST1
Agt	4,22	growth factor	Inhibited	-2,332 / 3,85E-24	ADAM23,ADIPOQ,ADM,AGT,AGTR2,ANGPT1,ATF3,ATP1B1, BGN,Calm1 (includes others), CAT, Ccl2, CCL3L3, CCL5, CCND2, CDK1,CIT, COL3A1, COL4A1, CP, CTSS, CXCL2, Cyp2c44, CYP2E1, Cyp4a14,DHFR,EDN1,F3,FDX1,FGF13, FGF2,FN1, FOS,GCH1,GJA1, GSS,GSTA3, GSTA5, HES1, HIF1A, HMGCS1,HMOX1,HSPA1A/HSPA1B,ICAM1,ID3,IDH1, IDI1,IGF1, IGFBP5,IL18, IL1B, IL6, LDLR, LSS,MAD2L1, MAPT, MGST1, MSMO1, MYC, NOX1, Nppb, NPR3,NPY,NR4A1, NRG1, PIK3R1, PPFIBP1, PPP1R3C,PTGS1,RGS2, RRAS,SGK1, SOD2, SOD3, SPP1, STAR, STC1, TGFB1, TGFB2, TIMP1, TNFRSF12A, TNFRSF1B, TUBB3, UGCG, VCAM1, VEGFC
SPP1	-4,35	cytokine	Inhibited	-2,527 / 9,62E-06	ADIPOQ,ANGPT1,ARG1,AURKA,CCL20,CCL5,CDC20,CXCL2, FN1,FOS,HMOX1,ICAM1,IL1B,IL6,KRT18,MYC,PIK3R1, S100A4, S100A6,SEPW1, SPP1,TGFB1,TIMP1, TM7SF2,VAT1, VIM

Csf2, colony stimulating factor 2; Nkx2-3, NK2 homeobox 3; Foxm1, forkhead box M1; Cyp2e1, cytochrome P450, family 2, subfamily e, polypeptide 1; Agt, angiotensinogen; and Spp1, secreted phosphoprotein 1.

Table 3. Shortlist of significantly modulated upstream regulators during the intermediate stage of ASML cell rat liver colonization.

From the advanced stage of liver colonization, four genes were selected for detailed analysis. These genes included Versican (Vcan), which showed a reduced expression but activated its downstream genes, as well as myelocytomatosis oncogene (Myc), which exhibited increased expression and also activated a considerable number of downstream genes. The genes CCAAT/enhancer-binding protein beta (Cebpb) and transforming growth factor, beta 1 (Tgfb1), on the other hand, were reduced in expression and as a result inhibited their respective genes (**Table 4**).

Upstream regulator (advanced stage)	Exp. fold change	Molecule type	Predicted activation state	Activation z-score/ p-value of overlap	Target molecules in Ingenuity Pathway Analysis dataset
Vcan	-4,25	other	Activated	2,823 / 5,37E-18	ADM,AEBP1,ANG,ASS1,C1R,C1S,Calm1, CASP1, Ccl2, CCL20,CEBPB, CIDEA,CPE,CXCL2,CYBA,FABP5,FAS, FST, ICAM1,LGALS9B, Mecom, METRNL,NFKB1, NFKBIA,PLA2G2A, PRDX5, RBP1, SERPING1, Slpi, SOD2, TGFB1, TIMP1, VCAM1, VCAN,VEGFA, Wfdc17/Wfdc18
Myc	2,57	trans-cription regulator	Activated	2,907 / 3,06E-20	ADK,ADM,ALB,ALDH18A1,ARG1,ASS1,AURKB,BCL6,BIN1,BIRC5, CASP1, CCNA2,CCNB1,CCND2,CD151,CD19, CDC20,CDCA7, CEBPD, CITED1, CKS2,COL2A1,COL3A1,COL5A2,CPD,CPT1A,CSPG4,CSRP2,CTSB,CTSD,D DIT3, DDX39B,DHFR,DUSP5,EBI3,EDN1,EFEMP1, EMP1, EPHA2, FABP5, FAS,FGFR1,FMOD,FOS, FOXE1, FTH1,G6PD,GAA,GADD45B, GADD45G, GAMT,Gar1,GBP2,GBP4,GCLC, GJA1,H19,HES1,HIVEP2,HLA-A, HMOX1, ICAM1, ID1, IDH1, IDH2, IER3, INHBA, ITGA6, JUN, KDR,KLF10, KLF4, KLF6,KRT7,Ptma,LUM,LYZ,MCM7,MGP,MKI67,Mt1,MYC,MYL9, MYLPF, NFKBIA, Nppb, NPY, OPRK1, PDCD4, PLA1A, PLK1, PLP1, PLS3, POLD1, PPL,Ppp1r15a,PSAT1,PTN,RBP1,SCAMP5,SHMT1,SHMT2, SLC22A4, SLC7A5, SMN1/SMN2, SOD2,SPN,STMN1, TAF1D, TF, TGFB1, THBS1, TIMP1,TMSB10/TMSB4X,TXNRD1,VCAM1,VEGFA,VEGFC, VIM, WISP1
Cebpb	-2,51	trans-cription regulator	Inhibited	-3,299 / 1,84E-21	Abcb1b,AKR1B10,AKR1C3,ALB,APLN,ARG1,BLNK,CCL2,Ccl2,CCL3L3 CCNA2,CCND2,CD14,CDC45,CDH3,CEBPB,CEBPD,COL5A2, CP, CPT1A, CSF3,CTSC,CXCL2,CXCR4,CYP11A1,CYP1A1,CYP27B1,DDIT3, DGAT2, DHFR, FAS, FBLN1, FGFR2,FHL2,FOS,FZD1,HDC,HLA-A, HP, ICAM1, ID1,IER3,IFITM3,IKBKE,IL1B,IL6,JUN, KRT18,MGP,MYC,NDRG4, NFKBIZ, NUPR1,PDK4,PEA15, PLA2G4A,PLAC1,PTGS1, SCD, SLC12A2, TF,TGFB1, TMEM176A, TNFAIP6, TNFRSF1A, TRIB3, TUBB3, VCAN, VIM, XDH
Tgfb1	-2,48	growth factor	Inhibited	-2,346 / 6,57E-59	ABCA1,ADAMTS4,ADK,ADM,ADORA1,AGTR2,ALB,ALDH18A1,APLN,AP OC2,AQP9,ARG1,ASS1,AXL,B3GALT2,BARD1, BCL3,BCL6, BGN, BIN1, BIRC5,BMP7,C1QA,C1QB,C1S,Calm1, CALML4, CAMP,CARS, CASP1, CAT,CBR3,CCL2,Ccl2,CCL20, CCL3L3,CCNA2,CCNB1, CCND2, CD14, CD36, CD68, CDC20, CDH11, CEBPB, CENPF,CITED2, CKS2, CLDN4, CMTM5, COL18A1, COL2A1, COL3A1, COTL1, CREB3, CSF1, CSPG4, CSRP2, CST3, CTGF,CTSB, CTSC, CTSD,CTSS,CX3CR1, CXCL2, CXCR4, CYBA,CYP11A1,CYP27B1, CYP3A7, DFNA5, DNMT3A, EDN1, ELF3, ELK3, ENPP1, EPHA2, ESPL1, EXT1, FABP5, FAM110B, FAS, FCER1G, FDXR, FGF2, FGF21, FGFR1,FGFR2,FOS,FSTL3,FTH1, FXYD5, FZD1, GADD45B, GATA3,GBP2,GCLC,GDF15,GJA1,GLCE,GLI1, Gsta4, GSTA5, GTPBP1, H6PD,HEBP1,HES1,HLA-DQB1, HMOX1, HPGD, HSPA1A / HSPA1B, HTRA1, ICAM1, ID1, IER3, IFRD1,IGF2, IGFBP2, IGFBP5, IGFBP6, IL11, IL13RA2, IL18,IL1B, IL33,IL6,IL6R,INHA, INHBA, IRAK3, ITGA1, ITGA6, ITGB6, JUN, KDR, KLF10,KLF15, KLF4, KRT18,KRT7,LITAF,LOXL1, LPAR1, MAOA,MFAP2,MGP, MKI67, MMP12, MSMO1, MTHFD2, MYBL1, MYC, MYD88,MYLK,MYLPF, MYO10, NAB2, NDC80, NDRG4, NFKBIA, NNMT, NOV, NPR1, NR4A1, NR4A3, NT5E,NUPR1,OSR2,P2RY6,PAPPA, PARP3, PDCD4,PDE4D,PGRMC1,PLA1A, PLA2G4A, PLAGL1, PLS3, PLXNC1, PNOC, POLD1, PPFIBP2, PPP1R13B, PPP1R3C, PRC1,PTGS1, PTK2B, PTPN6,RAB31, RACGAP1, RAPGEF3, RASGRP3, RASL11B,RASSF1, RBPMS, RHOD, S100A11, S100A4, SBNO2, SCD, SDC4, SEMA3A, SEMA3B, SFTPC, SHMT1, SHOC2, SLC7A5, SMC4, SNAI2,SOD2, SOD3, SPC25,SPEG,SPHK1,SRFBP1,TBX3,TCF12,TGFB1, TGM2, THBS1, TIMP1, TJP2, TLR2, TLR4,TNFAIP6, TNFRSF12A,Tpm2,TUBB2A,TUBB3, TXNRD1, VCAM1, VCAN,VEGFA, VEGFC,VIM, WFS1, WISP1,WNT11, WT1, XDH

Vcan, Versican; Myc, myelocytomatosis oncogene; Cebpb, CCAAT/enhancer-binding protein beta; and Tgfb1, transforming growth factor, beta 1.

Table 4. Shortlist of significantly modulated upstream regulators during the advanced stage of ASML cell rat liver colonization

http://dx.doi.org/10.5772/64335

Upstream regulator (terminal stage)	Exp. fold change	Mole-cule type	Predicted activation state	Activation z-score / p-value of overlap	Target molecules in Ingenuity Pathway Analysis dataset
Csf2	-2,81	Cyto-kine	Activated	2,752 / 3,11E-35	See Table 3
Foxm1	2,54	Transcription reg.	Activated	2,751 / 2,02E-11	See Table 3
Tsc2	3,08	other	Inhibited	-2,551 / 1,78E-12	A2M,ACSS2,ANXA1,ATF3,B3GALT2,BIRC5,Ccl2,CCND2,CCND3,DDIT3, DYNC1I1,EGR1,GPNMB, HMGCS2,HMOX1,IRS1,MGP, NSDHL, PDGFRA, PDGFRB,PRELP,RASSF4,S100A11,S100A6,SCD,SLC2A1, SMPDL3A, SOD2, TAGLN, TMEM176A, TMEM176B, VAMP8
Tnf	3,53	Cyto-kine	Inhibited	-2,209 / 3,74E-86	A2M,A4GALT,Abcb1b,ABCC3,ACP5,ACSL1,ADAMTS4,ADM,ADORA1,ADORA2A,AEBP1,AGT, AGTR1, AKR1B1, AKR1B10,ALB,ANGPT2, ANGPTL4, ANXA1,AOC3,APCS,APOA1,APOC2,APOC4,APOE,AQP1,AQP3,AQP9, ARG1,ARHGDIB,ARL6IP5,ARRDC3,ASGR1,ASS1,ATF3,AXIN2, B4GALNT1, B4GALT1, BACE1, BCL2A1, BCL3, BCL6, BID, BIK, BIRC5, BMP2, BTG2, BUB1B, C5AR1,CASP8,CAT, CCDC80,CCL19, CCL2,Ccl2, CCL20, CCL3L3, CCL4, CCL5,Ccl6,CCND2,CCND3,CCR1,CCR5,CCR6,CD14,CD163, CD247, CD40,CD82, CDH1, CDH11, CDH2, CEBPD, CFB, CFD, CFLAR, CH25H, CLDN4, COL1A2,COL3A1, COTL1, CPT1A,CREB3, CREB3L3, CSF1, CSF3, CTGF, CTSK, CTSS, CTSZ, CXCL12, CXCL13, CXCL2, Cxcl9, CXCR4, CYBA, CYBB,CYLD, CYP1A1, CYP1B1, CYP26B1,CYP2C8,CYP2E1,CYP7B1, CYTIP, DCBLD2, DCHS1, DCN, DDIT3,DENND2D, DPP4,DPYS,DUSP1, DUSP2, DUSP5, DUSP9,EBI3,EDN1,EDNRB, EFNA1, EGFR,EGR1, EGR2, EIF2AK2, ELF3, ELK3, EMP1, ENPP3, ENTPD5, EPHA2, ERG, ESM1,EXT1, F3,FABP1, FABP4, FADS1, FAM132A, FAM198B, FAS, FCER1G,FCGR2B, FDPS, FGF2, FGFR1, FGG, FOSL1,FOXE1,FRMD6,FRZB, G0S2,GADD45B,GCH1, GCLC, GDF15,GDNF, GPD1, GPR176, GPRC5B,GPX1, Gsta4, GSTP1, H19, HDC, HERC1,HES1,HID1,HK3,HLA-DRA,HMOX1,HP,HPGD,HSD11B1, HSD17B7, HSPA1A/ HSPA1B,ICAM1, ICAM2, ICOS, ID1, ID3,IDH2, IER2, IER3, IFIH1, IFIT3, IGF1, IGF2, IGFBP1, IGFBP2, IGFBP3, IGFBP5, IKBKE, IL11, IL16, IL18, IL1B, IL1R2, IL23A, IL24,IL3RA, IL6,INHA,INPP5D,IRAK3,IRF5, IRS1, ITGA6, ITGB2, ITGB6,JAG1, KDR, KIF20A, LAMC1,LBP,LCAT,LCN2, LDLR, LGALS8, LOX, LPAR6, LPL, LSS, LTB, LXN,LY96, LYVE1, MAFF, MALL, MAN1C1,MAP3K8,MBL2, MCAM, MEF2C,MET,MFHAS1, MGMT, MGP, MGST1, MMD, MMP12, MSLN, MST1, Mt1,MVP, Mx1/Mx2, MYLK, NCF1, NEFH, NFKB1,NFKB2, NFKBIA, NFKBIZ, NINJ1, NNMT, NOS3, NOTCH4, NOX1, NPM3, Nppb, NQO1, NR0B2, NR1I2, NR4A1, NRP1, OAS1, OCLN, OLR1, OPTN, ORM1, P2RX5,PCK1, PCSK6,PDE2A, PDGFA, PDGFRA, PDIA4, PENK, PER2, PIM3, PLA2G3, PLA2G4A, PLAUR, PLK2, PLK3, PLOD2, PLP1, PLVAP, POMC, POSTN,PPARG, PPP1R3C, Prl2c2, PRNP, PRSS23, PSMB9, PTGS1, PTPRC, PTPRN,RAB32,RARRES2, RBP1, RFTN1,RGCC, RGS1, RGS2, RGS20, RGS4, RGS5, RGS9, RND1, ROBO1, S100A8, S100A9,SCD,SDC2,SDC4, SEMA3C,SEPP1,SERPINA3, SERPINB1, SERPIND1,SERPINE1,SERPINE2,SGK1,SHBG,SLC10A1,SLC11A1, SLC11A2, SLC1A4, SLC22A4, SLC27A5, SLC2A1, SLC2A2, SLC7A2,SLC7A8, Slco1a1, Slco1a4, SMPD1, SMPD2, SMPDL3A, SNN,SOAT1,SOD2, SOD3, SPARC, SPHK1, SPP1, SPSB1, SQSTM1,ST3GAL6,STMN1,SYNPO,TAGLN, TBXAS1, TF,TGFB1,TGFB2,TGFB3,TGM2,THBS1,THBS2,TIMP1,TK1,TLR2, TLR3, TMEM176B, TNF, TNFRSF11B, TNFRSF1A,TNFRSF21, TNNC1, TPST1, TRAF3,TRPC6,TXNIP,TXNRD1,UBD,VCAM1,VMP1,XIAP, ZC3H12A

Csf2, colony stimulating factor 2; Foxm1, forkhead box M1; Tsc2, tuberous sclerosis 2; and Tnf, tumor necrosis factor.

Table 5. Shortlist of significantly modulated upstream regulators during the terminal stage of ASML cell rat liver colonization.

From the terminal stage of liver colonization, again four genes were selected for detailed analysis. These included two genes, which had been listed before (Csf2 and Foxm1) that caused the same pattern of expression and resulting influence as in the intermediate stage of liver colonization (decreased expression but subsequent activation in the case of Csf2 and increased expression resulting in subsequent activation in the case of Foxm2). The other two regulators (tuberous sclerosis 2 (Tsc2) and tumor necrosis factor (Tnf)) were both increased in expression and were predicted to inhibit a large number of downstream genes (see **Table 5**).

2.3. Changes in mRNA expression after recultivation in vitro

For assessing the influence of the environment on ASML tumor cells, ASML cells were also recultivated in vitro for 3, 6, and 9 days after they had been reisolated from rat liver after a colonization period for 21 days. As a result, genes were found to be downregulated in vitro or upregulated at varying degrees. Some examples are given in **Figure 5**. As can be seen, the genes desmoglein 4 (Dsg4), tRNA methyltransferase 10A (Trmt10a), and stathmin 2 (Stmn2) were decreased more than 1000-fold, more than 100-fold, and more than 3-fold, respectively. In contrast, the genes apolipoprotein C-II (Apoc2), ectonucleotide pyrophosphatase/phosphodiesterase 1 (Enpp1), and Keratin 18 (Krt18) were increased more than 3-fold (Apoc2 and Enpp1) and more than 100-fold (Krt18). The differences between the cultivation periods of 3, 6, and 9 days were very low and thus negligible.

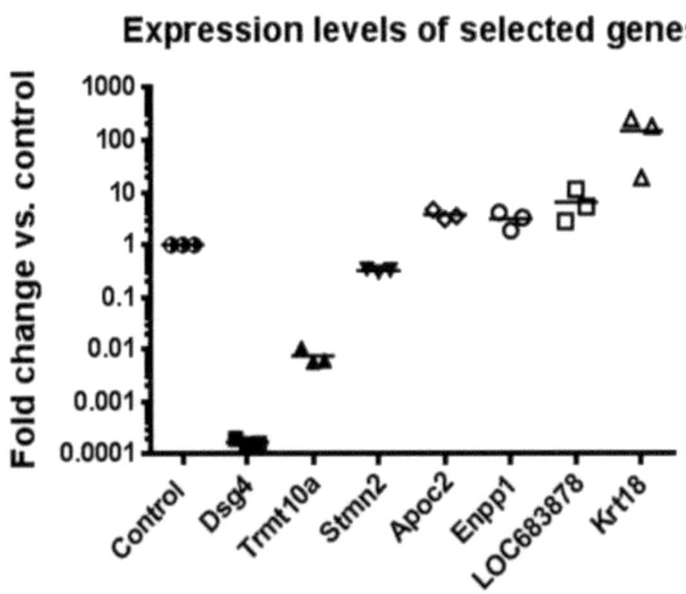

Figure 5. Changes in mRNA expression after recultivation in vitro: ASML cells were also recultivated in vitro for 3, 6, and 9 days after they had been reisolated from rat liver after a colonization period for 21 days. As a result, some genes were downregulated or upregulated in vitro, at varying degrees. Seven examples are given in comparison to control.

2.4. miRNA modulation of ASML cells colonizing rat liver

Concomitantly with the mRNA species, all known miRNA molecules were analyzed in the respective batches of reisolated ASML cells. As for the distribution of mRNAs, the modulation

http://dx.doi.org/10.5772/64335

of miRNA expression was detailed for the two same categories, i.e. the fold changes in miRNA expression and the respective stage of liver colonization, as shown in **Figure 6**.

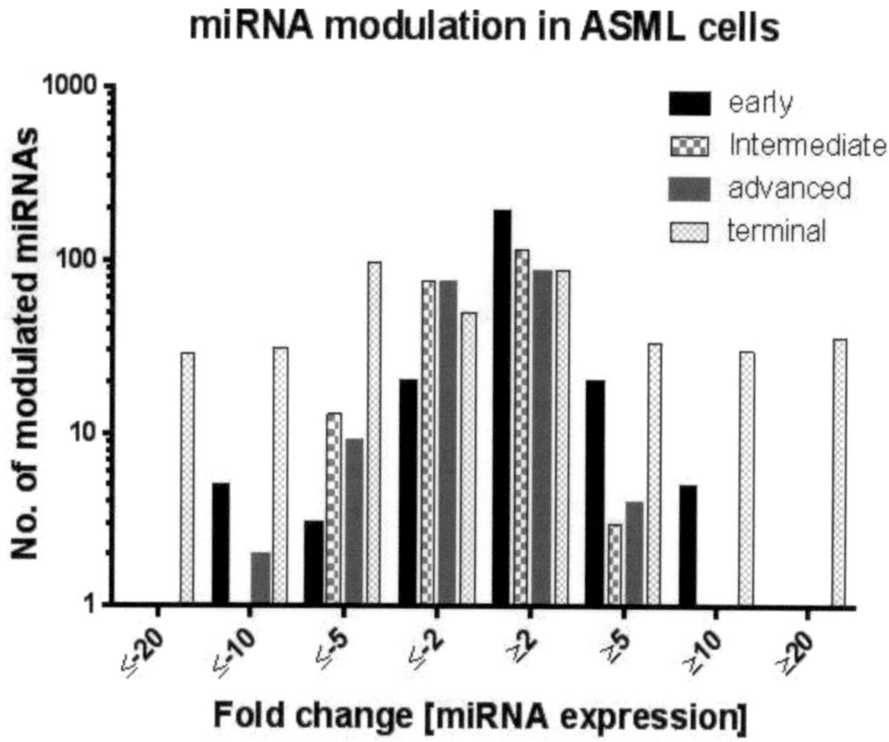

Figure 6. miRNA modulation of rat pancreatic cancer cells colonizing rat liver: Given is the fold change of mRNA expression of reisolated ASML cells during early, intermediate, advanced, and terminal stages of liver colonization relative to control cells growing in vitro.

Because of the lower number of existing miRNAs as compared to mRNAs, the distribution looks not as bell shaped as for mRNAs in **Figure 1**. This is also due to a considerable number of miRNAs, which show a more than 20-fold regulation (both, positive and negative) in the terminal stage of liver colonization.

An example for the influence of miRNAs is given in **Figure 7**. The miRNA 29b-3p is known for its effect on extracellular matrix proteins, as on collagens [17]. Downregulation of miRNA 29b-3p was observed in ASML cells during the whole period of liver colonization. This is shown in **Figure 7A**, with the nadir of miRNA 29b-3p expression appearing on day 3 (less than 10-fold of control level), and some recovery thereafter to a plateau of expression ranging from fivefold to threefold reduced levels, as related to control expression in vitro. This reduction was associated with distinctly increased expression of the collagens Col4a2 (collagen, type IV, alpha 2), Col3a2, Col1a2, Col1a1, and Col4a1. Col5a3 showed only a minor increase in expression, but Col5a2 (collagen, type V, alpha 2) showed reduced expression, as was true for Tgfb3 (transforming growth factor, beta 3) (**Figure 7B**).

A

B

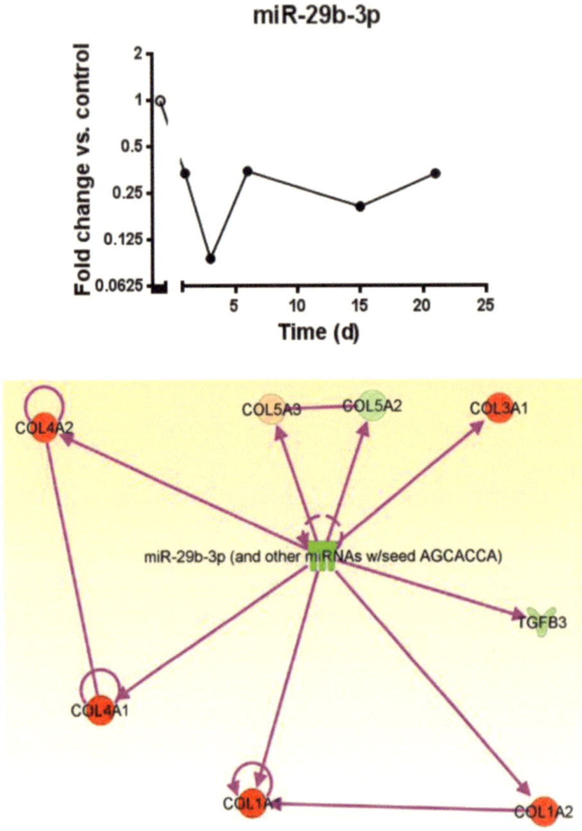

Figure 7. Influence of miRNA 29b-3p on gene expression: Shown is the expression of miRNA 29b-3p in ASML cells during liver colonization (**A**). In addition, the influence on mRNAs is given in terms of upregulation or downregulation (**B**). For color code, see **Figure 3**.

This analysis shows that certain extracellular matrix proteins, as the collagen family, are highly regulated by their respective miRNA. Further experiments are needed to reveal the mechanistic role of these proteins during liver colonization and to address the question whether they can be diagnostic or therapeutic targets.

Author details

Khamael M.K. Al-Taee, Hassan Adwan and Martin R. Berger*

*Address all correspondence to: m.berger@dkfz.de

Toxicology and Chemotherapy Unit, German Cancer Research Center (DKFZ), Heidelberg, Germany

References

[1] Ryan DP, Hong TS, Bardeesy N. Pancreatic adenocarcinoma. N Engl J Med. 2014;371(22):2140–2141.

[2] Sahin IH, Lowery MA, Stadler ZK, Salo-Mullen E, Iacobuzio-Donahue CA, Kelsen DP, et al. Genomic instability in pancreatic adenocarcinoma: a new step towards precision medicine and novel therapeutic approaches. Expert Rev Gastroenterol Hepatol. 2016:1–13.

[3] Siegel R, Ma J, Zou Z, Jemal A. Cancer statistics, 2014. CA Cancer J Clin. 2014;64(1):9–29.

[4] Schenk M, Schwartz AG, O'Neal E, Kinnard M, Greenson JK, Fryzek JP, et al. Familial risk of pancreatic cancer. J Natl Cancer Inst. 2001;93(8):640–644.

[5] Waddell N, Pajic M, Patch AM, Chang DK, Kassahn KS, Bailey P, et al. Whole genomes redefine the mutational landscape of pancreatic cancer. Nature. 2015;518(7540):495–501.

[6] Everhart J, Wright D. Diabetes mellitus as a risk factor for pancreatic cancer. A meta-analysis. JAMA 1995;273(20):1605–1609.

[7] Petersen GM, Hruban RH. Familial pancreatic cancer: where are we in 2003? J Natl Cancer Inst. 2003;95(3):180–181.

[8] Whitcomb DC, Gorry MC, Preston RA, Furey W, Sossenheimer MJ, Ulrich CD, et al. Hereditary pancreatitis is caused by a mutation in the cationic trypsinogen gene. Nat Genet. 1996;14(2):141–145.

[9] Ueki T, Walter KM, Skinner H, Jaffee E, Hruban RH, Goggins M. Aberrant CpG island methylation in cancer cell lines arises in the primary cancers from which they were derived. Oncogene. 2002;21(13):2114–2117.

[10] Wilentz RE, Geradts J, Maynard R, Offerhaus GJ, Kang M, Goggins M, et al. Inactivation of the p16 (INK4A) tumor-suppressor gene in pancreatic duct lesions: loss of intranuclear expression. Cancer Res. 1998;58(20):4740–4744.

[11] Hruban RH, Petersen GM, Ha PK, Kern SE. Genetics of pancreatic cancer. From genes to families. Surg Oncol Clin N Am. 1998;7(1):1–23.

[12] Fuchs CS, Colditz GA, Stampfer MJ, Giovannucci EL, Hunter DJ, Rimm EB, et al. A prospective study of cigarette smoking and the risk of pancreatic cancer. Arch Intern Med. 1996;156(19):2255–2260.

[13] Gupta S, Vittinghoff E, Bertenthal D, Corley D, Shen H, Walter LC, et al. New-onset diabetes and pancreatic cancer. Clin Gastroenterol Hepatol. 2006;4(11):1366–1372; quiz 01.

[14] Dunne RF, Hezel AF. Genetics and Biology of Pancreatic Ductal Adenocarcinoma. Hematol Oncol Clin North Am. 2015;29(4):595–608.

[15] Eyol E, Murtaga A, Zhivkova-Galunska M, Georges R, Zepp M, Djandji D, et al. Few genes are associated with the capability of pancreatic ductal adenocarcinoma cells to grow in the liver of nude rats. Oncol Rep. 2012;28(6):2177–2187.

[16] Al-Taee KK, Ansari S, Hielscher T, Berger MR, Adwan H. Metastasis-related processes show various degrees of activation in different stages of pancreatic cancer rat liver metastasis. Oncology research and treatment. 2014;37(9):464–470.

[17] Kwon JJ, Nabinger SC, Vega Z, Sahu SS, Alluri RK, Abdul-Sater Z, et al. Pathophysiological role of microRNA-29 in pancreatic cancer stroma. Sci Rep 2015;5:11450.

Chapter 7

Minimal Invasive Surgery of Metastatic Bone Tumor

Hyun Guy Kang and San Ha Kang

Additional information is available at the end of the chapter

http://dx.doi.org/10.5772/64341

Abstract

Bone is one of the most common metastatic areas in the cancer patient. Bone metastasis is the major cause to deteriorate the quality of life due to severe pain, walking difficulty, paraplegia, and pathologic fracture. To maintain patient's general condition and continue scheduled medical treatment, various minimally invasive surgical methods have been developed. The percutaneous methods including alcohol or bone cement (polymethyl methacrylate [PMMA]) injection, laser or radiofrequency ablation, cryosurgery, and MRI-HIFU have shown favorable outcomes in the spine, pelvis, and other flat bones. Using only these percutaneous methods have high risk of pathologic fracture in the long bone of extremity, which needs some metallic fixation. Therefore, the new surgical method and instrument involving percutaneous internal fixation with PMMA bone cement injection have been introduced. The PMMA bone cement injection is effective in the metastat ic bone tumor, providing reliable mechanical augmentation of destructive bone, durable local tumor suppression, and effective pain relief. The hollow-perforated screw and nail (multihole injection screw and nail) has central canal and multiple side holes to facilitate injection of bone cement to the bone lesion. An optimal customized surgical option according to the patient's circumstances should be planned.

Keywords: metastatic bone tumor, minimal invasive surgery, hollow-perforated screw, percutaneous fixation and injection, palliative management

1. Introduction

Metastatic bone cancer is the most common malignancy in the bone tumor. The life expectancy of patients has been increasing considerably over the recent years since the development of cancer management, but the occurrence chance of bone metastasis also increased. The incidence rate ranges from 20% to 85%, varying by type of cancers. Bone metastasis is the major cause to deteriorate the life quality of patients due to severe pain, walking difficulty, and pathologic fracture. Pathologic fracture is induced in around 10% of bone metastasis, and is life-threatening to patients.

The treatment of metastatic bone tumor includes the combination of modality including medication, radiation therapy, and surgery to reduce pain and prevent bone destruction. Recently, the use of bisphosphonate and denosumab was reported as an inhibition of osteolytic microenvironment factors. Radiation therapy is the most frequently used and effective method for palliation but has limitation of bone strengthening.

Generally, patients need operation for the prevention of pathologic fracture, especially on the weight-bearing bones like vertebrae, pelvis, and femur as well as long tubular bone of extremity. The early surgical management before the fracture is important and has many benefits: avoiding terrible pain and complications, relatively easy surgery, reducing rehabilitation time and life-threatening condition. The surgical methods for bony metastasis include curettage and bone cement (PMMA, polymethyl methacrylate) augmentation, internal fixation with plate or intramedullary (IM) nail, arthroplasty, and prosthesis reconstruction. The surgical treatment method is chosen by multidisciplinary teamwork. The most appropriate surgical option should be selected under the consideration of patient's age and life expectancy, general condition, response of medical treatment, and even preoperative life quality, because major surgery lead to stop or delay of chemotherapy and radiation therapy, and many accompanied complications.

Recently, various minimally invasive surgical methods that can be performed without general anesthesia and large incision have been introduced for metastatic bone tumor: ethanol injection, cryoablation, radiofrequency (RF) ablation, cementoplasty, etc. The percutaneous bone cement (PMMA, polymethyl methacrylate) injection is known as cementoplasty or osteoplasty, and has been shown favorable outcomes in the vertebral body and the flat bones such as pelvis, scapula, and sternum. However, solitary bone cement injection without metallic fixation at the long bone still has high risk of pathologic fracture.

A new novel surgical technique will be introduced in the concept of percutaneous metallic fixation and simultaneous bone cement injection. For this technique, the unique implant, multihole injection screw and nail, is developed. This implant has a hollow in the center and perforated side holes allowing the material injection to the bony lesion. This minimally invasive surgical method showed good result in the respect of pain relief, mechanical stability, surgical risk, rehabilitation period, hospital stay, surgical cost, and local tumor suppression. The injection material can be various, including chemotherapeutic agent, anti-osteolytic agent, and accelerate bone healing agent as well as PMMA bone cement. Recently, the MR-guided focused ultrasound surgery (MRgFUS) is introduced. MRgFUS is an external ablation which showed effectiveness in reducing pain from bone metastases. However, MRgFUS lacks restoration for mechanical stability.

This chapter will introduce the diverse developing minimally invasive surgical methods and suggest future direction for better management of patients with metastatic bone tumor.

http://dx.doi.org/10.5772/64341

2. Various methods of minimally invasive surgery for metastatic bone tumor

2.1. Alcohol ablation (ethanol injection)

Alcohol ablation is a simple and inexpensive technique for tumor ablation. The ablation involves cellular dehydration and ischemia that lead to endothelial necrosis and vascular thrombosis. Before the injection of the alcohol, a mixture of iodinated contrast material (25%) and lidocaine 1% (75%) is introduced to examine area of the alcohol diffusion, and patient will be put under local anesthesia. Alcohol ablation has been a treatment for bone metastases rather than primary bone tumor. However, the method has a risk of failure or complications as the alcohol may uncontrollably diffuse into the tumor and surrounding soft tissues [1].

2.2. Laser ablation

Laser ablation is the application of thermal energy converted from light energy. Thermal energy will be diffused into the tumor tissue, inducing cellular coagulation necrosis through denaturation of cellular protein. For this technique, a neodymium: yttrium aluminum garnet (Nd:YAG) type generator or diode is used at lower power for thermal effect (photocoagulation) or at higher frequency (vaporization and cavitation).

The procedure time is short (about 10 minutes) and the extent of tumor necrosis is related to the amount of deposited energy, up to 15 mm in diameter for 1200 J. In the case of photocoagulation, laser ablation has been a useful method to treat benign primary bone tumor osteoid osteoma because of its accuracy, reliability, and accessibility. However, photocoagulation is not appropriate to treat large lesions [1].

The current use of laser ablation for metastatic bone cancer is limited; the laser technology cannot cover large lesion and takes long time to be done percutaneously.

2.3. Radiofrequency (RF) ablation

Radiofrequency ablation is a procedure to damage tumor cell through heat generated from an active electrode inserted into the tumor. For effective treatment, the procedure is performed at a temperature between 60°C and 100°C for 5–10 minutes.

Different size of a single tip electrode, which ranges from less than 15 mm up to 50 mm in diameter, determines the removable size of tumor. To treat larger volume of tumor, additional electrode should be inserted: internally cooled electrodes for cooling system and pulsed mode, perfused electrode, which increases tissue conductivity, or umbrella-shaped electrode and multipolar arrays which increases electrode tip coverage.

Radiofrequency ablation has been widely used to treat soft tissue cancer including hepatocellular carcinoma and thyroid cancer. In the skeleton, this method is used both as curative treatment for benign bone tumor such as osteoid osteoma, and palliative treatment for metastatic bone tumor [1]. **Figure 1** illustrates an operation case for bone metastasis by RF ablation.

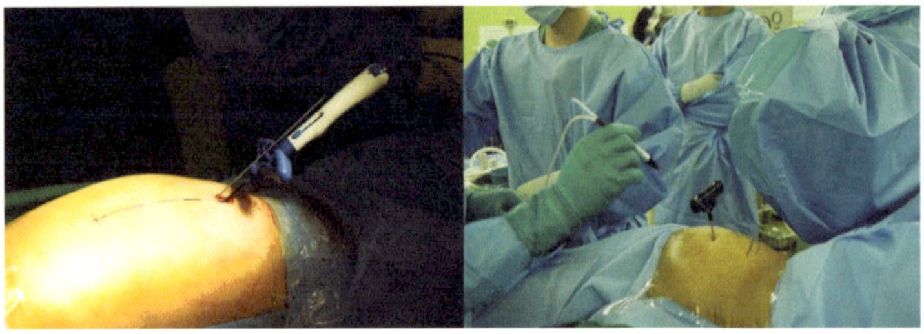

Figure 1. RF ablation can be applied for the pelvic bone metastasis.

2.4. Cryoablation

Liquid nitrogen has been used as an intraoperative adjuvant method in the open bone tumor surgery. For the percutaneous application, technical progress was made for probe manufacturing, and utilization of argon gas as a cryogen. The argon gas freezes the tumor tissues at −100°C around the active probe, forming ice balls around the probe. Temperature below −20°C leads to cellular necrosis causing protein denaturation and rupture of cell membranes.

In general, the size of the necrosis is likely to be smaller than the ice ball and its maximum is up to 3 cm in diameter. The forming ice ball can be monitored by ultrasonography or computer tomogram but cannot be detected by fluoroscopy. Processes of the cryoablation are categorized into three phases: a first freezing phase (10 minutes), a thawing phase with helium gas (5 minutes), and a second freezing phase (10 minutes). Cryoablation is commonly used to treat prostate cancer. Treating metastatic bone tumor using cryoablation, however, may not be a good choice; the method fails to cover its big sizes, takes a long time, and is unable to perform moving tip technique [1]. **Figure 2** illustrates a treatment for femoral neck metastasis by cryoablation.

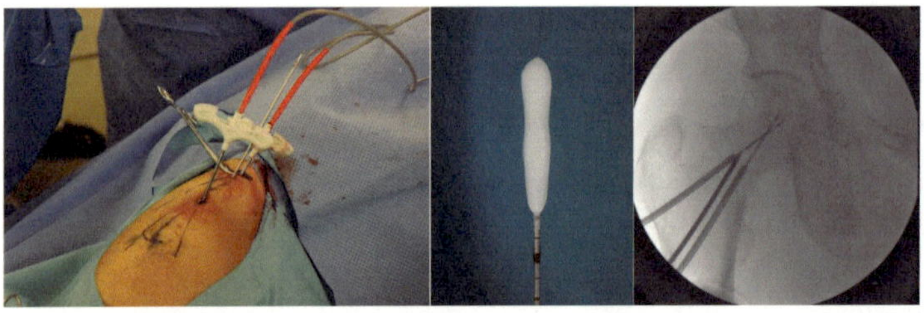

Figure 2. Cryosurgery with probe type rod is applied for femoral neck metastasis.

2.5. MRI-HIFU (high-intensity focused ultrasound) ablation

HIFU induces coagulation necrosis of the tumors by focusing high heat transformed from ultrasound produced by a transducer on tumors.

http://dx.doi.org/10.5772/64341

HIFU ablation has been a treatment for uterine myoma as well as palliation of bone metastases and sarcomas. The biggest advantage of HIFU ablation is its noninvasive procedure (however, the development of its interstitial applicators is in progress). In addition, HIFU ablation can eliminate tumors clearly and promptly: about 15 mm in diameter along the axis of the beam and about 1.5 mm in transverse diameter. Its procedure is conducted under MR or US guidance [1].

3. Polymethyl methacrylate (PMMA) bone cement injection

Percutaneous bone cement injection is known as a cementoplasty or an osteoplasty. The PMMA has been used in orthopedic surgery from 1945 including joint replacement surgery, spinal compression fractures, chronic osteomyelitis with antibiotics and tumors. The structure of methyl methacrylate monomer allows polymerization at room temperature to produce solid PMMA. The avidity of the polymer to dissolve in monomer aids this reaction. The composition of PMMA is shown in **Figure 3** and **Table 1**.

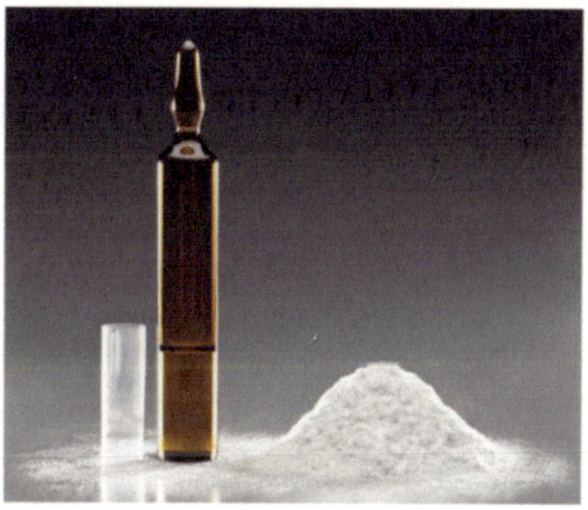

Figure 3. The PMMA bone cement is activated by mixing powder and liquid components.

Percutaneous vertebroplasty was originally developed as a treatment for angiomas, but its application to the osteoporotic spine has been shown to provide significant and prolonged relief of pain. It controls the symptoms of compression fractures by recreating mechanical stability. The technique involves the percutaneous transpedicular injection of low viscosity biomaterial into the vertebral body guided by an image intensifier.

Percutaneous bone cement injection for the metastatic bone tumor has been shown favorable outcomes in the vertebral body and the flat bones such as pelvis, scapula, and sternum. The PMMA has been one of the most useful agents in the treatment of bone tumors since it provides immediate mechanical stability and reduces bone pain. The reason for pain improvement after percutaneous cementoplasty (PC) procedure is due to tumor suppression, microfracture recovery, nerve ending sacrifice, mechanical strengthening, etc. When the heat is generated from solidification of bone cement, cytotoxic effect causes the destruction of tumor. The PMMA can also have a mass effect by interrupting circulation to the tumor. Nonetheless, the risk of pathologic fracture is still high when PC is solely performed in long tubular bones such as femur, tibia, and humerus without metal fixation [2].

Composition	Function
Powder compositions	
Polymer	Polymethyl methacrylate
Copolymers (e.g., methacrylate-methyl methacrylate)	Alter physical properties of the cement
Barium sulfate or zirconium dioxide	Radio-opacifiers
Antibiotics	Antimicrobial prophylaxis
Dye (e.g., chlorophyll)	Distinguish cement from bone
Liquid compositions	
Monomer	Methyl methacrylate monomer
N,N-dimethyl-p-toluidine (DMPT)	Initiates cold curing of polymer
Benzoyl peroxide	Reacts with DMPT to catalyze polymerization
Hydroquinone	Stabilizer preventing premature polymerization
Dye (e.g., chlorophyll)	Distinguish cement from bone

Table 1. Bone cement composition.

3.1. Percutaneous cementoplasty for pelvic bone metastasis

The pelvic bone is a connecting area between spine and femur. The acetabulum of pelvis is a direct contact area with femoral head and important for weight bearing. When the metastatic tumor occurred at the acetabulum, the percutaneous PMMA injection will be a good option [3].

3.1.1. Surgical technique

The PC is performed under regional spinal anesthesia. A patient is positioned in lateral decubitus position. A sterile field is prepared and skin is punctured with 10 or 11 gauge osteoplasty needle at the 10 cm posterior from anterior superior iliac spine. The needle is advanced from posterior to anterior at an angle about 70° from the horizontal plane. The osteoplasty needle is usually used over two needles to reduce intraosseous pressure at the time of bone cement injection: the bone cement is injected through a single needle, until bloody fluids, and injected bone cement regurgitate through the other needles. Empty syringe will aspirate the unnecessary fluids and then bone cement is injected through all needles. Under fluoroscopic guidance, with anterior-posterior and oblique views of a pelvis, the PV needle penetrates the outer cortex and the tip is positioned in the lesion. The low-viscosity radiopaque PMMA is mixed and transferred to a 30 ml or 50 ml syringe, depending on the number of cement pack (20 g per a pack). Then, PMMA is transferred again into several 1 ml syringes. With the frequent check of oblique fluoroscopic view to avoid sciatic nerve injury by leakage,

http://dx.doi.org/10.5772/64341

bone cement is injected as much as possible. If injection is not easily accomplished, a stylet is used to push PMMA through the lumen of needle. The bone cement injection is usually conducted within 3–4 minutes after making the cement mixture.

PMMA injection has to start slowly to prevent venous leakage with careful C-arm fluoroscopy monitoring. If the bone cement flows rapidly to the regional vein on the fluoroscopy, the injection has to be delayed to achieve thicker mixed bone cement. **Figures 4** and **5** show the operative process of percutaneous cementoplasty.

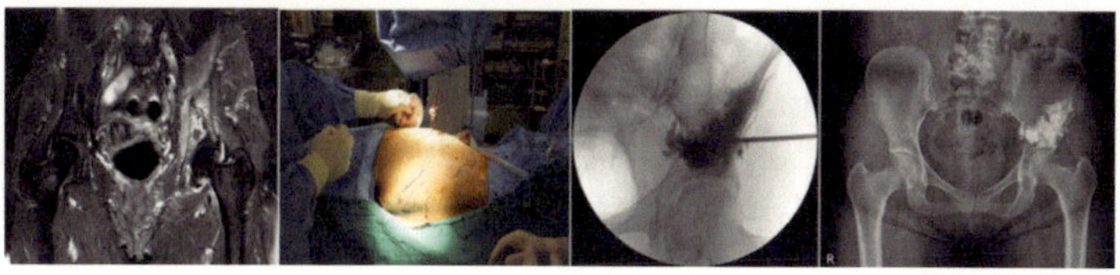

Figure 4. A 54-year-old female has left pelvic bone metastasis of breast cancer. Bloody osteolytic lesion managed by PMMA bone cement injection.

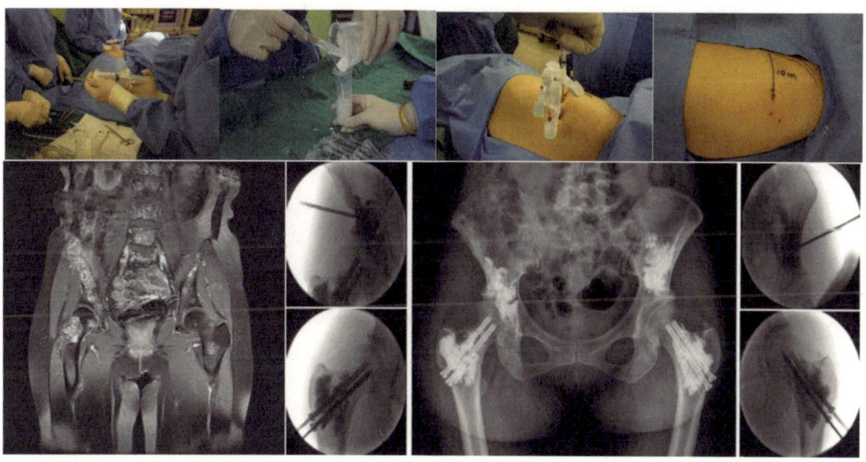

Figure 5. Intraoperative photographs showing preparation of bone cement and start of injection through one needle for intraosseous pressure decompression. Multiple bone metastases are frequently involved around hip joint and these can be treated with one time surgery by minimally invasive surgery.

The anesthesiologist is asked to monitor temporary change of blood pressure, pulse rate, and respiration due to toxicity and volatility smell of PMMA. In the case of a larger lesion encroaching most of the ilium, another VP needle can be employed in the same way.

3.2. Evaluation of percutaneous PMMA bone cement injection

F-18-FDG PET-CT is known for good detectability of bone metastases in several types of cancers, and became widely used for treatment response evaluation and recurrence detection.

The quantitative PET-CT values, SUVmax, and SUVmean showed significant uptake decrease after PMMA injection procedure, which means less glucose uptake and reflects tumor suppression. However, most control lesions were aggravated in the same individual patient.

Previous studies report that after bone cement injection, tumor volume is reduced and histology showed tumor necrosis, which support our hypothesis. Bone scan (BS) is known for good detectability, therapy response monitoring, and long-term follow-up of bone metastases. BS is advantageous for whole skeletal metastases detection [4]. BS and F-18-FDG PET-CT have complementary value as BS can detect osteoblastic metastasis well, and both are good imaging modality to detect bone metastasis.

Interpatient study was unable to be performed due to the differences in patient status (primary tumor, treatment, etc). So we performed comparison study of PS lesion and control lesion in the same patient. In our study, as shown in **Figure 6**, BS showed improved or stable state after PMMA injection procedure, which means local tumor suppression. However, most control lesions showed aggravated state [5].

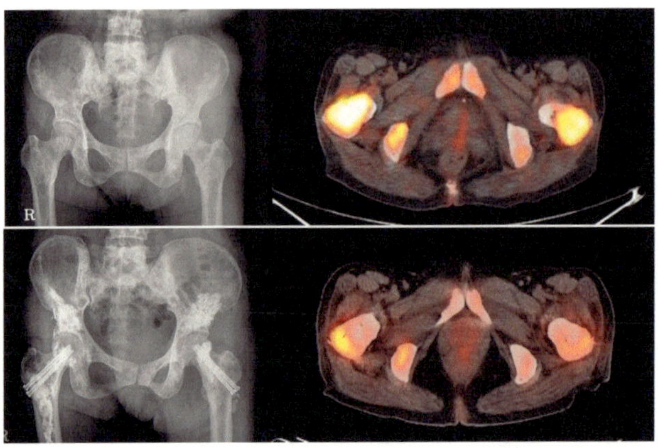

Figure 6. PET-CT evaluation after combined percutaneous cement injection surgery showed effective tumor suppression in the metastatic bone tumor. Before (above) and after (below) operation.

4. Percutaneous internal fixation and PMMA bone cement injection for long bone metastasis

4.1. Femoral neck metastasis

The femur neck is very vulnerable area to fractures due to senile osteoporosis and metastatic bone cancer [6]. The conservative treatment of metastatic tumors in the femoral neck is difficult because of the frequency of intractable pain and impending or established pathological fracture. Any of the aforementioned methods of treatment may be considered but do not significantly contribute to the stability of the femoral neck. Usually, the patients are treated by either joint replacement or internal fixation for pain palliation. The bipolar hip arthroplasty is a mainstay for femur neck metastasis but is too much a burden to the advanced terminal cancer patient. Recently, a new novel surgical technique for the treatment of femoral neck metastasis using hollow-perforated screws (HPSs) and bone cement was introduced [5–7].

4.1.1. Hollow-perforated screw

The hollow-perforated screw (HPS), as illustrated in **Figure 7**, is a newly developed device, modified from a 6.5-mm cannulated screw (Multihole Injection Screw; SOLCO, Seoul, Korea). The screw allows to achieve greater fixation capable of injecting material into the weak bone area simultaneously through its multiple side holes.

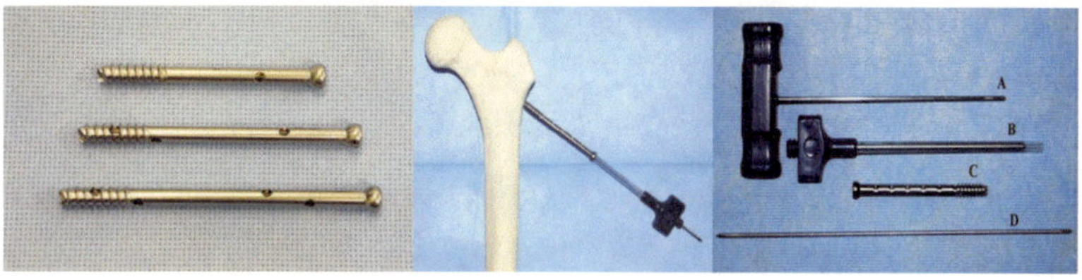

Figure 7. The hollow-perforated screws have multiple holes for injection. The equipment facilitates percutaneous fixation and simultaneous bone cement injection for femur neck.

4.1.2. Surgical technique

The procedure is performed in the lateral decubitus position under spinal anesthesia. The femoral neck anteversion is drawn with the guidance of C-arm fluoroscopy. Two or three 2.2-mm guide pins are inserted to the femoral neck as the same pattern of cannulated screw fixation in the femoral neck fracture. The length of the inserted guide pin is measured and a small skin incision is made for cannulated drilling. After the cannulated drilling, two or three multihole injection screws are introduced over the guide pins. After checking the location of all screws fluoroscopically, the osteoplasty needles are inserted into the canal of screw. These osteoplasty needles are driven into the silicone tube before insertion, which is made temporarily by segmentally cutting a hemovac line for preventing leakage of injected materials at the connecting site with the screw. The guide pin is removed and low-viscosity PMMA bone cement

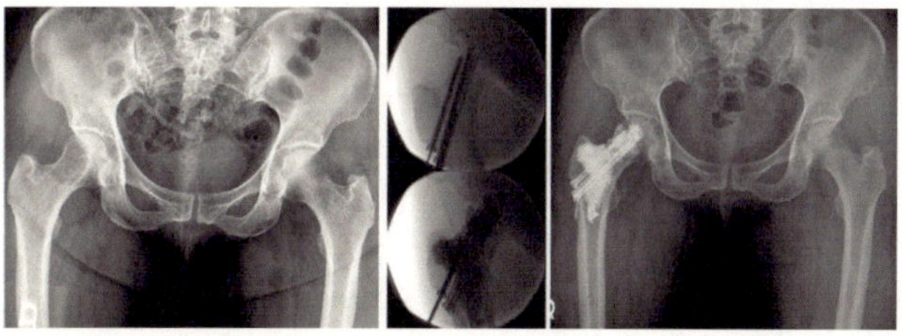

Figure 8. A 58-year-old female has impending fracture of right femoral neck metastasis by lung cancer. Percutaneous fixation and PMMA bone cement injection are effective methods for prevention of pathologic fracture.

is injected through 1 ml syringes. **Figure 8** shows preoperative and postoperative photographs by percutaneous fixation and PMMA bone cement injection and **Figure 9** shows detailed surgical procedures.

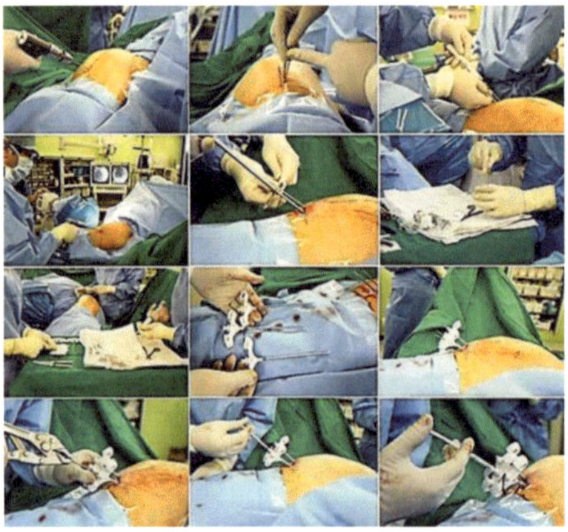

Figure 9. Detailed surgical procedure demonstrated for femoral neck metastasis.

4.2. Percutaneous flexible nail fixation and bone cement injection for humerus

The rigid conventional intramedullary nailing method has been widely used for treatment of traumatic fracture as well as long bone metastasis. When surgeons place rigid nail to the humeral lesion, general anesthesia, locked screws, and sometimes curettage and cementing are required. The current study reported the palliative surgical treatment of metastatic humeral lesions using percutaneous Ender nailing along with bone cement augmentation under regional anesthesia in patients with high-risk advanced cancer [4].

4.2.1. Surgical technique

After interscalene or axillary regional anesthesia, the patient is placed in the supine position so that fluoroscopy cannot be disturbed. The entry points of the Ender nails (4.5-mm diameters; Smith & Nephew plc, London, UK) are the greater tubercle of the humeral head for proximal and diaphyseal lesions, and the lateral condyle for supracondylar lesions. Ender nails that are long enough to pass the intramedullary metastatic lesion are selected. When the Ender nail is completely seated, the tip at the entry point should be buried beneath the cortex to prevent soft tissue irritation. The osteoplasty needles are directly inserted into the medullary cavity by hand-push or hammering in a percutaneous and transcortical manner. Over two needles are commonly used for decompression of intramedullary pressure during bone cement injection and coverage of larger or skipped lesions. The entry point of the needle is selected at the most easily accessible area to the lesion, which is apart from the neurovascular bundles. After identifying the location of the needles by fluoroscopy, low viscous bone cement is injected through one needle and sequential through other needles.

4.3. Percutaneous flexible nail fixation and bone cement injection for femur and tibia

The small diameter of intramedullary flexible nail fixation provides the space for percutaneous bone cement injection. The combinational percutaneous surgery with flexible nail insertion and bone cement injection can be useful to long bone metastasis patients who cannot undergo conventional intramedullary nailing due to poor life expectancy and multiple surgical demanding fracture risk areas. Although the pathologic fracture can be progressed more by weak stability of flexible nail than by rigid conventional nail, in the selective patient condition, this surgical method is effective to maintain bedside care and reduce further osteolytic progression. Patients with subtrochanteric lesion, pathologic fractures, or joint destructive lesions are excluded.

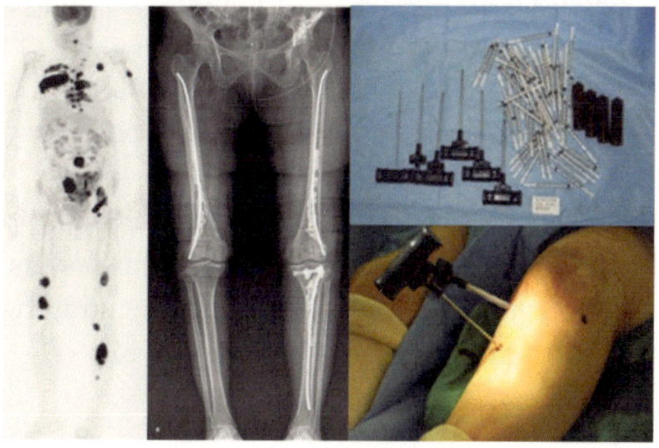

Figure 10. The four areas (left pelvis, both femurs, and left tibia) can be treated at once.

The Ender nail fixation in the humerus, femur, and tibia has some limitation for the bone cement injection. Each osteoplasty needle has to penetrate skin and bone cortex for placing to the intramedullary perimetal area [8]. **Figure 10** shows percutaneous flexible nail fixation and bone cement injection.

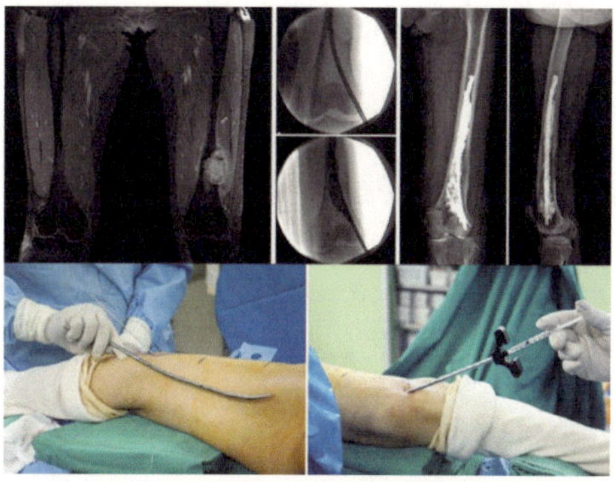

Figure 11. The multihole injection nail was developed for simultaneous bone cement injection in the course of nail insertion without adding cortical punctures.

Very recently, the multihole injection nail (SOLCO, Seoul, Korea) has developed into a hollow titanium flexible nail with the tip of multiple side holes. The bone cement could be injected deeply in the course of a percutaneous fixation without adding bone cortex holes. The advantages of this new implant include immediate achievement of stable fixation and effective pain relief, deeper injection of drugs or bone cements, a short recovery time, and high emotional satisfaction from simple operation [9]. The use of the multihole injection nail is shown in **Figure 11**.

4.4. Closed intramedullary (IM) nailing with percutaneous cement augmentation

The rigid IM nailing is widely used for metadiaphyseal lesions of the long bones and for trochanteric and subtrochanteric lesions of the femur in particular. Immediate bony stability and pain relief may be achieved with low morbidity. IM nailing may be undertaken using an open or closed technique. Closed IM nailing tends to be used when there are minimal bone destruction and displacement of the fragments. It may combine with percutaneous cement augmentation. Closed nailing with cement augmentation has many advantages over only closed nailing. First, intra- and post-operative bleeding is reduced as cement fills the space around the nail. Second, the cement gives early mechanical stability by preventing further destruction of bone and supporting the bone that remains; this results in further relief of pain. Third, filling the canal with cement at the time of nailing may limit the intramedullary spread of tumor [10]. Its operative procedures are shown in **Figure 12**.

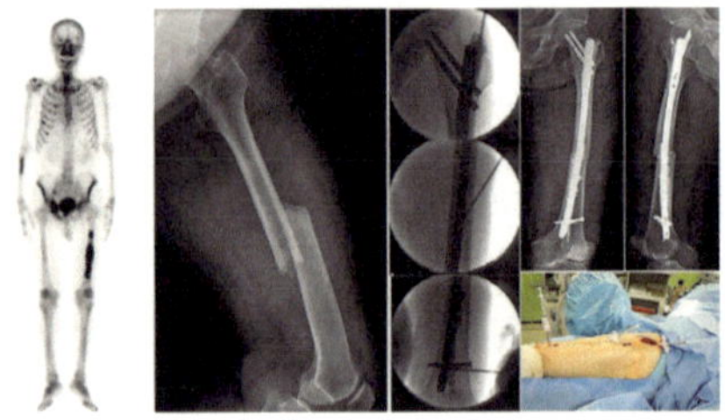

Figure 12. The combined percutaneous bone cement injection with the conventional intramedullary nailing leads more effective in the symptom relief and local tumor suppression.

5. Chemotherapeutic agent-loaded bone cement

Beyond the injection of bone cement only, there is growing interest on therapeutic effects on mixture of bone cement and chemotherapeutic agents. Many studies suggested that antineoplastic agent–loaded bone cement not only prevents tumor recurrences with better local tumor control but also decreases the number of distant metastases [11].

According to the literature, percutaneous injection with a mixture of gemcitabine and PMMA bone cement was applied to two patients of femoral neck metastasis from lung cancer [7]. In vitro test reported that the antineoplastic agents, such as cisplatin laden bone cement, hinder

http://dx.doi.org/10.5772/64341

the growth of giant tumor cells, colon cancer cells, lung cancer cells, and breast cancer cells [11]. But further studies are needed to investigate efficacy of the chemotherapeutic agents incorporated into bone cement.

6. Bisphosphonate-added bone cement

Bisphosphonates (BPs) are antiresorptive drugs widely used to treat bone diseases such as osteoporosis, bone metastases, and hypercalcemia of malignancy, to prevent bone loss, and to increase bone density [12, 13]. Several studies demonstrate that BPs with bone cement have effects on increasing mechanical property and reducing bone resorption.

BPs in combination with bone cement play a key role in mechanisms of reducing a risk of bone resorption. BP-enriched bone cement can regulate important mediators involved in osteoclastogenesis, such as RANKL synthesis by osteoblast, and may modulate OPG, a decoy receptor of RANKL absorption, thus preventing RANK activation. In addition, two BPs alendronate and pamidronate mixed with calcium phosphate bone cement showed satisfactory results in mechanical properties. Both of them raise osteoblast proliferation and differentiation while restraining osteoclastogenesis and osteoclast function [14]. BP-combined cement can be a promising drug device as a local approach, preventing osteoporotic vertebral defect [13].

However, there is a paucity of clinical cases on clear efficacy of BP-laden bone cementoplasty and further studies are needed.

7. Conclusion

The metastatic bone cancer takes the highest frequency of more than 95% of malignant bone tumors and has adverse influences on quality of life in patient with advanced disease. Moreover, metastatic bone tumor usually reveals in multiple areas. An optimal customized surgical option according to patient's circumstances should be planned, in order to achieve durable skeletal stability, effective pain relief, least surgical morbidity, less hospital stay, and local tumor suppression.

Author details

Hyun Guy Kang[1*] and San Ha Kang[2]

*Address all correspondence to: ostumor@ncc.re.kr

1 Orthopaedic Oncology Clinic, National Cancer Center, Gyeonggi-do, Republic of Korea

2 Bouve College of Health Sciences, Northeastern University, MA, USA

References

[1] Moser T, Buy X, Goyault G, Tok CH, Irani F, Gangi A. Image-guided ablation of bone tumors: review of current techniques. J Radiol. 2008;89:461-471.

[2] Webb JCJ, Spencer RF. The role of polymethylmethacrylate bone cement in modern orthopaedic surgery. J Bone Joint Surg. 2007;89(B):851-857.

[3] Hyun Guy Kang, Min Wook Joo, June Hyuk Kim, Seok Ki Kim, Patrick P. Lin, Han Soo Kim. P536-Percutaneous cementoplasty for pelvic bone metastasis in patients with advanced cancer. In: American Academy of Orthopaedic Surgeons (AAOS) 2013 Annual Meeting; March 19–23, 2013; Chicago, Illinois. 2013.

[4] June Hyuk Kim, Hyun Guy Kang, Jung Ryul Kim, Patrick P. Lin, Han Soo Kim. Minimally invasive surgery of humeral metastasis using flexible nails and cement in high-risk patients with advanced cancer. Surg Oncol. 2011;20(1):e32-e37.

[5] Yong-il Kim, Hyun Guy Kang, Seok-ki Kim, June Hyuk Kim, Han Soo Kim. Clinical outcome prediction of percutaneous cementoplasty for metastatic bone tumor using 18F-FDG PET-CT. Ann Nucl Med. 2013;27(10):916-923.

[6] Patrick P. Lin, Hyun Guy Kang, Yong-il Kim, June Hyuk Kim, Han Soo Kim. Minimally invasive surgery for femoral neck fractures using bone cement infusible hollow-perforated screw in high-risk patients with advanced cancer. Surg Oncol. 2015;24(3): 226-231.

[7] Kang HG, Roh YW, Kim HS. The treatment of metastasis to the femoral neck using percutaneous hollow perforated screws with cement augmentation. J Bone Joint Surg. 2009;91(B):1078-1082.

[8] Yong-il Kim, Hyun Guy Kang, Tae Sung Kim, Seok-ki Kim, June Hyuk Kim, Han Soo Kim. Palliative percutaneous stabilization of lower extremity for bone metastasis using flexible nails and bone cement. Surg Oncol. 2014;23(4):192-198.

[9] Hyun Guy Kang, June Hyuk Kim, Yong-il Kim, Patrick P. Lin, Han Soo Kim. Percutaneous surgical management of femur neck metastasis using hollow perforated screws (Multi-hole Injection System) for introducing bone cement in advanced lung cancer patients. In: European Musculo-Skeletal Oncology Society (EMSOS) 2015; April 29th – May 1st 2015; Athens, Greece. 2015.

[10] Kim Y-I, Kang HG, Kim JH, Kim S-K, Lin PP, Kim HS. Closed intramedullary nailing with percutaneous cement augmentation for long bone metastases. J Bone Joint Surg. 2016;98(B):703-709.

[11] Hakan Özben, Levent Eralp, Gökhan Baysal, Ayflegül Cort, Nazli Fiarkalkan, Tomris Özben. Cisplatin loaded PMMA: mechanical properties, surface analysis and effects on Saos-2 cell culture. Acta Orthop Traumatol Turc. 2013;47(3):184-192.

http://dx.doi.org/10.5772/64341

[12] Tomasz Mazurkiewicz, Łukasz Matuszewski, Anna Matuszewska, Magdalena Jaszek. Implanted bisphosphonates in bone cement affect bone markers in rat serum. Int Orthop. 2013;37(5):969-974.

[13] Elise Verron, Marie-Line Pissonnier, Julie Lesoeur, Verena Schnitzler, Borhane Hakim Fellah, Hugues Pascal-Moussellard, Paul Pilet, Olivier Gauthier, Jean-Michel Bouler. Vertebroplasty using bisphosphonate-loaded calcium phosphate cement in a standardized vertebral body bone defect in an osteoporotic sheep model. Acta Biomater. 2014;10(11):4887-4895.

[14] Panzavolta S, Torricelli P, Bracci B, Fini M, Bigi A. Alendronate and pamidronate calcium phosphate bone cements: setting properties and in vitro response of osteoblast and osteoclast cells. J Inorg Biochem. 2009;103(1):101-106.

Section 2

Circulating Tumor Cells

Chapter 8

The Selection Strategy for Circulating Tumor Cells (CTCs) Isolation and Enumeration: Technical Features, Methods, and Clinical Applications

Jason Chia-Hsun Hsieh and Tyler Ming-Hsien Wu

Additional information is available at the end of the chapter

http://dx.doi.org/10.5772/64812

Abstract

The key aim of the proposed chapter is to provide readers a brief description for the most important parts of the field of circulating tumor cells (CTCs): the core techniques, including negative and positive selection-based CTC isolation, and the differences between them. Most importantly, we will also review the clinical applications and important findings in clinical trials. The evidence-based review will not only help clinicians use CTCs to predict recurrence and foresee the disease-related outcomes but also to inspire the researchers in this field to conduct further investigations.

Keywords: circulating tumor cells, negative selection, cancer, stem cell, liquid biopsy

1. Introduction of circulating tumor cells (CTCs)

1.1. Brief history of CTC researches

Circulating tumor cells (CTCs) are cells shedding from primary tumor(s) into the adjacent vasculature and are floating around in the circulation throughout the human body. The cells, as seeds for the subsequent initiation of distant site metastases, are responsible for the cancer-related deaths [1]. For the first time, CTCs were described via the observation in the blood of cancer patient by Dr. Thomas Ramsden Ashworth, who postulated that "cells identical with those of the cancer itself being seen in the blood may tend to throw some light upon the mode of origin of multiple tumors existing in the same person" in 1869 [2]. In 1906, Goldmann reported that visible venous invasion by cancer in approximately 20% of 500 necropsies and microscopic invasion of vasculature in nearly 10% [3]. In very early 1900s, several reports of observation of free cancer cells by morphology have been discussed in patients with melanoma, gastric cancer [4–6], and lung cancer [7]. However, long being in the technical limitation on isolation of these rare cells in circulation, the realization of CTCs isolated from living cancer patients and analysis of their clinical impacts began since 1930s [8–10]. One of the first systemic surveys in 40 living cancer patients was done by Pool and Dunlop in 1934 [11]. In this period, morphology and cytochemical characteristics remained the most important method to identify "abnormal" or "atypical" cells. Tumor cell embolization was observed [12] and widely accepted to be one of the major mechanisms for dissemination of cancer [13, 14]. Since 1986 with the development of polymerase chain reaction (PCR), investigators began to utilize these nucleic acid-based detection methods to help identify CTCs, including circulating tumor mutated DNA and mRNAs [15–23]. In early 2000s, semi-automated devices appeared and facilitate the advances of CTC testing in clinical study enrolling healthy subjects and patients with various types of cancer [24–26], given the fact that numerous previous methods were relatively operator-dependent and often lacked of validated sensitivity, specificity, coefficient of variation and reproducibility [22, 27–31]. In 2004, CellSearch™ (Veridex, Janssen Diagnostics, USA) got approval from United States (US) Food and Drug Administration (FDA) for testing in patients with breast, colorectal, and prostate cancer [32, 33]. Since 2012, a rapid exploration of number of CTC isolation devices having nearly fully automated design emerged [34–40].

Recently, CTC studies are focusing on devices harboring high sensitivity, high specificity, reduced sample requirement, label-free isolation, and the ability to catch living CTCs for in-vitro culture. Owing to the less invasive nature than conventional cancer tissue biopsy, CTCs, as serum circulating tumor DNA (ctDNA) and microRNA (miRNA), are termed to be "liquid biopsies."

1.2. Natures of CTCs

It has been a long time after CTCs were noticed and efficiently captured by many methods; however, little is known about the behavior of CTCs [41]. Investigators have observed some phenomenon about what CTCs look like, how CTCs shed, migrate, live, defense human immune system, and initiate distant metastases.

First, CTCs were believed to be larger than normal blood cells, which contributed the development size-based isolation strategy. Marrinucci et al. [42] supported that the fact of CTCs being larger than white blood cells and having high nuclear to cytoplasmic ratios with voluminous cytoplasm. In addition, the morphology of CTCs is highly similar to that of cells from original biopsied cancer tissues. Numerous devices were developed on the basis of this characteristics and collect cells with larger size (often >15 μm), including dielectrophoresis (DEP) [43, 44], optically induced dielectrophoretic (ODEP) [45] force-dependent devices, and filter-based systems [46–61]. However, other investigators found that the size of real CTCs could be greatly differed from cell lines [62], and might even vary interindividually and intraindividually [63, 64]. The size criteria of CTC definition remain in debate.

Second, CTCs exist in almost all staged cancer and could be detected in the course of the disease [27]. In 1995, Hansen et al. analyzed the blood samples drawn from surgical fields during 61 oncologic surgeries and 93.4% samples found tumor cells [65], which suggest one of the possible routes of early dissemination of cancer cells. In 2000, Yamashita et al. found that signals of CTCs (carcinoembryonic antigen messenger RNA, CEA mRNA) from preoperatively negative to postsurgically positive might suggest a specific type of surgery could contribute to the cancer cell dissemination [66]. Similar results were reported by other investigators to support the findings in various types of cancer (but breast cancer mainly) [67–73]. Although CTCs were found in early-stage cancer patients, the cells do not result in metastasis all the times. The clearance of human immune systems and inadequate "soil" of distant organs are one of the plausible explanations. To look on the bright side, CTCs in very early stage cancer could help early diagnosis of cancer and prevent overwhelming dissemination and cancer death [74].

Third, CTCs would form cell clusters, clumps, or circulating tumor microemboli (CTM) and were found to highly correlate to cancer progression [75–79] and resistance to systemic anticancer therapies [78, 80], which was established on the basis of many animal model and preclinical reports [81–85]. Recently, Sarioglu et al. [86] designed a Cluster-Chip for efficient capture of CTC clusters and enable the detailed characterization of the biological properties and role of CTC clusters in metastasis [86]. Studies of cancer metastasis have emphasized the novel concept of "seed and soil" as a key determinant of metastatic propensity [87]. This model matches the importance of mutated genetic drivers within tumor cells conferring proliferative and invasive properties, with that of the microenvironment of the distant organ or "niche," which may facilitate metastasis occurrence. However, the physical characteristics of single CTCs and CTC clusters may also contribute to metastatic propensity, especially as they impact the ability of epithelial tumor cells to survive the loss of cell adherence and shear forces in the blood stream, i.e., different survival signals among the cancer cell "seeds" may be important. For instance, in a mouse endogenous pancreatic cancer model, noncanonical Wnt signaling is elevated within CTCs, where it appears to suppress anoikis [88], while in a subcutaneous tumor xenograft model, the admixture of tumor and stromal cells within microemboli may contribute to stromal-derived survival signals [77, 89, 90].

Fourth, CTCs could also be detected in cancer patients who underwent curative surgery, indicating minimal residual disease in the circulation [91–99] and suggesting the correlation to disease recurrence in the following months [92, 95, 100, 101]. van Dalum et al. [99] found that the presence of CTC in blood drawn pre and one and two years after surgery, but not postsurgery is associated with shorter Relapse-free survival (RFS) and OS for stages I–III breast cancer, which could partially answer the question of how frequent and how long oncologists should follow patients' CTCs up and the timing of CTC testing after curative surgery. This phenomenon indicates that postsurgical adjuvant therapy might be required in specific population on the basis of CTC testing which remains uncertain to date.

Fifth, the captured CTCs according to their method of isolation, sometimes are alive for in-vitro culture [48, 61, 102, 103] and might play a very important role to continuously obtain primary cancer cell lines in the near future. Furthermore, CTC-derived cell lines and xenografts might reveal new therapeutic targets and can be used for drug screening [104, 105]. The phenomenon is the main difference of CTCs from ctDNA possibly being released from dead cancer cells. In addition, living CTCs can also colonize their tumors of origin, in a process that is call "tumor self-seeding." Kim et al. [106] successfully revealed the self-seeding phenomenon in breast cancer, colon cancer, and melanoma tumors in mice model, which was predominantly mediated by CTCs with aggressive features, including those with bone, lung, or brain metastatic tropism. The cancer-derived cytokines IL-6 and IL-8 acted as CTC attractants and the markers MMP1/collagenase-1 and the actin cytoskeleton component fascin-1 as mediators of CTC infiltration into mammary tumors. The important findings of tumor self-seeding phenomenon could explain the relationships between tumor size, anaplasia, vascularity and prognosis, and local recurrence seeded by disseminated cells following ostensibly complete tumor excision.

Sixth, CTCs could represent a merged status of a whole tumor mass, including static and active parts with expression of specific functional markers [107–110] and could serve as a multifunctional biomarker [108, 111]. Functional analyses on CTCs might provide the possibility to identify the biological characteristics of metastatic cancer cells, including the identification of metastasis-initiating cells [104].

1.3. CTCs in cancer progression

1.3.1. Cancer migration, invasion, epithelial-mesenchymal transition (EMT), mesenchymal-epithelial transition (MET) and cancer stem cells (CSCs)

As mentioned above, Hansen et al. [65] found that CTCs exist in the 93% blood samples drawn from surgical fields. That correlated to one of the two common routes of cancer migration: hematologic and lymphatic spreading. In clinical aspect, tumor migration and invasion means tumor growth or progression and can be analyzed via the time from disease-free status to recurrence or time from baseline to enlargement of tumor size. Early in 1999, Palmieri et al. have found a significant correlation among clinical stages, tumor progression, and presence of circulating cancer-associated antigens in stages I–III melanoma patients [112]. In other cancer types, investigators widely agreed with the observation that the higher CTCs signals indicate to higher cancer stage and recurrence rate, suggesting larger number of CTCs might promote cancer progression [113–117]. However, not only CTC count but also the specific properties of cancer cells matter. Two of them have been widely reported are epithelial-mesenchymal transitions (EMTs) or stem-like properties of CTCs [118].

In many animal species, EMTs normally occur during critical phases of embryonic development. The formation of mesenchymal cells (nonepithelial) that are loosely embedded in an extracellular matrix from a primitive epithelium is an important feature of most metazoans [119]. During this transition, mesenchymal cells acquire a morphology that is appropriate for migration in an extracellular environment and settlement in areas that are involved in organ formation, which involves interactions between epithelial and mesenchymal cells. Mesenchymal cells can also participate in the formation of epithelial organs through mesenchymal-epithelial transition (MET) [119]. CTCs may also undergo phenotypic EMT changes, which allow them to travel to the site of metastasis formation without getting affected by conventional treatment [118, 120, 121]. The acquired molecular changes by CTCs undergoing EMT that facilitates cancer progression and resistance to conventional therapies [122, 123]. EMT markers, including vimentin, twist, ZEB1, ZEB2, snail, slug, and N-cadherin in CTCs, primary HCC tumors and adjacent nontumoral liver tissues were evaluated by Li et al. [123] and the twist and vimentin expression levels in CTCs could be promising biomarkers for evaluating metastasis and prognosis in liver cancer patients. Most importantly, CTCs would abandon their epithelial properties (EpCAM) [88, 124] and escape from CTC capture by positive selection strategy (will discuss below) and become one of the main downsides of the strategy of CTC isolation. Several investigators have noticed that phenomenon and suggested that there is an urgent need for optimizing CTCs detection methods through the inclusion of EMT markers [120, 125–129]. Deeper understanding of those processes is of fundamental importance for the development of new strategies of early cancer detection and effective cancer treatment approaches that will be translated into clinical practice [122].

Stemness features of CTCs, sometimes termed as circulating cancer stem cells (CSCs), have also been getting noticed as EMT of CTCs in recent years. The CSC hypothesis claims that a small subset of cells within a tumor has the ability of both tumor initiation and sustaining tumor growth [130–132]. These cells with expression of stemness markers are capable of forming floating spheres in serum-free medium, a property associated with stem cells and are able to differentiate into an aberrant cell phenotype constituting tumor heterogeneity [133]. Among all the possible molecular markers of stemness feature, CD133, CD44, ICAM-1, and CXCR4 are common used antibodies for labeling the subpopulation from other CTCs and actually technically available [134–136]. These are not the only markers to identify CSCs and depend on cancer types. Sun et al. [137] found that stem cell-like phenotypes (labeled with CD133 and ABCG2) in EpCAM-positive CTCs, and a preoperative CTC of more than 2 cells/7.5 ml blood is a novel predictor for tumor recurrence in HCC patients after surgery, especially in patient subgroups with AFP levels of less than 400 ng/ml or low tumor recurrence risk. Many other studies in various types of cancer have come across with the similar conclusions, including breast, colorectal, gastric, liver, and NSCLC, etc. [120, 123, 138–145].

Therefore, the subpopulation of CTCs, CSCs, and CTC with EMT features is probably the one of the key determinants of future CTC and cancer metastasis investigations.

1.4. The impact of CTCs on multidrug resistance

In 2011, Gradilone et al. reported an interesting study aiming to test the hypothesis that drug-resistant CTCs might have predictive value in metastatic breast cancer (MBC) and possibly retain stem-like properties [146]. As the study presented, the extraction of mRNA from CTCs for multiple drug resistance proteins (MRPs) analysis are most commonly used protocol. They also found the expression status of MRP1 and MRP2 in CTCs was found to correlate to response to anthracyclines (doxorubicin or epirubicin) [147]. In 2013, Nadal et al. found an interesting phenomenon that a relative enrichment of cytokeratin CK(+)/CD133(+) CTCs in triple negative and HER2-amplified tumors was found. While CK(+)/CTCs decreases after chemotherapy when analyzing the whole population, CK(+)/CD133(+) CTCs were enriched in posttreatment samples in nonluminal BC subtypes. These findings suggest the potential role of CD133 as a promising marker of chemoresistance in nonluminal BC patients [148]. Similar results were also reported in recent years and the authors have come across with the same conclusion that multiple drug resistance profiling (MRPs mainly, sometimes with CD133 [148], ALDH1 [149], and ERCC1 [150]) of CTCs could predict the responses to given chemotherapies [146, 148, 150–152].

One direct proof of CTC exhibiting drug resistance comes from a study in 2014. Pavese et al. observed that CTC and DTC cell lines, established from mice bearing human prostate cancer orthotopic implants, exhibit increased cellular invasion in vitro, increased metastasis in mice, and express increased EMT biomarkers. In addition, CTC cell lines are selectively resistant to growth inhibition by mitoxantrone-like agents. The findings are important and suggested that CTC formation is accompanied by phenotypic progression without obligate reversion. Their increased metastatic potential, selective therapeutic resistance, and differential expression of potential therapeutic targets provide a rational basis to test further interventions [153].

Therefore, developing an in-vitro chemosensitivity test on CTCs is not impossible though it required large-scale clinical trials to test and validate. Yu et al. applied pharmacogenomic (PGx) modeling testing on CTCs, while PGx testing was used on cancer tissue to predict the efficacy of chemotherapeutic agents in preclinical cancer models, and reported the feasibility in 2014. In the report, clinical benefit was seen for study participants treated with chemotherapy regimens predicted to be effective versus chemotherapy regimens predicted to be ineffective with regard to progression-free (10.4 months versus 3.6 months; $P < 0.0001$; HR, 0.14) and overall survival (17.2 months versus 8.3 months; $P < 0.0249$; HR, 0.29) [151]. In another study, thymidylate synthase expression in CTCs could possibly serve as a new tool to predict 5-fluorouracil resistance in metastatic colorectal cancer patients [152]. Other than conventional imaging studies evaluating two-dimensional tumor size every 8–12 weeks for routine tumor assessment during anticancer therapy, CTCs could possibly serve as a rapid responding biomarker to real-time change of cancer cells, including the early response or resistance to given therapeutic drugs [154–156].

2. The strategies for CTC isolation and enumeration

There are hundreds of methods/protocols reported to be able to efficiently detect or isolate CTCs. In a simple way to discuss here, we have several common strategies of CTC isolation could be worthy of development in the future. The first one is **label-free isolation strategy**, including size-based, physical properties-based, morphology-based isolation strategy; the second one is **positive selection strategy**, including positively identification of cancer-specific markers on nucleus or cell surface, or specific DNA mutation(s), mRNA(s) overexpression; and the third one is **negative selection strategy**, consisting of depletion of red and white blood cells by any means. Finally, the fourth one is combination of two or more strategies mentioned above.

2.1. Label-free isolation strategy

Several novel studies using size as a key criterion of CTC identification were reported [157–160]. Early in 2004, ISET system was used for a well-designed clinical trial evaluating 44 patients with primary liver cancer and without metastases, 30 patients with chronic active hepatitis, 39 with liver cirrhosis, and 38 healthy individuals, and all participants were followed up for a mean period of 1 year. Both the presence ($P = 0.01$) and number ($P = 0.02$) of CTCs and microemboli were significantly associated with a shorter overall survival. Beta-catenin mutations could be found in 3 of 60 CTCs which might be suggesting their impact on the initiation of cancer cells invasion [161]. Similar positive findings by size-based CTC isolation were reported in melanoma [162–164], gastric cancer [76, 165], prostate cancer [166, 167], lung cancer [168–170], pancreatic cancer [103], liver cancer [127], sarcoma [171], and breast cancer [172]. Separation by physical properties, i.e., gravity, density gradients, using microfluidic technology [45, 46, 56, 60, 173–186], or microfiltration [53, 172, 187, 188] were also reported to be able to capture CTCs efficiently.

By means of label-free isolation, combined molecular analysis could be easily performed after CTC isolation owing to no chemicals exposure and less procedures done during isolation. For instance, Zheng et al. [189] reported a novel device designed based on membrane microfilter device to isolate CTCs and then send them to PCR-based genomic analysis by performing on-membrane electrolysis with embedded electrodes reaching each of the individual 16,000 filtering pores. Immunocytochemistry and FISH assays following label-free isolation were reported to be successfully performed directly on the filter system [157, 176, 190, 191]. Interestingly, some investigators compared the isolation efficiency of ISET and CellSearch™ systems [76, 93] and one team concluded that a combination of ISET plus CellSearch™ would have better performance in CTC detection in NCSCL patients than ISET or CellSearch™ alone [93].

There are several disadvantages of physical methods should be noticed. First, the isolation process based on physical properties can cause the deformation and damage of CTCs by filter pores [192]. Second, larger size cells could not always be cancer cells and the isolated population often mixed up with megakaryocytes, which are very common to see in the circulation of cancer patients just underwent chemotherapy. Third, small-size CTCs would be inevitably missed by this isolation strategy.

2.2. Positive versus negative selection-based CTC isolation

2.2.1. Positive selection methods

Positive selection strategy is the most commonly used method of CTC isolation in the literature. CellSearch™ is the most evidenced and the only one device having class III approval from US FDA since 2004; therefore, hundreds of clinical trials chose to apply the device for CTC testing for validation [114, 193–204], mainly in patients with breast, colorectal, and prostate cancer. Other representative positive selection platforms are magnetic-activated cell sorting system (MACS) and Isoflux. The main process of positive selection is to label targets cells by anti-CK (AE1/AE3) antibody with ferric beads and immunofluorescence dye. The approximate sensitivity of detection is 10^{-7} (CTCs/hematologic cells). Another system, MACS used 50–100 nm-sized ferric beads. However, lower sensitivity and lower recovery rate of CTCs were observed. The device was firstly introduced in 1998 [205] and then CTCs obtained by the system could correlated with breast cancer stages [206] and could correlate with progression-free survival in colorectal cancer patients [207]. These systems are all based on immunomagnetic beads technology for CTC isolation and have long been limited by relatively low efficiency of antibody conjugation due to tumor heterogeneity [192]. This limitation further causes the difficulty of molecular analysis [208]. Fortunately, the technique of single CTC isolation and analysis has been much more mature in recent years [166, 209, 210]. However, fewer sampling (CTCs) could greatly contribute to the bias for prediction of target population behavior (the whole tumors in the body). Another downside of positive selection strategy was the limitation of EpCAM-dependent nature. Hyun et al. [124] demonstrated that EMT-induced breast cancer cells maintained in prolonged mammosphere culture conditions possess increased EMT markers and cancer stem cell markers, as well as reduced cell mass and size by quantitative phase microscopy. In addition, EpCAM expression is dramatically decreased in these cells. Moreover, CTCs isolated from breast cancer patients using a label-free microfluidic flow fractionation device had differing expression patterns of EpCAM, indicating that affinity approaches reliant on EpCAM expression may underestimate CTC number and potentially miss critical subpopulations.

In addition to conventional immunomagnetic bead separation methods, density separation and flow cytometry or cell sorting systems have been postulated to be potential tools of CTC isolation and identification considering their high sensitivity and purity since 1998 [27]. This method could be seen as a combination of negative selection strategy and a positive confirmation with surface markers, such as EpCAM or cytokeratins. Later in 2011, leukapheresis and fluorescence-activated cell sorting (FACS) elutriation were also reported to be effective for large volume blood process for CTC isolation with molecular analysis [211]. Recently, many microscale on-chip sorting systems were developed considering the high purity of isolation for CTC culture or tumor related genetic analysis. In 2014, Kim et al. have postulated an on-chip multi-imaging flow cytometry system to obtain morphometric parameters of cell clusters such as cell number, perimeter, total cross-sectional area, number of nuclei, and size of clusters as "imaging biomarkers," with simultaneous acquisition and analysis of both bright-field and fluorescent images at 200 frames per second [212]. Moreover, laser scanning cytometry is also a novel innovation developed to help identify CTCs [213, 214]. These methods, are mainly based on flow cytometry and sorting techniques, which could possibly yield an extremely high purity of CTCs (more than 80%). However, one of the drawbacks of the cytometric systems is operator-dependent and multiple quality and internal controls are often required when setting a criterion of CTC identification. Another downside of conventional sorting systems is cell damage and decreased viability after sorting process.

Recently, by the advances of nanotechnology, nanoplates [215], nanowires [216], for positively trapping of CTCs are becoming hot devices with theoretically higher sensitive capturing efficiency than conventional ones. These techniques are often developed by biomedical engineers who are good at medicine, biology and engineering; however, the devices seem to be still in proof-on-concept phase. Hopefully, these new devices would facilitate the development of easy hands-on CTC testing and validation in clinical trials in the near future. In brief, positive selection methods hold the greatest clinical application to date.

2.2.2. *Negative selection methods*

Negative selection methods are developed on the basis of the disadvantages of positive selection methods-losing non-EpCAM or CK-expressing CTCs and relatively poor recovery rate. The principle of negative selection strategy is to remove all the cells other than CTCs as its first step. Owing to the sequence of isolation has changed, in the negative depletion processing, the cancer information was preserved as possible, which makes the phenomenon that the number of CTCs isolated by a negative method would generally (but not always) larger than those by a positive one. In addition, by the CD45 depletion procedures, CTCs without expression of epithelial markers could be isolated though further clarification of the clinical significance of these cell populations is required [217]. The nature of the isolation strategy increased the sensitivity, recovery rate of CTCs but decrease the specificity with inevitable "background noises."

In the developing history of the negative selection methods, Naume et al. [29, 218] have proposed to use CD45 (a common antigen of leukocytes) coated beads to remove white blood cells from tumor cells and red blood cells depleted by lysis buffer or density separation processing for CTC isolation. Based on the concepts, Balasubramanian et al. [219] also successfully demonstrated positive staining images for cytokeratin-positive CTC identification after negative selection processes in 32 cancer blood samples. Among all the negative selection systems, one of the representative systems is epithelial immunospot (EPISPOT) [220–224]. By the procedures, CTCs in the blood sample are enriched by anti-CD45 immunomagnetic beads. The isolated CTCs are then cultured in tissue culture plates precoated with antibodies which capture cathepsin D, MUC1, or CK19 protein [225]. After the incubation period, cells are washed out and the released protein spots are detected by the incubation with a fluorochrome-conjugated antibody and counted. Each spot corresponds to one viable CTC. The device focused on the expression of CK19-expressing cells, which were found to be detectable in up to 65 and 70% of colorectal cancer and breast cancer patients, respectively, and correlated with status of metastasis and poor survival in breast cancer [226, 227]. However, a single sample processing in EPISPOT system requires three days for analysis, which prohibits of its clinical use considering the time-consuming problem.

Nevertheless, the background cells in a negatively isolated sample are often mixed with numerous white blood cells and red blood cells if the process is not well-performed, thus prohibit the following molecular analyses. For this disadvantages of conventional negative selection method, a better depletion process for red and white blood cells depletion are warranted. Another device developed by Wu et al. [228], CanPatrol™ CTC enrichment, they reported a recovery rate more than 80%. Interestingly, FISH assay could be successfully performed for ALK gene rearrangement from CTC samples; however, further validation in prospective clinical trials was still required.

Similarly, Lin et al. [229–231] postulated a protocol and a device (PowerMag) to perform red blood cell lysis and immunomagnetic beads conjugation for CD45-positve cells and identify EpCAM-positive cells (defined as CTCs) from the blood samples. The protocol was proven to effectively isolate CTCs from patients with colorectal, head and neck cancer and thyroid cancer. Furthermore, the CTCs isolated by this negative selection method are further proven to be alive and are capable of being cultivated for at least several weeks [229].

2.3. Other methodologies

In addition to pure positive and negative or label-free methods, some investigators proposed their prototypes for CTC isolation. For example, Qin et al. [50] performed CTC isolation by the size and deformability based separation from castrate resistant prostate cancer patients using resettable cell traps. Compared with CellSearch™, the method could capture more than 10 times of CTCs for subsequent analyses. Basically, it is a label-free method and could be rapidly processed.

Synchrotron X-ray microimaging techniques, high-resolution images of individual flowing tumor cells, and nanotechnology were also proposed to help identification of CTCs. Positively charged gold nanoparticles (AuNPs) which were inappropriate for incorporation into human red blood cells were selectively incorporated into tumor cells to enhance the image contrast, which was reported by Jung et al. [232]. This new technology for in vivo imaging of CTCs would contribute to improve cancer diagnosis and cancer therapy prognosis. Moreover, new chemical materials using a refined carbon-coated pure iron-based immunomagnetic nanoparticle-enriched assay, and nested-RT-PCR was also reported to successfully isolate CTCs efficiently.

Furthermore, not only for general population of CTCs, Hosseini et al. [233] postulated an integrated nano-electromechanical chip (NELMEC) to isolate CTCs and CTCs with EMT features from white blood cells. These new technologies hold great promising on automation, which might greatly ameliorate current problems in CTC field.

2.3.1. Comparison of different strategies

In comparison between positive selection strategy and negative selection methods, the former is most commonly used CTC isolation platform and widely validated by prospective clinical trials. Several articles of meta-analysis confirmed the clinical impacts of CTCs obtained by CellSearch™ [107, 234–237]. However, it is relatively costly and device-dependent. Interestingly, some investigators compared the ISET and CellSearch™ systems for their performance on CTC isolation [76, 93] and one team concluded that a combination of ISET plus CellSearch™ would have better performance in CTC detection in NCSCL patients than ISET or CellSearch™ alone [93]. That intriguing conclusion supports the combination method in the following eras; however, a long processing time of combined platforms also causes cell damage or loss which is a problem the combined systems should be noticed.

In comparison between positive selection method and label-free strategy, Konigsberg et al. [238] compared the efficiency of CTC isolation of MACS (positive selection system) with

http://dx.doi.org/10.5772/64812

OncoQuick (label-free system) and found EpCAM-negative CTCs cannot be detected by EpCAM-dependent enrichment methods. EpCAM-independent enrichment technologies seem to be superior to detect the entire CTC population.

Enrichment strategy	System	Detection markers	Pros	Cons
Positive selection	CellSearch	EpCAM, CKs, CD45, DAPI	FDA cleared; reliable; reproducible; visual identification; clinical relevance in metastatic breast, colorectal and prostate cancer; semi-automated processing; capable of detecting smaller CTCs; standardized kits	EpCAM-positivity dependent, expensive; cells losing EpCAM could not be detected; limited number of markers
	CTC chip	EpCAM, CKs, CD45, DAPI	High detection rate; visual identification	EpCAM-positivity dependent, cells losing EpCAM could not be detected; require clinical trial validation
	Ariol system	EpCAM, CKs, CD45, DAPI	High detection rate (versus CellSearch)	EpCAM-positivity dependent
	Laser-scanning cytometer		Automated microscopic procedure; high detection rate	EpCAM-positivity dependent
	Adna test	EpCAM, MUC1, mucin-1, HER2	High sensitivity; rapid processing	No morphology confirmation; EpCAM and MUC1-positivity dependent
Negative selection	EPISPOT assay	CD45, CK19, mucin-1, cathepsin-D	Can detect viable CTCs	Lack of enough clinical trials for validation
	PowerMag	CD45 depletion for 4 repeated times, EpCAM, Hoechst	Clinically validated in several cancer types; viable CTCs	Background noise, subjective judgment of CTCs, labor-intensive; limited markers can be used for a sample
	Negative + flow cytometry, FACS	CD45, EpCAM, CKs, CD133, CD44, Syto62	High sensitivity for multiple markers, high purity of isolation	Controls, cell aggregations, laser compensation, operator-dependent
Label-free (size)	CTC-filtering devices;	Size, CKs, Her2/neu, ALDH1, CD44, CD24	Rapid processing; multiplexed imaging and genetic analysis	Limited by size of CTCs variation
	ISET	Size, CKs, EGFR, VE-cadherin, ki67	Rapid processing; non-antigen dependent; able to isolate CTM; cell illustrated by IHC staining, able to	Size-dependent (may miss cells less than 8 μm); require more clinical validation trials; manual processing

Enrichment strategy	System	Detection markers	Pros	Cons
			perform FISH, DNA/RNA analysis	
	DEP force	Size, surface electricity, viability	Rapid processing, can isolate single cell very precisely	Low throughput; time-consuming
	ODEP force	Size, surface electricity, viability	Rapid processing, can isolate single cell very precisely; can differ viable from dead cells	Relatively low throughput
	Tracheal carina-inspired bifurcated (TRAB) microfilter system	Size	High recovery rate, acceptable purity; viable isolation	Require clinical trial validation
Label-free (gradient)	Ficoll + RT-PCR	CK-19, HER2, h-MAM, CEA, maspin, GABA A, B726P	High sensitivity	No morphology confirmation; not really capture CTCs
	Ficoll + RT -qPCR	CK-19, BST1, PTPRC	High sensitivity; quantification	No morphology confirmation; not really capture CTCs
	OncoQuick	CCNE2, DKFZp762E1312, EMP2	High sensitivity; quantification	No morphology confirmation; not really capture CTCs
		MAL2, PPIC and SLC6A8, hMAM, and EpCAM	High sensitivity; quantification	No morphology confirmation; not really capture CTCs

Table 1. Overview of analytical methodologies for the detection and molecular characterization of CTCs.

Another report addressed the differences between positive and label-free method was reported by Qin et al. [50]. They designed a micropore filtration platform (using resettable cell traps) to perform CTC isolation by the characteristic of CTCs (size and deformability) from patients with castrate resistant prostate cancer. Compared with CellSearch™, the method could capture CTCs 10 times more than CellSearch™ can achieve. The method was also proven to be able to perform subsequent molecular analyses.

Interestingly, some investigators compared the isolation efficiency of ISET and CellSearch™ systems [76, 93] and one team concluded that a combination of ISET plus CellSearch™ would have better performance in CTC detection in NCSCL patients than ISET or CellSearch™ alone [93].

One question which is often and needed to be asked is that how to choose a best platform for upcoming studies and trials. Before answering the question, the readers/investigators should fully understand the differences, pros and cons among these methods. Then you should choose a platform wisely according to future directions of investigations (i.e., clinical trial, CTC culture, patient-derived xerograft model from CTCs) (i.e., genetic analysis, single cell, physical properties) and the requirements of the study materials (i.e., cells with high purity, with high cell numbers, viability, expression with specific marker, etc.). **Table 1** demonstrated the brief comparison among novel platforms. In our opinion, for genetic analysis and future personalized medicine, we need a large number of CTCs captured for cultivate, whole genome or transcriptome sequencing and avoid sampling errors by hyper-selection of few cells to represent the whole populations of cancer. Therefore, negative selection as first step is currently most suitable strategy among all the methods.

3. The main elements in negative selection plus microfluidic CTCs isolation

3.1. Immunomagnetic beads-based methods

The method is in fact derived from conventional cytological diagnostics for bone marrow and hematologic malignancies. However, when investigators attempted to apply this method to CTC filed, they faced a big problem—the CTCs were so rare to identify in thousands of blood smear slides. Therefore, an alternative method was to exam samples after series of centrifugation, density separation (i.e., in buffy coat or peripheral blood mononuclear cells, PBMC layer), and red blood cells removal. The vast majority of the following detection techniques of CTCs in these prepared samples has long been based on sensitive immunocytochemical (ICC) analysis using antibodies against different epithelial antigens [29, 31, 239–242]. Whether positive selection or negative selection procedures using immunomagnetic beads before ICC analysis are both helpful and critical for efficient CTC identification [29, 31]. Zigeuner et al. [31] found that immunomagnetic cell enrichment significantly improves the sensitivity of detection of CTCs cells added to mononuclear cells compared to immunocytochemistry method.

Although the exact procedures of immunomagnetic beads separation protocol was variable with the beads and antibiotics but they have general principles and we would take the procedures of Dynabeads as an example (modified from Naume et al.'s work in 1997 [29]). The main procedures are preparation of beads, incubation with samples and beads, using a magnetic field or column (depends on chosen systems) for target cells isolation by washing out other cells which did not conjugated with beads. If the target cells are those we do not want to analyze, the procedure is defined to be a negative selection. Conversely, if the cells are the targets in the study, it is a positive selection.

3.1.1. Preparation of the magnetic beads

Rat antimouse (RAM) IgGl-coated M280 Dynabeads coupled to BerEP4 mAb (Product No. 112.07), M450 Dynabeads coated with an anti-CD45 mAb that recognizes all isoforms of CD45 (Product No. 111.19), and Neodynium Magnetic Particle Concentrators were sup plied by Dynal (Oslo, Norway). Coating of the M280 Dynabeads with antiepithelial mAb was performed according to the manufacturer's instructions. Briefly, the RAM M280 Dynabeads were incubated with either BerEP4, 9189, or MOC31 mAbs at a concentration of 1/u.g/107 beads for 30 min at 4°C under gentle rotation, followed by three magnet washes in PBS/0.1% HSA and then stored at 4°C. Before use, the Dynabeads were washed once with separation medium.

3.1.2. Positive immunomagnetic separation technique

A total of 1 × 10^7 peripheral blood mononuclear cells (PBMNC) were resuspended in cold separation medium to a concentration of 2 ×10^7 MNC/ml (0.5 ml volume) and incubated with RAM IgGl M280 Dynabeads coated with either BerEP4 317G5, or MOC31 mAb. The bead concentration varied from 2.5 to 40 × 10^6 b/ml, as described in individual experiments. The bead/cell suspension was incubated under gentle rotation for 30 min at 4°C. The sample was then diluted to 3 ml and placed against a magnet for 7 min to recover the rosetted cells, followed by two additional washes as follows. The supernatant was removed, and the rosetted cells were resuspended in 3 ml separation medium, followed by treatment with the magnet (7 min). To facilitate ICC TC detection, the positive LMS product was finally resuspended to contain 5–7 × 10^6 beads/ml, and 0.5 ml aliquots were centrifuged onto each cytospin slide for further immunocytochemical analysis.

3.1.3. Negative immunomagnetic separation technique

A total of 1 × 10^7 peripheral blood mononuclear cells (PBMNC) were resuspended in cold separation medium to a concentration of 2 × 10^7 MNC/ml (0.5 ml volume) and incubated with anti-CD45-conjugated M450 Dynabeads at a bead/cell ratio of 2.5:1, 5:1, or 10:1. The bead/cell suspension was incubated under gentle rotation for 45 min. The solution was then diluted to about 30 ml, and the magnet was applied for 5 min, with initial rotation of the tubes onto the magnet to reduce trapping of tumor cells. The supernatant was collected and centrifuged at 450*g* for 10 min, counted, and resuspended in 10% FBS in PBS to 1 × 10^6 cells/ml. Then, cytospins containing 5 × 10^5 cells were prepared. All the slides were air-dried overnight and stained by immunocytochemistry.

3.2. Microfluidic-based methods for the high purity CTC isolation

In novel era of huge advances of microfluidic devices as mentioned in the section of "Label-free isolation strategy" [45, 46, 56, 60, 173–186]. In fact, the vast majority of microfluidic devices were designed based on EpCAM- or CK-identifying mechanism, which is positive selection method. The CTC-Chip [25, 243], and the herringbone chip [244, 245] have been proven effective to isolate CTCs with both high CTC purity (50–62%) [25, 245] and high recovery rate (90–95%) [244, 245]. There are several microfluidic devices designed to use positive selection strategy for proof-of-concept purpose [34, 57, 59, 124, 184, 210, 246–269] and for specific cancer in clinical trials, (e.g., breast [270, 271], pancreas [272, 273], ovarian [274], prostate [275], esophageal cancer [270], gastric [271], colorectal cancer [276], cancer of unknown primary [277]) and for mutational analysis [278]. Moreover, combined preparation using positive, negative, or label-free selection methods with microfluidic devices for better performance is also feasible and have been reported [93].

However, there are several drawbacks or limitations of microfluidic devices reported [267]. First of all, reports in literature, however, have revealed that EpCAM or CKs are not expressed in all cancer cells (e.g., sarcoma, melanoma, or CTCs bearing EMT), and therefore some kinds of CTCs cannot be targeted via the positive selection-based microfluidic device [279]. Secondly, several microfluidic chips could identify with microtubes or micropoles with or without EpCAM conjugation. It seems to be difficult to release captured CTCs from the chips. The efficiency of identification will not be equal to recovered cells for further molecular or genetic analysis. Thirdly, almost more than 80% of microfluidic devices are still in proof-of-concepts phase and comes from a single team or laboratory. It might be because that the advances of new innovation always come up faster than validation reports. However, we do need well-designed and well-conducted prospective clinical studies to critically elucidate the clinical impacts of the microfluidic devices. The investigators could consider to learn from the developing history of CellSearch™ system.

3.3. Perspective for future of CTC technology: combinations of several methods

Our perspectives for future CTC isolation is mainly combined methodologies instead of conventional ones based on a single isolation strategy.

Yamamoto et al. [49] displayed a combination of size-based filtration plus a magnetic column method for CTC isolation. The combined use of the column and filter decreased the required time for the spiked cancer cell capture, and the recovery rate of the spiked cancer cells from blood was significantly higher using the combination process (80.7%) than that using the filter alone (64.7%). Moreover, the recovered CTCs are more abundant by the combination process. Another combination was ISET and CellSearch™ systems [76, 93] and the combination had better performance in CTC detection in non-small cell lung cancer (NCSCL) patients than ISET or CellSearch™ alone [93]. Furthermore, density separation plus flow cytometry or cell sorting systems have been postulated to be potential tools of CTC isolation and identification considering their high sensitivity and purity since 1998 [27]. This method could be seen as a combination of negative selection strategy and a positive confirmation with surface markers, such as EpCAM or cytokeratins. Later in 2011, leukapheresis plus fluorescence-activated cell sorting (FACS) elutriation were also reported to be effective for large volume blood process for CTC isolation with molecular analysis [211]. These studies illustrated the possibility and better efficacy the combination can achieve, therefore, in our opinion, to find a suitable combination of CTC isolation protocols considering the balance of efficiency, time, sample and costs is very important in the future CTC field.

Intriguingly, several liquid biopsies, as aforementioned, could be combined to be tested in a single sample and at the same time. To realize the goals and minimize the blood sample required, Chudziak et al. [248] reported a novel device, Parsortix system, could negatively select CTCs and perform cfDNA analysis simultaneously. The system recovered more CTCs than CellSearch™ system in the comparison.

4. The applications of CTC testing in clinical cancer researches

As aforementioned, CTC testing are designed to help the diagnosis, early detection and monitoring for response and disease status of cancer patients. Clinical trials to evaluate and validate are inevitable during the developing of any CTC testing. Here, we introduce several important clinical validated studies for the clinical impacts of CTC testing in different cancer types.

4.1. Breast cancer

One meta-analysis reported by Liao et al. [107], 14 studies with 2336 patients were enrolled and found that presence of CTCs in peripheral blood was significantly associated with the size of tumor [OR 0.68, 95% confidence interval (CI) (0.54, 0.87), $P = 0.002$], tumor grade [OR 0.71, 95% CI (0.55, 0.91), $P = 0.006$], estrogen receptor (ER) status [OR 0.72, 95% CI (0.57, 0.91), $P = 0.007$], and progesterone receptor (PR) of tumor status [OR 0.78, 95% CI (0.61, 0.98), $P = 0.04$]. In addition, the presence of CTCs is highly correlated with tumor size, tumor grade, ER, and PR status in patients with breast cancer. Although the analysis did not consider the method of isolation which might be one of the downsides and biases of the analysis, the results suggested a trend of physical (tumor size), functional (tumor grade) and status of drugable targets (ER, PR status), which are very useful clinically.

In Zhao et al. [234] performed a meta-analysis collecting 24 trials with 4013 breast cancer patients and 1333 controls. Poor overall survival was found to be associated with the positive CTC detection (HR = 3.00 [95% CI 2.29–3.94], $P < 0.0001$) and recurrence-free survival as well (HR = 2.67 [95% CI 2.09–3.42], $P < 0.0001$). CTC-positive breast cancers were significantly associated with high histological grade (HR = 1.21 [95% CI 1.09–1.35], $P < 0.0001$), tumor size (>2 cm) (HR = 1.12 [95% CI 1.02–1.22], $P = 0.01$), and nodal status (≥1) (HR = 1.10 [95% CI 1.00–1.21], $P = 0.037$). The studies, different to that of Liao et al. [107], mentioned about prognostic values of CTC testing. However, the two reports did not mention about the isolation methods and might neglect the biases from CTC number is highly correlated to the method of isolation.

For the purpose of technical standardization, Janni et al. [235] conducted a pooled analysis of individual data from 3173 patients with nonmetastatic (stages I–III) breast cancer from five breast cancer institutions. The prevalence and numbers of CTCs were assessed at the time of primary diagnosis with the FDA-cleared CellSearch System. Results confirmed that ≥1 CTC(s) were detected in 20.2% of the patients and CTC-positive patients had larger tumors, increased lymph node involvement, and a higher histologic tumor grade than did CTC-negative patients (all $P < 0.002$). Multivariate Cox regressions confirmed that the presence of CTCs was an independent prognostic factor for disease-free survival [HR, 1.82; 95% confidence interval (CI), 1.47–2.26], distant disease-free survival (HR, 1.89; 95% CI, 1.49–2.40), breast cancer-specific survival (HR, 2.04; 95% CI, 1.52–2.75), and overall survival (HR, 1.97; 95% CI, 1.51–2.59). The study addressed the clinical impacts of CellSearch™ system in breast cancer patients and it has confirmed the positive results from a large pooled database.

For a subset in breast cancers, Rack et al. [91] addressed the role of CTCs isolated by CellSearch™ in a prospective trial enrolling 2026 early average-to-high risk breast cancer patients and found an independent prognostic relevance of CTCs both before and after adjuvant chemotherapy. The study successfully proved the prognostic role of CTCs in adjuvant settings. The next direction of future studies should be designed to answer the question that whether if extended adjuvant therapy is needed and whether if the extended therapy did reduce the risk of recurrence or not.

For the role of CTCs in a novel and specific therapy in breast cancer, Paoletti et al. [280] reported that heterogeneous mechanisms of resistance to fulvestrant, including estrogen receptor alpha gene (ESR1) mutation. CTC enumeration, phenotyping, and genotyping might identify patients who would benefit from fulvestrant dose escalation versus switching to alternative therapies. The CTCs could possibly help find the resistance genes during the therapy and warn the clinicians to change therapy in time before the tumor already gets progression.

In triple negative breast cancer (TNBC) who lacks of drugable targets (hormone therapy) in breast cancer, Hall et al. (2015) enrolled 44 TNBC patients using CellSearch™ for CTC testing and found that ≥1 CTC in each sample was identified in 30% of patients completing neoadjuvant chemotherapy (NACT). Multivariate analysis demonstrated that detection of ≥1 CTC predicted decreased RFS (log-rank $P = 0.03$, HR 5.25, 95% CI 1.34–20.56) and OS (log-rank $P = 0.03$, HR 7.04, 95% CI 1.26–39.35). The results suggested a modification of clinical management for TNBC patients with positive CTC detection after NACT, including extension of NACT or adding another anti-cancer therapy before tumor recurs.

4.2. Lung cancer

In a meta-analysis reported in 2013, pooled results from a total of 20 studies, comprising 1576 nonsmall cell lung cancer (NSCLC) patients showed that CTCs were associated with lymph node metastasis (OR = 2.06; 95% CI: 1.18–3.62; $Z = 2.20$; $P = 0.027$) and tumor stage (OR = 1.95; 95% CI: 1.08–3.54; $Z = 2.53$; $P = 0.011$). CTCs were significantly associated with shorter overall survival (relative risk [RR] = 2.19; 95% CI: 1.53–3.12; $Z = 4.32$; $P < 0.0001$) and progression-free/disease-free survival (RR = 2.14; 95% CI: 1.36–3.38; $Z = 3.28$; $P < 0.0001$) [281]. Another study reported the ability to recurrence prediction after curative surgery is positive [282].

For small cell lung cancer, a relatively aggressive subtype with poor prognosis population, a total of seven papers covering 440 SCLC patients were combined in the final analysis. The meta-analysis revealed that CTCs were significantly associated with shorter overall survival (HR = 1.9; 95% CI: 1.19–3.04; $Z = 2.67$; $P < 0.0001$) and progression-free survival (HR = 2.6; 95% CI: 1.9–3.54; $Z = 6.04$; $P < 0.0001$) [283].

Interestingly, in a molecular era nowadays, cancer therapy often relies on genetic or molecular information from cancer tissues, CTCs as well. Das et al. [105] checked the status of ERCC1 expression on captured and found that low expression of ERCC1 on CTCs correlates with progression-free survival (PFS) in patients with metastatic NSCLC receiving platinum-based therapy. ERCC1 expression was conventionally checked on NSCLC cancer tissue to predict the response to platinum therapy, which has been the first line standard chemotherapy in patients without active EGFR mutation responding to tyrosine kinase inhibitors (TKIs). The impacts of the study suggested that analysis of ERCC1 expression on CTCs in lung cancer patients could predict the chemotherapy responses. It is a predictive role could possible direct therapy in the future if the findings were confirmed in another large-scale phase III clinical trials. In addition. Yanagita et al. [284] evaluated CTCs and cfDNA in EGFR-mutant NSCLC patients treated with erlotinib until progression. Among the enrolled 60 patients, rebiopsy was performed in 35/44 patients (80%), with paired CTC/cfDNA analysis in 41/44 samples at baseline and 36/44 samples at progression. T790M was identified in 23/35 (66%) of tissue biopsies and 9/39 (23%) of cfDNA samples. At diagnosis, high levels of cfDNA but not high levels of CTCs correlated with progression-free survival. Therefore, cfDNA and CTCs are complementary, noninvasive assays for evaluation of acquired resistance to first-line EGFR TKIs. Recently, *ALK* rearrangement on CTCs are successfully performed and compared with cancer tissues [51, 285]. Chromosome instability and *ROS-1* rearrangement on CTCs were also proved to be successful [51]. Immune cells analysis, tumor-associated macrophages (TAMs) accompanied with CTCs analysis were also proven to be possible and CTCs are competent to specifically manipulate TAMs to increase cancer invasiveness, angiogenesis, immunosuppression and possibly lipid catabolism in lung cancer patients [286]. These studies pointed to the driven mutation detection and would directly benefit to NSCLC patients under targeted therapies.

4.3. Gastrointestinal tract cancer

In 2014, a meta-analysis comprised 26 studies with peripheral blood samples of 1950 cases for final analysis. The pooled results showed that gastric cancer (GC) patients with detectable CTCs (including circulating miRNAs) had a tendency to experience shortened RFS (HR = 2.91, 95% CI [1.84–4.61], I2 = 52.18%). As for patient deaths, we found a similar association of CTC (including circulating miRNAs) presence with worse OS (HR = 1.78, 95% CI [1.49–2.12], I2 = 30.71%, $n = 30$). Additionally, subgroup analyses indicated strong prognostic powers of CTCs, irrespective of geographical, methodological, detection time and sample size differences of the studies [287]. In addition, the role of EMT status on CTCs correlates with poor treatment outcomes was also revealed. CTCs expressing CD44 were also found to be prognostic and indicated to malignant behaviors of gastric cancer [288].

For pancreatic cancer, a prospective study addressing the role of CTCs, CTMs in 63 pancreatic ductal adenocarcinoma (PDAC) patients before treatment using anti-EpCAM (epithelial cell adhesion molecule)-conjugated supported lipid bilayer-coated microfluidic chips. CTM was an independent prognostic factor of overall survival (OS) and progression free survival (PFS). Patients were stratified into unfavorable and favorable CTM groups on the basis of CTM more or less than 30 per 2 ml blood, respectively. Patients with baseline unfavorable CTM, compared with patients with favorable CTM, had shorter PFS (2.7 versus 12.1 months; $P < 0.0001$) and OS (6.4 versus 19.8 months; $P < 0.0001$). Differences persisted if we stratified patients into early and advanced diseases. The number of CTM before treatment was an independent predictor of PFS and OS after adjustment for clinically significant factors. Therefore, in conclusion, the number of CTM, instead of CTCs, before treatment is an independent predictor of PFS and OS in patients with PDAC [272].

In molecular analysis to predict treatment response, Abdallah et al. [152] found that thymidylate synthase expression in circulating tumor cells can be useful tool as a 5-FU resistance predictor biomarker in patients with colorectal cancer while other studies elucidate the prognostic and predictive roles of CTCs [198, 289–291]. Recently, *KRAS* and *BRAF* were successfully detected on CTCs by high-resolution melt (HRM) and allele-specific PCR (ASPCR) and *KRAS*-codon 12/13- and *BRAF*-codon 600-specific assays. Comparing tumor tissues and CTCs mutation status using HRM, Mohamed Suhaimi et al. [292] reported that a 84.1% concordance in KRAS genotype (P = 0.000129) and a 90.9% (P = 0.174) concordance in BRAF genotype. Another report utilized ISET system plus PCR for KRAS codons 12 and 13 mutation with a 71% concordance between cancer tissue and CTCs from colorectal cancer patients [293]. In gastrointestinal stroma tumor, Li et al. [294] conducted a trial to elucidate the role of CTCs expressing ANO1(DOG1) in GIST. ANO1s were more frequently detected in unresectable patients. Tumor size, mitotic count, and risk level were associated with ANO1 detection in resectable GIST patients. The presence of ANO1 significantly correlated with poor disease-free survival (15.3 versus 19.6 months, P = 0.038). Most patients turned ANO1-negative after surgery and inversely, all 21 patients with recurrence turned ANO1-positive with high ANO1 expression levels. Moreover, in the neoadjuvant setting, decline of ANO1 expression level correlated with the response of imatinib. In the near future, these results would possibly promote the genetic analysis on mutation-driven cancer therapies although they have not become routine screen tools in CRC patients to date.

4.4. Head and neck cancer

Grobe et al. [92] used CellSearch™ for CTC isolation in 80 oral cavity cancer patients and found that 12.5% patients harbored CTCs in peripheral blood, whereas in 20.0% patients DTCs in bone marrow could be detected. Significant correlations could be found for CTCs and tumor size (P = 0.04), nodal status and DTCs (P = 0.02), and distant metastasis with CTCs (P = 0.004) and DTCs (P = 0.005). Univariate and multivariate analyses revealed that CTCs and DTCs were significant and independent predictors of recurrence-free survival (P < 0.001) as well as in other findings in HNSCC, including the ability of prediction 6-month death [231]. In 2015, Oliveira-Costa et al. reported that immunohistochemistry was performed in cancer tissues and in CTCs by immunofluorescence and Nanostring. Correlation was shown between PD-L1 and tumor size and lymph node metastasis, HOXB9 and tumor size, BLNK and perineural invasion, and between ZNF813 and perineural invasion. PD-L1 positivity was an independent prognostic factor in this cohort (P = 0.044, HH = 0.426) in OSCC patients [295]. The results could possibly apply to current immune-oncology studies.

Wu et al. [296] reported a meta-analysis conducted a computerized retrieval of literatures. Twenty-two retrieved studies were eligible for systematic review, of which nine conformed for the diagnostic test meta-analysis and five for the prognostic analysis. Subgroup analysis showed 24.6% pooled sensitivity and 100% pooled specificity of detections by using positive selection strategy, which moreover presented low heterogeneity. The presence of CTC was significantly associated with shorter disease free survival (DFS, HR 4.62, 95% CI 2.51–8.52). The presence of CTC indicates a worse DFS.

4.5. Liver cancer

Early in 2004, Vona et al. have reported that the presence ($P = 0.01$) and number ($P = 0.02$) of CTCs and microemboli (CTMs) were significantly associated with a shorter survival [161]. Fan et al. [297] reported a meta-analysis consisting of 23 trials and found that CTC positivity was significantly associated with RFS (HR 3.03, 95% CI: [1.89–4.86]; $P < 0.00001$) and overall survival (OS) (HR 2.45, 95% CI: [1.73–3.48]; $P < 0.00001$). CTC positivity were also significantly associated with TNM Stage (RR 1.30, 95% CI: [1.02–1.65]; $P = 0.03$), Tumor size (RR 1.36, 95% CI: [1.09–1.69]; $P = 0.006$), Vascular invasion (RR 1.99, 95% CI: [1.43–2.77]; $P < 0.0001$), Portal vein tumor thrombus (RR 1.73, 95% CI: [1.42–2.11]; $P = 0.0001$), Serum alpha-fetoprotein (AFP) level (RR 2.05; $P = 0.01$) [297]. Sun et al. found that Stem cell-like phenotypes are observed in EpCAM $^+$ CTCs, and a preoperative CTCs of ≥2 is a novel predictor for tumor recurrence in hepatocellular carcinoma (HCC) patients after surgery, especially in patient subgroups with AFP levels of ≤400 ng/ml or low tumor recurrence risk. EpCAM+ CTCs could serve as a real-time parameter for monitoring treatment response and a therapeutic target in HCC recurrence [137]. The prognostic value of overall survival of CTCs in HCC patients has been also revealed [298].

4.6. Genitourinary tract cancer

Rink et al. (2012) found that using CellSearch™, CTC were detected in 23 of 100 patients (23%) with nonmetastatic urothelial carcinoma of urinary bladder. CTC-positive patients had significantly higher risks of disease recurrence and cancer-specific and overall mortality (P values ≤ 0.001). After adjusting for effects of standard clinicopathologic features, CTC positivity remained an independent predictor for all end points (hazard ratios: 4.6, 5.2, and 3.5, respectively; P values ≤ 0.003). HER2 positivity was found in 3 of 22 patients (14%). There was concordance between CTC, primary tumors, and lymph node metastases in all CTC-positive cases (100%).

4.7. Skin cancer and melanoma

Conventionally, melanoma cells lack of cytokeratin or EpCAM expression and CTCs by definition are very difficult to identify. However, investigators broke through the strait by combination with CTCs plus cfDNA. Salvianti et al. [299] enrolled 84 melanoma patients and 68 healthy controls for CTC and cell-free DNA (cfDNA) testing to assess the diagnostic performance of a tumor-related methylated cfDNA marker in melanoma patients and to compare this parameter with the presence of CTCs. The percentage of cases with methylated RASSF1A promoter in cfDNA was significantly higher in each class of melanoma patients (in situ, invasive and metastatic) than in healthy subjects ($P < 0.001$). The concentration of RASSF1A methylated cfDNA in the subjects with a detectable quantity of methylated alleles was significantly higher in melanoma patients than in controls. When the CTCs plus RASSF1A cfDNA are jointly considered, a higher sensitivity of the detection of positive cases in invasive and metastatic melanomas could be obtained. A similar finding was obtained to suggest combine cfDNA (GNAQ/GNA11 mutations) and CTCs to identify uveal melanoma patients with poor prognosis [300]. In another reports, a phase III trial of adjuvant immunotherapy after complete resection of stage IV melanoma, quantitative real-time reverse-transcriptase polymerase chain reaction (qPCR) for expression of CTC-specific MART-1, MAGE-A3, and PAX3 mRNA biomarkers were found to be not associated with known prognostic factors or treatment arm. In multivariate analysis, pretreatment CTC (>0 versus 0 biomarker) status was significantly associated with disease-free survival (DFS; HR 1.64, $P = 0.002$) and overall survival (OS; HR 1.53, $P = 0.028$). Serial CTC (>0 versus 0 biomarker) status was also significantly associated with DFS (HR 1.91, $P = 0.02$) and OS (HR 2.57, $P = 0.012$) [301]. The report suggested CTCT could be a new risk factor other than any conventional known factors, which might change the staging systems if the evidence gets solid and validated.

4.8. Other cancers

For ovarian cancer, Romero-Laorden et al. [302] performed a meta-analysis enrolling 14 studies. Results showed the presence of CTCs and DTCs is associated with adverse clinicopathological characteristics and poor clinical outcomes in ovarian cancer patients. They noticed that different CTC number obtained by different devices could not be compared. Using size-based isolation strategy (MetaCell®) in 118 ovarian cancer patients, CTCs might have add-on values on current staging system and the cells could be cultivated after isolation [303, 304]. Furthermore, in another meta-analysis, eight studies of 1184 ovarian cancer patients were included in the final analysis. In the PB group, it showed that patients with positive CTCs had significantly shorter overall survival (OS) and disease-free survival (DFS) than patients with negative CTCs (HR, 2.09; CI, 1.13–3.88 and HR, 1.72; CI, 1.32–2.25, respectively). The same result was shown with DTCs in the BM group (HR, 1.61; CI, 1.27–2.04 and HR, 1.44; CI, 1.15–1.80, respectively) [305].

For carcinoma of unknown primary (CUP), Matthew et al. [306] used a real-time, single-cell multiplex immunophenotyping of CTCs to inform diagnosis of tissue of origin in CUP patients. CellSearch™ plus multiplexed Q-dot or DyLight conjugated antibodies were used for cytokeratin 7 (CK7), cytokeratin 20 (CK20), thyroid transcription factor 1 (TTF-1), estrogen receptor (ER), or prostate-specific antigen (PSA) expression. The feasibility of staining multiple markers in CTCs presented in this work suggested CTCs could possibly have a non-inferior role as that of cancer tissues in diagnostics.

5. Unanswered questions in the field of CTCs, technically and clinically

The unanswered question is that the optimal protocol or device has not been found or validated. Many investigators have clearly realized that the number of CTCs cannot easily compare with that counted by another system, but some are not. Recently, Fina et al. [307] compared two CTC isolation methods in a clinical trial. AdnaTest EMT-1/ and EMT-2/Stem CellSelect/Detect kits, and ScreenCell Cyto devices were both performed for all samples.

Higher CTC detection rates were obtained with the AdnaTest approach when using for CTC-enrichment antibodies against ERBB2 and EGFR in addition to MUC1 and the classical epithelial surface marker EPCAM (13% versus 48%). When the physical properties of tumor cells were exploited, CTCs were detected at higher percentages than with positive-selection-based methods. The results supported that different approaches for CTC detection probably identify distinct tumor cell subpopulations. Technical standardization before clinical validity would be the most urgent issue we have to solve.

6. Concluding remarks

We suggest the investigators to combine different isolation methods to achieve the most optimal performance of CTC isolation and clinical trials for solid validation. The cooperation among medical oncologists and biomedical engineers are critically important for the future advances in CTC field. Genetic or molecular analysis, such as PCR for epigenetics or mutation of specific gene(s) or next-generation sequencing for whole genome, whole exon, or chosen targeted genes will be the major directions for personalized cancer therapies. The advances of microfluidic devices will quickly solve the conventional problems of time-consuming, sample-consuming, operator-dependent, and marker-dependent limitations.

Author details

Jason Chia-Hsun Hsieh[1*] and Tyler Ming-Hsien Wu[1,2,3]

*Address all correspondence to: wisdom5000@gmail.com

1 Circulating Tumor Cells Lab, Division of Hematology-Oncology, Department of Internal Medicine, Chang Gung Memorial Hospital, Linkou, Taiwan and Department of Chemical and Materials Engineering, Chang Gung University, Taoyuan, Taiwan

2 Graduate Institute of Biochemical and Biomedical Engineering, Chang Gung University, Taoyuan, Taiwan

3 Department of Chemical Engineering, Ming Chi University of Technology, New Taipei City, Taiwan

References

[1] G.P. Gupta, J. Massague, Cancer metastasis: building a framework, Cell, 127 (2006) 679–695.

[2] T.R. Ashworth, A case of cancer in which cells similar to those in the tumours were seen in the blood after death, Aust Med J, 14 (1989) 146–147

[3] E. Goldmann, Relation of cancer cells to blood vessels andducts, Lancet, 1 (1906) 23.

[4] R.A. Sellwood, S.W. Kuper, J.I. Burn, E.N. Wallace, Circulating cancer cells, Br Med J, 1 (1964) 1683–1686.

[5] W.R. McCune, E.P. Galleher, C. Wood, Circulating "cancer cells", JAMA, 189 (1964) 852.

[6] S. Roberts, A. Watne, G.R. Mc, G.E. Mc, W.H. Cole, Technique and results of isolation of cancer cells from the circulating blood, AMA Arch Surg, 76 (1958) 334–346.

[7] H. Marcus, Krebszellen im strömenden Blut (Cancerous cells in the circulating blood.), Z Krebsforsch, 16 (1919) 217.

[8] H.C. Engell, Cancer cells in the circulating blood; a clinical study on the occurrence of cancer cells in the peripheral blood and in venous blood draining the tumour area at operation, Acta Chir Scand Suppl, 201 (1955) 1–70.

[9] T.M. Scheinin, A.P. Koivuniemi, Large benign cells in circulating blood and their significance in the identification of cancer cells, Cancer, 15 (1962) 972–977.

[10] S. Roberts, O.L.L. Jonasson, G.R. Mc, G.E. Mc, W.H. Cole, Clinical significance of cancer cells in the circulating blood: two- to five-year survival, Ann Surg, 154 (1961) 362–371.

[11] E.H. Pool, G.R. Dunlop, Cancer cells in the blood stream, Am J Cancer, 21 (1934) 99–102.

[12] S. Warren, O. Gates, The fate of intravenously injected tumor cells, Am J Cancer, 27 (1936) 485–492.

[13] J. Ewing, Neoplastic diseases, 4th ed. Philadelphia: W.B. Saunders, 1940.

[14] O. Saphir, The fate of carcinoma emboli in the lung, Am J Pathol 23 (1947) 245–253.

[15] D. Billadeau, L. Quam, W. Thomas, N. Kay, P. Greipp, R. Kyle, M.M. Oken, B. Van Ness, Detection and quantitation of malignant cells in the peripheral blood of multiple myeloma patients, Blood, 80 (1992) 1818–1824.

[16] K. Pittman, S. Burchill, B. Smith, J. Southgate, J. Joffe, M. Gore, P. Selby, Reverse transcriptase-polymerase chain reaction for expression of tyrosinase to identify malignant melanoma cells in peripheral blood, Ann Oncol, 7 (1996) 297–301.

[17] F.W. Cremer, K. Kiel, C. Sucker, J. Wacker, A. Atzberger, R. Haas, H. Goldschmidt, M. Moos, A rationale for positive selection of peripheral blood stem cells in multiple myeloma: highly purified CD34+ cell fractions of leukapheresis products do not contain malignant cells, Leukemia, 11 (Suppl 5) (1997) S41–S46.

[18] M. Kawakami, T. Okaneya, K. Furihata, O. Nishizawa, T. Katsuyama, Detection of prostate cancer cells circulating in peripheral blood by reverse transcription-PCR for hKLK2, Cancer Res, 57 (1997) 4167–4170.

[19] M. Probst-Kepper, A. Schrader, J. Buer, J. Grosse, M. Volkenandt, H.J. Illiger, B. Metzner, J. Kadar, S. Duensing, B. Hertenstein, A. Ganser, J. Atzpodien, Detection of melanoma cells in peripheral blood stem cell harvests of patients with progressive metastatic malignant melanoma, Br J Haematol, 98 (1997) 488–490.

[20] K. Peck, Y.P. Sher, J.Y. Shih, S.R. Roffler, C.W. Wu, P.C. Yang, Detection and quantitation of circulating cancer cells in the peripheral blood of lung cancer patients, Cancer Res, 58 (1998) 2761–2765.

[21] J.E. Hardingham, D. Kotasek, R.E. Sage, M.C. Eaton, V.H. Pascoe, A. Dobrovic, Detection of circulating tumor cells in colorectal cancer by immunobead-PCR is a sensitive prognostic marker for relapse of disease, Mol Med, 1 (1995) 789–794.

[22] J.E. Hardingham, D. Kotasek, B. Farmer, R.N. Butler, J.X. Mi, R.E. Sage, A. Dobrovic, Immunobead-PCR: a technique for the detection of circulating tumor cells using immunomagnetic beads and the polymerase chain reaction, Cancer Res, 53 (1993) 3455–3458.

[23] I. Leotsakos, P. Dimopoulos, E. Gkioka, P. Msaouel, A. Nezos, K.G. Stravodimos, M. Koutsilieris, C.A. Constantinides, Detection of circulating tumor cells in bladder cancer using multiplex PCR assays, Anticancer Res, 34 (2014) 7415–7424.

[24] W.J. Allard, J. Matera, M.C. Miller, M. Repollet, M.C. Connelly, C. Rao, A.G. Tibbe, J.W. Uhr, L.W. Terstappen, Tumor cells circulate in the peripheral blood of all major carcinomas but not in healthy subjects or patients with nonmalignant diseases, Clin Cancer Res, 10 (2004) 6897–6904.

[25] S. Nagrath, L.V. Sequist, S. Maheswaran, D.W. Bell, D. Irimia, L. Ulkus, M.R. Smith, E.L. Kwak, S. Digumarthy, A. Muzikansky, P. Ryan, U.J. Balis, R.G. Tompkins, D.A. Haber, M. Toner, Isolation of rare circulating tumour cells in cancer patients by microchip technology, Nature, 450 (2007) 1235–1239.

[26] I. Van der Auwera, D. Peeters, I.H. Benoy, H.J. Elst, S.J. Van Laere, A. Prove, H. Maes, P. Huget, P. van Dam, P.B. Vermeulen, L.Y. Dirix, Circulating tumour cell detection: a direct comparison between the CellSearch System, the AdnaTest and CK-19/mammaglobin RT-PCR in patients with metastatic breast cancer, Br J Cancer, 102 (2010) 276–284.

[27] E. Racila, D. Euhus, A.J. Weiss, C. Rao, J. McConnell, L.W. Terstappen, J.W. Uhr, Detection and characterization of carcinoma cells in the blood, Proc Natl Acad Sci USA, 95 (1998) 4589–4594.

[28] A.A. Ross, B.W. Cooper, H.M. Lazarus, W. Mackay, T.J. Moss, N. Ciobanu, M.S. Tallman, M.J. Kennedy, N.E. Davidson, D. Sweet, et al., Detection and viability of tumor

cells in peripheral blood stem cell collections from breast cancer patients using immunocytochemical and clonogenic assay techniques, Blood, 82 (1993) 2605–2610.

[29] B. Naume, E. Borgen, K. Beiske, T.K. Herstad, G. Ravnas, A. Renolen, S. Trachsel, K. Thrane-Steen, S. Funderud, G. Kvalheim, Immunomagnetic techniques for the enrichment and detection of isolated breast carcinoma cells in bone marrow and peripheral blood, J Hematother, 6 (1997) 103–114.

[30] U. Bilkenroth, H. Taubert, D. Riemann, U. Rebmann, H. Heynemann, A. Meye, Detection and enrichment of disseminated renal carcinoma cells from peripheral blood by immunomagnetic cell separation, Int J Cancer, 92 (2001) 577–582.

[31] R.E. Zigeuner, R. Riesenberg, H. Pohla, A. Hofstetter, R. Oberneder, Immunomagnetic cell enrichment detects more disseminated cancer cells than immunocytochemistry in vitro, J Urol, 164 (2000) 1834–1837.

[32] Available at: http://www.fda.gov/MedicalDevices/ProductsandMedicalProcedures/DeviceApprovalsandClearances/Recently-ApprovedDevices/ucm081239.htm. Clearance Date: January 21, 2004 (Approved Evaluation of Automatic Class III Designation).

[33] M. Cristofanilli, Circulating tumor cells, disease progression, and survival in metastatic breast cancer, Semin Oncol, 33 (2006) S9–S14.

[34] J.M. Park, M.S. Kim, H.S. Moon, C.E. Yoo, D. Park, Y.J. Kim, K.Y. Han, J.Y. Lee, J.H. Oh, S.S. Kim, W.Y. Park, W.Y. Lee, N. Huh, Fully automated circulating tumor cell isolation platform with large-volume capacity based on lab-on-a-disc, Anal Chem, 86 (2014) 3735–3742.

[35] P. Gogoi, S. Sepehri, Y. Zhou, M.A. Gorin, C. Paolillo, E. Capoluongo, K. Gleason, A. Payne, B. Boniface, M. Cristofanilli, T.M. Morgan, P. Fortina, K.J. Pienta, K. Handique, Y. Wang, Development of an automated and sensitive microfluidic device for capturing and characterizing circulating tumor cells (CTCs) from clinical blood samples, PLoS One, 11 (2016) e0147400.

[36] C.M. Svensson, R. Hubler, M.T. Figge, Automated classification of circulating tumor cells and the impact of interobsever variability on classifier training and performance, J Immunol Res, 2015 (2015) 573165.

[37] D.E. Campton, A.B. Ramirez, J.J. Nordberg, N. Drovetto, A.C. Clein, P. Varshavskaya, B.H. Friemel, S. Quarre, A. Breman, M. Dorschner, S. Blau, C.A. Blau, D.E. Sabath, J.L. Stilwell, E.P. Kaldjian, High-recovery visual identification and single-cell retrieval of circulating tumor cells for genomic analysis using a dual-technology platform integrated with automated immunofluorescence staining, BMC Cancer, 15 (2015) 360.

[38] C.M. Svensson, S. Krusekopf, J. Lucke, M. Thilo Figge, Automated detection of circulating tumor cells with naive Bayesian classifiers, Cytometry A, 85 (2014) 501–511.

[39] M. Zhao, P.G. Schiro, J.S. Kuo, K.M. Koehler, D.E. Sabath, V. Popov, Q. Feng, D.T. Chiu, An automated high-throughput counting method for screening circulating tumor cells in peripheral blood, Anal Chem, 85 (2013) 2465–2471.

[40] T.M. Scholtens, F. Schreuder, S.T. Ligthart, J.F. Swennenhuis, J. Greve, L.W. Terstappen, Automated identification of circulating tumor cells by image cytometry, Cytometry A, 81 (2012) 138–148.

[41] S.M. Leong, K.M. Tan, H.W. Chua, D. Tan, D. Fareda, S. Osmany, M.H. Li, S. Tucker, E.S. Koay, Sampling circulating tumor cells for clinical benefits: how frequent?, J Hematol Oncol, 8 (2015) 75.

[42] D. Marrinucci, K. Bethel, M. Luttgen, R.H. Bruce, J. Nieva, P. Kuhn, Circulating tumor cells from well-differentiated lung adenocarcinoma retain cytomorphologic features of primary tumor type, Arch Pathol Lab Med, 133 (2009) 1468–1471.

[43] P.R. Gascoyne, S. Shim, Isolation of circulating tumor cells by dielectrophoresis, Cancers (Basel), 6 (2014) 545–579.

[44] S. Shim, K. Stemke-Hale, A.M. Tsimberidou, J. Noshari, T.E. Anderson, P.R. Gascoyne, Antibody-independent isolation of circulating tumor cells by continuous-flow dielectrophoresis, Biomicrofluidics, 7 (2013) 11807.

[45] S.B. Huang, M.H. Wu, Y.H. Lin, C.H. Hsieh, C.L. Yang, H.C. Lin, C.P. Tseng, G.B. Lee, High-purity and label-free isolation of circulating tumor cells (CTCs) in a microfluidic platform by using optically-induced-dielectrophoretic (ODEP) force, Lab Chip, 13 (2013) 1371–1383.

[46] M.E. Warkiani, B.L. Khoo, L. Wu, A.K. Tay, A.A. Bhagat, J. Han, C.T. Lim, Ultra-fast, label-free isolation of circulating tumor cells from blood using spiral microfluidics, Nat Protoc, 11 (2016) 134–148.

[47] H. Li, P. Song, B. Zou, M. Liu, K. Cui, P. Zhou, S. Li, B. Zhang, Circulating tumor cell analyses in patients with esophageal squamous cell carcinoma using epithelial marker-dependent and -independent approaches, Medicine (Baltimore), 94 (2015) e1565.

[48] L. Xu, X. Mao, A. Imrali, F. Syed, K. Mutsvangwa, D. Berney, P. Cathcart, J. Hines, J. Shamash, Y.J. Lu, Optimization and evaluation of a novel size based circulating tumor cell isolation system, PLoS One, 10 (2015) e0138032.

[49] S. Yamamoto, J. Fei, M. Okochi, K. Shimizu, A. Yusa, N. Kondo, H. Iwata, H. Nakanishi, H. Honda, Efficient capturing of circulating tumor cells using a magnetic capture column and a size-selective filter, Bioprocess Biosyst Eng, 38 (2015) 1693–1704.

[50] X. Qin, S. Park, S.P. Duffy, K. Matthews, R.R. Ang, T. Todenhofer, H. Abdi, A. Azad, J. Bazov, K.N. Chi, P.C. Black, H. Ma, Size and deformability based separation of circulating tumor cells from castrate resistant prostate cancer patients using resettable cell traps, Lab Chip, 15 (2015) 2278–2286.

[51] E. Pailler, N. Auger, C.R. Lindsay, P. Vielh, A. Islas-Morris-Hernandez, I. Borget, M. Ngo-Camus, D. Planchard, J.C. Soria, B. Besse, F. Farace, High level of chromosomal instability in circulating tumor cells of ROS1-rearranged non-small-cell lung cancer, Ann Oncol, 26 (2015) 1408–1415.

[52] J.T. Kaifi, M. Kunkel, A. Das, R.A. Harouaka, D.T. Dicker, G. Li, J. Zhu, G.A. Clawson, Z. Yang, M.F. Reed, N.J. Gusani, E.T. Kimchi, K.F. Staveley-O'Carroll, S.Y. Zheng, W.S. El-Deiry, Circulating tumor cell isolation during resection of colorectal cancer lung and liver metastases: a prospective trial with different detection techniques, Cancer Biol Ther, 16 (2015) 699–708.

[53] X. Fan, C. Jia, J. Yang, G. Li, H. Mao, Q. Jin, J. Zhao, A microfluidic chip integrated with a high-density PDMS-based microfiltration membrane for rapid isolation and detection of circulating tumor cells, Biosens Bioelectron, 71 (2015) 380–386.

[54] J.F. Chen, H. Ho, J. Lichterman, Y.T. Lu, Y. Zhang, M.A. Garcia, S.F. Chen, A.J. Liang, E. Hodara, H.E. Zhau, S. Hou, R.S. Ahmed, D.J. Luthringer, J. Huang, K.C. Li, L.W. Chung, Z. Ke, H.R. Tseng, E.M. Posadas, Subclassification of prostate cancer circulating tumor cells by nuclear size reveals very small nuclear circulating tumor cells in patients with visceral metastases, Cancer, 121 (2015) 3240–3251.

[55] C.L. Chang, W. Huang, S.I. Jalal, B.D. Chan, A. Mahmood, S. Shahda, B.H. O'Neil, D.E. Matei, C.A. Savran, Circulating tumor cell detection using a parallel flow micro-aperture chip system, Lab Chip, 15 (2015) 1677–1688.

[56] Y. Tang, J. Shi, S. Li, L. Wang, Y.E. Cayre, Y. Chen, Microfluidic device with integrated microfilter of conical-shaped holes for high efficiency and high purity capture of circulating tumor cells, Sci Rep, 4 (2014) 6052.

[57] E. Sollier, D.E. Go, J. Che, D.R. Gossett, S. O'Byrne, W.M. Weaver, N. Kummer, M. Rettig, J. Goldman, N. Nickols, S. McCloskey, R.P. Kulkarni, D. Di Carlo, Size-selective collection of circulating tumor cells using Vortex technology, Lab Chip, 14 (2014) 63–77.

[58] V.K. Liadov, M.A. Skrypnikova, O.P. Popova, Isolation of circulating tumor cells in blood by means of "Isolation by SizE of Tumor cells (ISET)", Vopr Onkol, 60 (2014) 548–552.

[59] A. Lee, J. Park, M. Lim, V. Sunkara, S.Y. Kim, G.H. Kim, M.H. Kim, Y.K. Cho, All-in-one centrifugal microfluidic device for size-selective circulating tumor cell isolation with high purity, Anal Chem, 86 (2014) 11349–11356.

[60] T. Huang, C.P. Jia, Y. Jun, W.J. Sun, W.T. Wang, H.L. Zhang, H. Cong, F.X. Jing, H.J. Mao, Q.H. Jin, Z. Zhang, Y.J. Chen, G. Li, G.X. Mao, J.L. Zhao, Highly sensitive enumeration of circulating tumor cells in lung cancer patients using a size-based filtration microfluidic chip, Biosens Bioelectron, 51 (2014) 213–218.

[61] V. Bobek, R. Matkowski, R. Gurlich, K. Grabowski, J. Szelachowska, R. Lischke, J. Schutzner, T. Harustiak, A. Pazdro, A. Rzechonek, K. Kolostova, Cultivation of

circulating tumor cells in esophageal cancer, Folia Histochem Cytobiol, 52 (2014) 171–177.

[62] S. Park, R.R. Ang, S.P. Duffy, J. Bazov, K.N. Chi, P.C. Black, H. Ma, Morphological differences between circulating tumor cells from prostate cancer patients and cultured prostate cancer cells, PLoS One, 9 (2014) e85264.

[63] I. Nel, H.A. Baba, J. Ertle, F. Weber, B. Sitek, M. Eisenacher, H.E. Meyer, J.F. Schlaak, A.C. Hoffmann, Individual profiling of circulating tumor cell composition and therapeutic outcome in patients with hepatocellular carcinoma, Transl Oncol, 6 (2013) 420–428.

[64] I. Nel, U. Jehn, T. Gauler, A.C. Hoffmann, Individual profiling of circulating tumor cell composition in patients with non-small cell lung cancer receiving platinum based treatment, Transl Lung Cancer Res, 3 (2014) 100–106.

[65] E. Hansen, N. Wolff, R. Knuechel, J. Ruschoff, F. Hofstaedter, K. Taeger, Tumor cells in blood shed from the surgical field, Arch Surg, 130 (1995) 387–393.

[66] J.I. Yamashita, Y. Kurusu, N. Fujino, T. Saisyoji, M. Ogawa, Detection of circulating tumor cells in patients with non-small cell lung cancer undergoing lobectomy by video-assisted thoracic surgery: a potential hazard for intraoperative hematogenous tumor cell dissemination, J Thorac Cardiovasc Surg, 119 (2000) 899–905.

[67] T. Nakagawa, S.R. Martinez, Y. Goto, K. Koyanagi, M. Kitago, T. Shingai, D.A. Elashoff, X. Ye, F.R. Singer, A.E. Giuliano, D.S. Hoon, Detection of circulating tumor cells in early-stage breast cancer metastasis to axillary lymph nodes, Clin Cancer Res, 13 (2007) 4105–4110.

[68] M.P. Raynor, S.A. Stephenson, K.B. Pittman, D.C. Walsh, M.A. Henderson, A. Dobrovic, Identification of circulating tumour cells in early stage breast cancer patients using multi marker immunobead RT-PCR, J Hematol Oncol, 2 (2009) 24.

[69] R.M. Reddy, V. Murlidhar, L. Zhao, S. Grabauskiene, Z. Zhang, N. Ramnath, J. Lin, A.C. Chang, P. Carrott, W. Lynch, M.B. Orringer, D.G. Beer, S. Nagrath, Pulmonary venous blood sampling significantly increases the yield of circulating tumor cells in early-stage lung cancer, J Thorac Cardiovasc Surg, 151 (2016) 852–858.

[70] G. Sinha, Circulating tumor cells in early-stage breast cancer, J Natl Cancer Inst, 104 (2012) 1693–1694.

[71] M. Tewes, S. Kasimir-Bauer, A. Welt, M. Schuler, R. Kimmig, B. Aktas, Detection of disseminated tumor cells in bone marrow and circulating tumor cells in blood of patients with early-stage male breast cancer, J Cancer Res Clin Oncol, 141 (2015) 87–92.

[72] F. Miyazono, S. Natsugoe, S. Takao, K. Tokuda, F. Kijima, K. Aridome, S. Hokita, M. Baba, Y. Eizuru, T. Aikou, Surgical maneuvers enhance molecular detection of circulating tumor cells during gastric cancer surgery, Ann Surg, 233 (2001) 189–194.

[73] W.S. Chen, M.Y. Chung, J.H. Liu, J.M. Liu, J.K. Lin, Impact of circulating free tumor cells in the peripheral blood of colorectal cancer patients during laparoscopic surgery, World J Surg, 28 (2004) 552–557.

[74] M. Ilie, V. Hofman, E. Long-Mira, E. Selva, J.M. Vignaud, B. Padovani, J. Mouroux, C.H. Marquette, P. Hofman, "Sentinel" circulating tumor cells allow early diagnosis of lung cancer in patients with chronic obstructive pulmonary disease, PLoS One, 9 (2014).

[75] J.M. Hou, M.G. Krebs, L. Lancashire, R. Sloane, A. Backen, R.K. Swain, L.J. Priest, A. Greystoke, C. Zhou, K. Morris, T. Ward, F.H. Blackhall, C. Dive, Clinical significance and molecular characteristics of circulating tumor cells and circulating tumor micro-emboli in patients with small-cell lung cancer, J Clin Oncol, 30 (2012) 525–532.

[76] M.G. Krebs, J.M. Hou, R. Sloane, L. Lancashire, L. Priest, D. Nonaka, T.H. Ward, A. Backen, G. Clack, A. Hughes, M. Ranson, F.H. Blackhall, C. Dive, Analysis of circulating tumor cells in patients with non-small cell lung cancer using epithelial marker-dependent and -independent approaches, J Thorac Oncol, 7 (2012) 306–315.

[77] N. Aceto, A. Bardia, D.T. Miyamoto, M.C. Donaldson, B.S. Wittner, J.A. Spencer, M. Yu, A. Pely, A. Engstrom, H. Zhu, B.W. Brannigan, R. Kapur, S.L. Stott, T. Shioda, S. Ramaswamy, D.T. Ting, C.P. Lin, M. Toner, D.A. Haber, S. Maheswaran, Circulating tumor cell clusters are oligoclonal precursors of breast cancer metastasis, Cell, 158 (2014) 1110–1122.

[78] G. Kats-Ugurlu, E. Oosterwijk, S. Muselaers, J. Oosterwijk-Wakka, C. Hulsbergen-van de Kaa, M. de Weijert, H. van Krieken, I. Desar, C. van Herpen, C. Maass, R. de Waal, P. Mulders, W. Leenders, Neoadjuvant sorafenib treatment of clear cell renal cell carcinoma and release of circulating tumor fragments, Neoplasia, 16 (2014) 221–228.

[79] L. Lu, H. Zeng, X. Gu, W. Ma, Circulating tumor cell clusters-associated gene plakoglobin and breast cancer survival, Breast Cancer Res Treat, 151 (2015) 491–500.

[80] B. Molnar, A. Ladanyi, L. Tanko, L. Sreter, Z. Tulassay, Circulating tumor cell clusters in the peripheral blood of colorectal cancer patients, Clin Cancer Res, 7 (2001) 4080–4085.

[81] I.J. Fidler, The relationship of embolic homogeneity, number, size and viability to the incidence of experimental metastasis, Eur J Cancer, 9 (1973) 223–227.

[82] L.A. Liotta, M.G. Saidel, J. Kleinerman, The significance of hematogenous tumor cell clumps in the metastatic process, Cancer Res, 36 (1976) 889–894.

[83] P. Friedl, D. Gilmour, Collective cell migration in morphogenesis, regeneration and cancer, Nat Rev Mol Cell Biol, 10 (2009) 445–457.

[84] O. Ilina, P. Friedl, Mechanisms of collective cell migration at a glance, J Cell Sci, 122 (2009) 3203–3208.

[85] K.J. Cheung, V. Padmanaban, V. Silvestri, K. Schipper, J.D. Cohen, A.N. Fairchild, M.A. Gorin, J.E. Verdone, K.J. Pienta, J.S. Bader, A.J. Ewald, Polyclonal breast cancer

metastases arise from collective dissemination of keratin 14-expressing tumor cell clusters, Proc Natl Acad Sci USA, 113 (2016) E854–E863.

[86] A.F. Sarioglu, N. Aceto, N. Kojic, M.C. Donaldson, M. Zeinali, B. Hamza, A. Engstrom, H. Zhu, T.K. Sundaresan, D.T. Miyamoto, X. Luo, A. Bardia, B.S. Wittner, S. Ramaswamy, T. Shioda, D.T. Ting, S.L. Stott, R. Kapur, S. Maheswaran, D.A. Haber, M. Toner, A microfluidic device for label-free, physical capture of circulating tumor cell clusters, Nat Methods, 12 (2015) 685–691.

[87] I.J. Fidler, The pathogenesis of cancer metastasis: the 'seed and soil' hypothesis revisited, Nat Rev Cancer, 3 (2003) 453–458.

[88] M. Yu, A. Bardia, B.S. Wittner, S.L. Stott, M.E. Smas, D.T. Ting, S.J. Isakoff, J.C. Ciciliano, M.N. Wells, A.M. Shah, K.F. Concannon, M.C. Donaldson, L.V. Sequist, E. Brachtel, D. Sgroi, J. Baselga, S. Ramaswamy, M. Toner, D.A. Haber, S. Maheswaran, Circulating breast tumor cells exhibit dynamic changes in epithelial and mesenchymal composition, Science, 339 (2013) 580–584.

[89] D.G. Duda, A.M. Duyverman, M. Kohno, M. Snuderl, E.J. Steller, D. Fukumura, R.K. Jain, Malignant cells facilitate lung metastasis by bringing their own soil, Proc Natl Acad Sci USA, 107 (2010) 21677–21682.

[90] C. Alix-Panabieres, K. Pantel, Circulating tumor cells: liquid biopsy of cancer, Clin Chem, 59 (2013) 110–118.

[91] B. Rack, C. Schindlbeck, J. Juckstock, U. Andergassen, P. Hepp, T. Zwingers, T.W. Friedl, R. Lorenz, H. Tesch, P.A. Fasching, T. Fehm, A. Schneeweiss, W. Lichtenegger, M.W. Beckmann, K. Friese, K. Pantel, W. Janni, S.S. Group, Circulating tumor cells predict survival in early average-to-high risk breast cancer patients, J Natl Cancer Inst, 106 (2014).

[92] A. Grobe, M. Blessmann, H. Hanken, R.E. Friedrich, G. Schon, J. Wikner, K.E. Effenberger, L. Kluwe, M. Heiland, K. Pantel, S. Riethdorf, Prognostic relevance of circulating tumor cells in blood and disseminated tumor cells in bone marrow of patients with squamous cell carcinoma of the oral cavity, Clin Cancer Res, 20 (2014) 425–433.

[93] V. Hofman, M.I. Ilie, E. Long, E. Selva, C. Bonnetaud, T. Molina, N. Venissac, J. Mouroux, P. Vielh, P. Hofman, Detection of circulating tumor cells as a prognostic factor in patients undergoing radical surgery for non-small-cell lung carcinoma: comparison of the efficacy of the CellSearch Assay and the isolation by size of epithelial tumor cell method, Int J Cancer, 129 (2011) 1651–1660.

[94] C. Ren, P. He, J. Zhang, Z. Zheng, Y. Qiao, X. Zhao, Malignant characteristics of circulating tumor cells and corresponding primary tumor in a patient with esophageal squamous cell carcinoma before and after surgery, Cancer Biol Ther, 11 (2011) 633–638.

[95] M. Pesta, J. Fichtl, V. Kulda, O. Topolcan, V. Treska, Monitoring of circulating tumor cells in patients undergoing surgery for hepatic metastases from colorectal cancer, Anticancer Res, 33 (2013) 2239–2243.

[96] E. Magni, E. Botteri, P.S. Ravenda, M.C. Cassatella, E. Bertani, A. Chiappa, F. Luca, L. Zorzino, P.P. Bianchi, L. Adamoli, M.T. Sandri, M.G. Zampino, Detection of circulating tumor cells in patients with locally advanced rectal cancer undergoing neoadjuvant therapy followed by curative surgery, Int J Colorectal Dis, 29 (2014) 1053–1059.

[97] J. Inhestern, K. Oertel, V. Stemmann, H. Schmalenberg, A. Dietz, N. Rotter, J. Veit, M. Gorner, H. Sudhoff, C. Junghanss, C. Wittekindt, K. Pachmann, O. Guntinas-Lichius, Prognostic role of circulating tumor cells during Induction chemotherapy followed by curative surgery combined with postoperative radiotherapy in patients with locally advanced oral and oropharyngeal squamous cell cancer, PLoS One, 10 (2015) e0132901.

[98] W. Li, X. Zhou, Z. Huang, H. Zhang, L. Zhang, C. Shang, Y. Chen, Laparoscopic surgery minimizes the release of circulating tumor cells compared to open surgery for hepatocellular carcinoma, Surg Endosc, 29 (2015) 3146–3153.

[99] G. van Dalum, G.J. van der Stam, A.G. Tibbe, B. Franken, W.J. Mastboom, I. Vermes, M.R. de Groot, L.W. Terstappen, Circulating tumor cells before and during follow-up after breast cancer surgery, Int J Oncol, 46 (2015) 407–413.

[100] B. Biggers, S. Knox, M. Grant, J. Kuhn, J. Nemunatitis, T. Fisher, J. Lamont, Circulating tumor cells in patients undergoing surgery for primary breast cancer: preliminary results of a pilot study, Ann Surg Oncol, 16 (2009) 969–971.

[101] L.E. Lowes, M. Lock, G. Rodrigues, D. D'Souza, G. Bauman, B. Ahmad, V. Venkatesan, A.L. Allan, T. Sexton, The significance of circulating tumor cells in prostate cancer patients undergoing adjuvant or salvage radiation therapy, Prostate Cancer Prostatic Dis, 18 (2015) 358–364.

[102] V. Bobek, G. Kacprzak, A. Rzechonek, K. Kolostova, Detection and cultivation of circulating tumor cells in malignant pleural mesothelioma, Anticancer Res, 34 (2014) 2565–2569.

[103] V. Bobek, R. Gurlich, P. Eliasova, K. Kolostova, Circulating tumor cells in pancreatic cancer patients: enrichment and cultivation, World J Gastroenterol, 20 (2014) 17163–17170.

[104] K. Pantel, C. Alix-Panabieres, Functional studies on viable circulating tumor cells, Clin Chem, 62 (2016) 328–334.

[105] M. Das, J.W. Riess, P. Frankel, E. Schwartz, R. Bennis, H.B. Hsieh, X. Liu, J.C. Ly, L. Zhou, J.J. Nieva, H.A. Wakelee, R.H. Bruce, ERCC1 expression in circulating tumor cells (CTCs) using a novel detection platform correlates with progression-free survival (PFS) in patients with metastatic non-small-cell lung cancer (NSCLC) receiving platinum chemotherapy, Lung Cancer, 77 (2012) 421–426.

[106] M.Y. Kim, T. Oskarsson, S. Acharyya, D.X. Nguyen, X.H. Zhang, L. Norton, J. Massague, Tumor self-seeding by circulating cancer cells, Cell, 139 (2009) 1315–1326.

[107] Y. Liao, S.Y. Wang, X.Y. Meng, J. Yang, M.J. Shi, H.L. Liu, F.F. Chen, B. Xiong, Circulating tumor cells in breast cancer and its association with tumor clinicopathological characteristics: a meta-analysis, Med Oncol, 31 (2014) 343.

[108] T.A. Yap, D. Lorente, A. Omlin, D. Olmos, J.S. de Bono, Circulating tumor cells: a multifunctional biomarker, Clin Cancer Res, 20 (2014) 2553–2568.

[109] C. Alix-Panabieres, K. Bartkowiak, K. Pantel, Functional studies on circulating and disseminated tumor cells in carcinoma patients, Mol Oncol, 10 (2016) 443–449.

[110] B.J. Kirby, M. Jodari, M.S. Loftus, G. Gakhar, E.D. Pratt, C. Chanel-Vos, J.P. Gleghorn, S.M. Santana, H. Liu, J.P. Smith, V.N. Navarro, S.T. Tagawa, N.H. Bander, D.M. Nanus, P. Giannakakou, Functional characterization of circulating tumor cells with a prostate-cancer-specific microfluidic device, PLoS One, 7 (2012) e35976.

[111] B. Paiva, T. Paino, J.M. Sayagues, M. Garayoa, L. San-Segundo, M. Martin, I. Mota, M.L. Sanchez, P. Barcena, I. Aires-Mejia, L. Corchete, C. Jimenez, R. Garcia-Sanz, N.C. Gutierrez, E.M. Ocio, M.V. Mateos, M.B. Vidriales, A. Orfao, J.F. San Miguel, Detailed characterization of multiple myeloma circulating tumor cells shows unique phenotypic, cytogenetic, functional, and circadian distribution profile, Blood, 122 (2013) 3591–3598.

[112] G. Palmieri, M. Strazzullo, P.A. Ascierto, S.M. Satriano, A. Daponte, G. Castello, Polymerase chain reaction-based detection of circulating melanoma cells as an effective marker of tumor progression. Melanoma Cooperative Group, J Clin Oncol, 17 (1999) 304–311.

[113] I.H. Wong, Transcriptional profiling of circulating tumor cells: quantification and cancer progression (review), Oncol Rep, 10 (2003) 229–235.

[114] M. Cristofanilli, G.T. Budd, M.J. Ellis, A. Stopeck, J. Matera, M.C. Miller, J.M. Reuben, G.V. Doyle, W.J. Allard, L.W. Terstappen, D.F. Hayes, Circulating tumor cells, disease progression, and survival in metastatic breast cancer, N Engl J Med, 351 (2004) 781–791.

[115] T. Bauernhofer, S. Zenahlik, G. Hofmann, M. Balic, M. Resel, R. Pirchmoser, P. Regitnig, P. Ambros, N. Dandachi, H. Samonigg, Association of disease progression and poor overall survival with detection of circulating tumor cells in peripheral blood of patients with metastatic breast cancer, Oncol Rep, 13 (2005) 179–184.

[116] D.F. Hayes, M. Cristofanilli, G.T. Budd, M.J. Ellis, A. Stopeck, M.C. Miller, J. Matera, W.J. Allard, G.V. Doyle, L.W. Terstappen, Circulating tumor cells at each follow-up time point during therapy of metastatic breast cancer patients predict progression-free and overall survival, Clin Cancer Res, 12 (2006) 4218–4224.

[117] A. Poveda, S.B. Kaye, R. McCormack, S. Wang, T. Parekh, D. Ricci, C.A. Lebedinsky, J.C. Tercero, P. Zintl, B.J. Monk, Circulating tumor cells predict progression free

survival and overall survival in patients with relapsed/recurrent advanced ovarian cancer, Gynecol Oncol, 122 (2011) 567–572.

[118] B. Aktas, M. Tewes, T. Fehm, S. Hauch, R. Kimmig, S. Kasimir-Bauer, Stem cell and epithelial-mesenchymal transition markers are frequently overexpressed in circulating tumor cells of metastatic breast cancer patients, Breast Cancer Res, 11 (2009) R46.

[119] J.P. Thiery, Epithelial-mesenchymal transitions in tumour progression, Nat Rev Cancer, 2 (2002) 442–454.

[120] C. Raimondi, A. Gradilone, G. Naso, B. Vincenzi, A. Petracca, C. Nicolazzo, A. Palazzo, R. Saltarelli, F. Spremberg, E. Cortesi, P. Gazzaniga, Epithelial-mesenchymal transition and stemness features in circulating tumor cells from breast cancer patients, Breast Cancer Res Treat, 130 (2011) 449–455.

[121] M. Bourcy, M. Suarez-Carmona, J. Lambert, M.E. Francart, H. Schroeder, C. Delierneux, N. Skrypek, E.W. Thompson, G. Jerusalem, G. Berx, M. Thiry, S. Blacher, B.G. Hollier, A. Noel, C. Oury, M. Polette, C. Gilles, Tissue factor induced by epithelial-mesenchymal transition triggers a pro-coagulant state that drives metastasis of circulating tumor cells, Cancer Res, (2016). DOI: 10.1158/0008-5472.CAN-15-2263.

[122] M. Ksiazkiewicz, A. Markiewicz, A.J. Zaczek, Epithelial-mesenchymal transition: a hallmark in metastasis formation linking circulating tumor cells and cancer stem cells, Pathobiology, 79 (2012) 195–208.

[123] Y.M. Li, S.C. Xu, J. Li, K.Q. Han, H.F. Pi, L. Zheng, G.H. Zuo, X.B. Huang, H.Y. Li, H.Z. Zhao, Z.P. Yu, Z. Zhou, P. Liang, Epithelial-mesenchymal transition markers expressed in circulating tumor cells in hepatocellular carcinoma patients with different stages of disease, Cell Death Dis, 4 (2013) e831.

[124] K.A. Hyun, K.B. Goo, H. Han, J. Sohn, W. Choi, S.I. Kim, H.I. Jung, Y.S. Kim, Epithelial-to-mesenchymal transition leads to loss of EpCAM and different physical properties in circulating tumor cells from metastatic breast cancer, Oncotarget, 7 (2016) 24677-24687

[125] G. Barriere, M. Tartary, M. Rigaud, Epithelial mesenchymal transition: a new insight into the detection of circulating tumor cells, ISRN Oncol, 2012 (2012) 382010.

[126] S. Kasimir-Bauer, O. Hoffmann, D. Wallwiener, R. Kimmig, T. Fehm, Expression of stem cell and epithelial-mesenchymal transition markers in primary breast cancer patients with circulating tumor cells, Breast Cancer Res, 14 (2012) R15.

[127] Y.K. Liu, B.S. Hu, Z.L. Li, X. He, Y. Li, L.G. Lu, An improved strategy to detect the epithelial-mesenchymal transition process in circulating tumor cells in hepatocellular carcinoma patients, Hepatol Int, 10 (2016) 640-646.

[128] S. Wu, S. Liu, Z. Liu, J. Huang, X. Pu, J. Li, D. Yang, H. Deng, N. Yang, J. Xu, Classification of circulating tumor cells by epithelial-mesenchymal transition markers, PLoS One, 10 (2015) e0123976.

[129] G. Barriere, P. Fici, G. Gallerani, F. Fabbri, W. Zoli, M. Rigaud, Circulating tumor cells and epithelial, mesenchymal and stemness markers: characterization of cell subpopulations, Ann Transl Med, 2 (2014) 109.

[130] C.T. Jordan, M.L. Guzman, M. Noble, Cancer stem cells, N Engl J Med, 355 (2006) 1253–1261.

[131] J.E. Visvader, G.J. Lindeman, Cancer stem cells in solid tumours: accumulating evidence and unresolved questions, Nat Rev Cancer, 8 (2008) 755–768.

[132] T. Dittmar, C. Heyder, E. Gloria-Maercker, W. Hatzmann, K.S. Zanker, Adhesion molecules and chemokines: the navigation system for circulating tumor (stem) cells to metastasize in an organ-specific manner, Clin Exp Metastasis, 25 (2008) 11–32.

[133] M. Locke, M. Heywood, S. Fawell, I.C. Mackenzie, Retention of intrinsic stem cell hierarchies in carcinoma-derived cell lines, Cancer Res, 65 (2005) 8944–8950.

[134] L. Zhu, W. Zhang, J. Wang, R. Liu, Evidence of CD90+CXCR4+ cells as circulating tumor stem cells in hepatocellular carcinoma, Tumour Biol, 36 (2015) 5353–5360.

[135] S. Katoh, T. Goi, T. Naruse, Y. Ueda, H. Kurebayashi, T. Nakazawa, Y. Kimura, Y. Hirono, A. Yamaguchi, Cancer stem cell marker in circulating tumor cells: expression of CD44 variant exon 9 is strongly correlated to treatment refractoriness, recurrence and prognosis of human colorectal cancer, Anticancer Res, 35 (2015) 239–244.

[136] S. Liu, N. Li, X. Yu, X. Xiao, K. Cheng, J. Hu, J. Wang, D. Zhang, S. Cheng, S. Liu, Expression of intercellular adhesion molecule 1 by hepatocellular carcinoma stem cells and circulating tumor cells, Gastroenterology, 144 (2013) 1031–1041 e1010.

[137] Y.F. Sun, Y. Xu, X.R. Yang, W. Guo, X. Zhang, S.J. Qiu, R.Y. Shi, B. Hu, J. Zhou, J. Fan, Circulating stem cell-like epithelial cell adhesion molecule-positive tumor cells indicate poor prognosis of hepatocellular carcinoma after curative resection, Hepatology, 57 (2013) 1458–1468.

[138] M.A. Papadaki, G. Kallergi, Z. Zafeiriou, L. Manouras, P.A. Theodoropoulos, D. Mavroudis, V. Georgoulias, S. Agelaki, Co-expression of putative stemness and epithelial-to-mesenchymal transition markers on single circulating tumour cells from patients with early and metastatic breast cancer, BMC Cancer, 14 (2014) 651.

[139] F. Wang, Y.C. Li, L.P. Liu, H.M. Zhang, S. Tong, Circulating Tumor Cells and Tumor Stem Cells Detection in the Peripheral Blood Mononuclear Cells of Breast Cancer, J Clin Lab Anal, (2016). DOI: 10.1002/jcla.21911

[140] I. Tinhofer, M. Saki, F. Niehr, U. Keilholz, V. Budach, Cancer stem cell characteristics of circulating tumor cells, Int J Radiat Biol, 90 (2014) 622–627.

[141] I. Nel, P. David, G.G. Gerken, J.F. Schlaak, A.C. Hoffmann, Role of circulating tumor cells and cancer stem cells in hepatocellular carcinoma, Hepatol Int, 8 (2014) 321–329.

[142] M. Li, B. Zhang, Z. Zhang, X. Liu, X. Qi, J. Zhao, Y. Jiang, H. Zhai, Y. Ji, D. Luo, Stem cell-like circulating tumor cells indicate poor prognosis in gastric cancer, Biomed Res Int, 2014 (2014) 981261.

[143] N. Krawczyk, F. Meier-Stiegen, M. Banys, H. Neubauer, E. Ruckhaeberle, T. Fehm, Expression of stem cell and epithelial-mesenchymal transition markers in circulating tumor cells of breast cancer patients, Biomed Res Int, 2014 (2014) 415721.

[144] G. Pirozzi, V. Tirino, R. Camerlingo, A. La Rocca, N. Martucci, G. Scognamiglio, R. Franco, M. Cantile, N. Normanno, G. Rocco, Prognostic value of cancer stem cells, epithelial-mesenchymal transition and circulating tumor cells in lung cancer, Oncol Rep, 29 (2013) 1763–1768.

[145] D. Yuan, H. Xia, Y. Zhang, L. Chen, W. Leng, T. Chen, Q. Chen, Q. Tang, X. Mo, M. Liu, F. Bi, P-Akt/miR200 signaling regulates epithelial-mesenchymal transition, migration and invasion in circulating gastric tumor cells, Int J Oncol, 45 (2014) 2430–2438.

[146] A. Gradilone, G. Naso, C. Raimondi, E. Cortesi, O. Gandini, B. Vincenzi, R. Saltarelli, E. Chiapparino, F. Spremberg, M. Cristofanilli, L. Frati, A.M. Agliano, P. Gazzaniga, Circulating tumor cells (CTCs) in metastatic breast cancer (MBC): prognosis, drug resistance and phenotypic characterization, Ann Oncol, 22 (2011) 86–92.

[147] P. Gazzaniga, G. Naso, A. Gradilone, E. Cortesi, O. Gandini, W. Gianni, M.A. Fabbri, B. Vincenzi, F. di Silverio, L. Frati, A.M. Agliano, M. Cristofanilli, Chemosensitivity profile assay of circulating cancer cells: prognostic and predictive value in epithelial tumors, Int J Cancer, 126 (2010) 2437–2447.

[148] R. Nadal, F.G. Ortega, M. Salido, J.A. Lorente, M. Rodriguez-Rivera, M. Delgado-Rodriguez, M. Macia, A. Fernandez, J.M. Corominas, J.L. Garcia-Puche, P. Sanchez-Rovira, F. Sole, M.J. Serrano, CD133 expression in circulating tumor cells from breast cancer patients: potential role in resistance to chemotherapy, Int J Cancer, 133 (2013) 2398–2407.

[149] A. Gradilone, C. Raimondi, G. Naso, I. Silvestri, L. Repetto, A. Palazzo, W. Gianni, L. Frati, E. Cortesi, P. Gazzaniga, How circulating tumor cells escape from multidrug resistance: translating molecular mechanisms in metastatic breast cancer treatment, Am J Clin Oncol, 34 (2011) 625–627.

[150] J.D. Kuhlmann, P. Wimberger, A. Bankfalvi, T. Keller, S. Scholer, B. Aktas, P. Buderath, S. Hauch, F. Otterbach, R. Kimmig, S. Kasimir-Bauer, ERCC1-positive circulating tumor cells in the blood of ovarian cancer patients as a predictive biomarker for platinum resistance, Clin Chem, 60 (2014) 1282–1289.

[151] K.H. Yu, M. Ricigliano, M. Hidalgo, G.K. Abou-Alfa, M.A. Lowery, L.B. Saltz, J.F. Crotty, K. Gary, B. Cooper, R. Lapidus, M. Sadowska, E.M. O'Reilly, Pharmacogenomic modeling of circulating tumor and invasive cells for prediction of chemotherapy response and resistance in pancreatic cancer, Clin Cancer Res, 20 (2014) 5281–5289.

[152] E.A. Abdallah, M.F. Fanelli, M.E. Buim, M.C. Machado Netto, J.L. Gasparini Junior, E.S.V. Souza, A.L. Dettino, N.B. Mingues, J.V. Romero, L.M. Ocea, B.M. Rocha, V.S. Alves, D.V. Araujo, L.T. Chinen, Thymidylate synthase expression in circulating tumor cells: a new tool to predict 5-fluorouracil resistance in metastatic colorectal cancer patients, Int J Cancer, 137 (2015) 1397–1405.

[153] J.M. Pavese, R.C. Bergan, Circulating tumor cells exhibit a biologically aggressive cancer phenotype accompanied by selective resistance to chemotherapy, Cancer Lett, 352 (2014) 179–186.

[154] S.J. Cohen, C.J. Punt, N. Iannotti, B.H. Saidman, K.D. Sabbath, N.Y. Gabrail, J. Picus, M. Morse, E. Mitchell, M.C. Miller, G.V. Doyle, H. Tissing, L.W. Terstappen, N.J. Meropol, Relationship of circulating tumor cells to tumor response, progression-free survival, and overall survival in patients with metastatic colorectal cancer, J Clin Oncol, 26 (2008) 3213–3221.

[155] S. Yalcin, S. Kilickap, O. Portakal, C. Arslan, G. Hascelik, T. Kutluk, Determination of circulating tumor cells for detection of colorectal cancer progression or recurrence, Hepatogastroenterology, 57 (2010) 1395–1398.

[156] K. Pachmann, O. Camara, A. Kohlhase, C. Rabenstein, T. Kroll, I.B. Runnebaum, K. Hoeffken, Assessing the efficacy of targeted therapy using circulating epithelial tumor cells (CETC): the example of SERM therapy monitoring as a unique tool to individualize therapy, J Cancer Res Clin Oncol, 137 (2011) 821–828.

[157] I. Desitter, B.S. Guerrouahen, N. Benali-Furet, J. Wechsler, P.A. Janne, Y. Kuang, M. Yanagita, L. Wang, J.A. Berkowitz, R.J. Distel, Y.E. Cayre, A new device for rapid isolation by size and characterization of rare circulating tumor cells, Anticancer Res, 31 (2011) 427–441.

[158] E.S. Lianidou, A. Markou, Circulating tumor cells in breast cancer: detection systems, molecular characterization, and future challenges, Clin Chem, 57 (2011) 1242–1255.

[159] J.M. Park, J.Y. Lee, J.G. Lee, H. Jeong, J.M. Oh, Y.J. Kim, D. Park, M.S. Kim, H.J. Lee, J.H. Oh, S.S. Lee, W.Y. Lee, N. Huh, Highly efficient assay of circulating tumor cells by selective sedimentation with a density gradient medium and microfiltration from whole blood, Anal Chem, 84 (2012) 7400–7407.

[160] R. Harouaka, Z. Kang, S.Y. Zheng, L. Cao, Circulating tumor cells: advances in isolation and analysis, and challenges for clinical applications, Pharmacol Ther, 141 (2014) 209–221.

[161] G. Vona, L. Estepa, C. Beroud, D. Damotte, F. Capron, B. Nalpas, A. Mineur, D. Franco, B. Lacour, S. Pol, C. Brechot, P. Paterlini-Brechot, Impact of cytomorphological detection of circulating tumor cells in patients with liver cancer, Hepatology, 39 (2004) 792–797.

[162] V. De Giorgi, P. Pinzani, F. Salvianti, J. Panelos, M. Paglierani, A. Janowska, M. Grazzini, J. Wechsler, C. Orlando, M. Santucci, T. Lotti, M. Pazzagli, D. Massi, Appli-

cation of a filtration- and isolation-by-size technique for the detection of circulating tumor cells in cutaneous melanoma, J Invest Dermatol, 130 (2010) 2440–2447.

[163] P. Pinzani, C. Mazzini, F. Salvianti, D. Massi, R. Grifoni, C. Paoletti, F. Ucci, E. Molinara, C. Orlando, M. Pazzagli, B. Neri, Tyrosinase mRNA levels in the blood of uveal melanoma patients: correlation with the number of circulating tumor cells and tumor progression, Melanoma Res, 20 (2010) 303–310.

[164] C. Mazzini, P. Pinzani, F. Salvianti, C. Scatena, M. Paglierani, F. Ucci, M. Pazzagli, D. Massi, Circulating tumor cells detection and counting in uveal melanomas by a filtration-based method, Cancers (Basel), 6 (2014) 323–332.

[165] K. Kolostova, R. Matkowski, R. Gurlich, K. Grabowski, K. Soter, R. Lischke, J. Schutzner, V. Bobek, Detection and cultivation of circulating tumor cells in gastric cancer, Cytotechnology, 68 (2015) 1095-1102.

[166] C.L. Chen, D. Mahalingam, P. Osmulski, R.R. Jadhav, C.M. Wang, R.J. Leach, T.C. Chang, S.D. Weitman, A.P. Kumar, L. Sun, M.E. Gaczynska, I.M. Thompson, T.H. Huang, Single-cell analysis of circulating tumor cells identifies cumulative expression patterns of EMT-related genes in metastatic prostate cancer, Prostate, 73 (2013) 813–826.

[167] K. Kolostova, M. Broul, J. Schraml, M. Cegan, R. Matkowski, M. Fiutowski, V. Bobek, Circulating tumor cells in localized prostate cancer: isolation, cultivation in vitro and relationship to T-stage and Gleason score, Anticancer Res, 34 (2014) 3641–3646.

[168] M. Hosokawa, H. Kenmotsu, Y. Koh, T. Yoshino, T. Yoshikawa, T. Naito, T. Takahashi, H. Murakami, Y. Nakamura, A. Tsuya, T. Shukuya, A. Ono, H. Akamatsu, R. Watanabe, S. Ono, K. Mori, H. Kanbara, K. Yamaguchi, T. Tanaka, T. Matsunaga, N. Yamamoto, Size-based isolation of circulating tumor cells in lung cancer patients using a microcavity array system, PLoS One, 8 (2013) e67466.

[169] M. Hosokawa, T. Yoshikawa, R. Negishi, T. Yoshino, Y. Koh, H. Kenmotsu, T. Naito, T. Takahashi, N. Yamamoto, Y. Kikuhara, H. Kanbara, T. Tanaka, K. Yamaguchi, T. Matsunaga, Microcavity array system for size-based enrichment of circulating tumor cells from the blood of patients with small-cell lung cancer, Anal Chem, 85 (2013) 5692–5698.

[170] A. Fiorelli, M. Accardo, E. Carelli, D. Angioletti, M. Santini, M. Di Domenico, Circulating tumor cells in diagnosing lung cancer: clinical and morphologic analysis, Ann Thorac Surg, 99 (2015) 1899–1905.

[171] L.T. Chinen, C.A. Mello, E.A. Abdallah, L.M. Ocea, M.E. Buim, N.M. Breve, J.L.J. Gasparini, M.F. Fanelli, P. Paterlini-Brechot, Isolation, detection, and immunomorphological characterization of circulating tumor cells (CTCs) from patients with different types of sarcoma using isolation by size of tumor cells: a window on sarcoma-cell invasion, Onco Targets Ther, 7 (2014) 1609–1617.

[172] R. Riahi, P. Gogoi, S. Sepehri, Y. Zhou, K. Handique, J. Godsey, Y. Wang, A novel microchannel-based device to capture and analyze circulating tumor cells (CTCs) of breast cancer, Int J Oncol, 44 (2014) 1870–1878.

[173] M. Hosokawa, T. Hayata, Y. Fukuda, A. Arakaki, T. Yoshino, T. Tanaka, T. Matsunaga, Size-selective microcavity array for rapid and efficient detection of circulating tumor cells, Anal Chem, 82 (2010) 6629–6635.

[174] H.K. Lin, S. Zheng, A.J. Williams, M. Balic, S. Groshen, H.I. Scher, M. Fleisher, W. Stadler, R.H. Datar, Y.C. Tai, R.J. Cote, Portable filter-based microdevice for detection and characterization of circulating tumor cells, Clin Cancer Res, 16 (2010) 5011–5018.

[175] S.J. Tan, R.L. Lakshmi, P. Chen, W.T. Lim, L. Yobas, C.T. Lim, Versatile label free biochip for the detection of circulating tumor cells from peripheral blood in cancer patients, Biosens Bioelectron, 26 (2010) 1701–1705.

[176] L.S. Lim, M. Hu, M.C. Huang, W.C. Cheong, A.T. Gan, X.L. Looi, S.M. Leong, E.S. Koay, M.H. Li, Microsieve lab-chip device for rapid enumeration and fluorescence in situ hybridization of circulating tumor cells, Lab Chip, 12 (2012) 4388–4396.

[177] H.W. Hou, M.E. Warkiani, B.L. Khoo, Z.R. Li, R.A. Soo, D.S. Tan, W.T. Lim, J. Han, A.A. Bhagat, C.T. Lim, Isolation and retrieval of circulating tumor cells using centrifugal forces, Sci Rep, 3 (2013) 1259.

[178] K.A. Hyun, K. Kwon, H. Han, S.I. Kim, H.I. Jung, Microfluidic flow fractionation device for label-free isolation of circulating tumor cells (CTCs) from breast cancer patients, Biosens Bioelectron, 40 (2013) 206–212.

[179] M.X. Lin, K.A. Hyun, H.S. Moon, T.S. Sim, J.G. Lee, J.C. Park, S.S. Lee, H.I. Jung, Continuous labeling of circulating tumor cells with microbeads using a vortex micromixer for highly selective isolation, Biosens Bioelectron, 40 (2013) 63–67.

[180] E. Ozkumur, A.M. Shah, J.C. Ciciliano, B.L. Emmink, D.T. Miyamoto, E. Brachtel, M. Yu, P.I. Chen, B. Morgan, J. Trautwein, A. Kimura, S. Sengupta, S.L. Stott, N.M. Karabacak, T.A. Barber, J.R. Walsh, K. Smith, P.S. Spuhler, J.P. Sullivan, R.J. Lee, D.T. Ting, X. Luo, A.T. Shaw, A. Bardia, L.V. Sequist, D.N. Louis, S. Maheswaran, R. Kapur, D.A. Haber, M. Toner, Inertial focusing for tumor antigen-dependent and -independent sorting of rare circulating tumor cells, Sci Transl Med, 5 (2013) 179ra147.

[181] W. Sun, C. Jia, T. Huang, W. Sheng, G. Li, H. Zhang, F. Jing, Q. Jin, J. Zhao, G. Li, Z. Zhang, High-performance size-based microdevice for the detection of circulating tumor cells from peripheral blood in rectal cancer patients, PLoS One, 8 (2013) e75865.

[182] T.H. Kim, H.J. Yoon, P. Stella, S. Nagrath, Cascaded spiral microfluidic device for deterministic and high purity continuous separation of circulating tumor cells, Biomicrofluidics, 8 (2014) 064117.

[183] M.E. Warkiani, B.L. Khoo, D.S. Tan, A.A. Bhagat, W.T. Lim, Y.S. Yap, S.C. Lee, R.A. Soo, J. Han, C.T. Lim, An ultra-high-throughput spiral microfluidic biochip for the enrichment of circulating tumor cells, Analyst, 139 (2014) 3245–3255.

[184] K.A. Hyun, T.Y. Lee, S.H. Lee, H.I. Jung, Two-stage microfluidic chip for selective isolation of circulating tumor cells (CTCs), Biosens Bioelectron, 67 (2015) 86–92.

[185] J. Che, V. Yu, M. Dhar, C. Renier, M. Matsumoto, K. Heirich, E.B. Garon, J. Goldman, J. Rao, G.W. Sledge, M.D. Pegram, S. Sheth, S.S. Jeffrey, R.P. Kulkarni, E. Sollier, D. Di Carlo, Classification of large circulating tumor cells isolated with ultra-high throughput microfluidic vortex technology, Oncotarget, 7 (2016) 12748–12760.

[186] G.E. Hvichia, Z. Parveen, C. Wagner, M. Janning, J. Quidde, A. Stein, V. Muller, S. Loges, R.P. Neves, N.H. Stoecklein, H. Wikman, S. Riethdorf, K. Pantel, T.M. Gorges, A novel microfluidic platform for size and deformability based separation and the subsequent molecular characterization of viable circulating tumor cells, Int J Cancer, 138 (2016) 2894–2904.

[187] M.S. Kim, J. Kim, W. Lee, S.J. Cho, J.M. Oh, J.Y. Lee, S. Baek, Y.J. Kim, T.S. Sim, H.J. Lee, G.E. Jung, S.I. Kim, J.M. Park, J.H. Oh, O. Gurel, S.S. Lee, J.G. Lee, A trachea-inspired bifurcated microfilter capturing viable circulating tumor cells via altered biophysical properties as measured by atomic force microscopy, Small, 9 (2013) 3103–3110.

[188] J. Wang, W. Lu, C. Tang, Y. Liu, J. Sun, X. Mu, L. Zhang, B. Dai, X. Li, H. Zhuo, X. Jiang, Label-free isolation and mRNA detection of circulating tumor cells from patients with metastatic lung cancer for disease diagnosis and monitoring therapeutic efficacy, Anal Chem, 87 (2015) 11893–11900.

[189] S. Zheng, H. Lin, J.Q. Liu, M. Balic, R. Datar, R.J. Cote, Y.C. Tai, Membrane microfilter device for selective capture, electrolysis and genomic analysis of human circulating tumor cells, J Chromatogr A, 1162 (2007) 154–161.

[190] W. Xu, L. Cao, L. Chen, J. Li, X.F. Zhang, H.H. Qian, X.Y. Kang, Y. Zhang, J. Liao, L.H. Shi, Y.F. Yang, M.C. Wu, Z.F. Yin, Isolation of circulating tumor cells in patients with hepatocellular carcinoma using a novel cell separation strategy, Clin Cancer Res, 17 (2011) 3783–3793.

[191] F. Ge, H. Zhang, D.D. Wang, L. Li, P.P. Lin, Enhanced detection and comprehensive in situ phenotypic characterization of circulating and disseminated heteroploid epithelial and glioma tumor cells, Oncotarget, 6 (2015) 27049–27064.

[192] S.W. Lee, K.A. Hyun, S.I. Kim, J.Y. Kang, H.I. Jung, Continuous enrichment of circulating tumor cells using a microfluidic lateral flow filtration chip, J Chromatogr A, 1377 (2015) 100–105.

[193] D.J. Gallagher, M.I. Milowsky, N. Ishill, A. Trout, M.G. Boyle, J. Riches, M. Fleisher, D.F. Bajorin, Detection of circulating tumor cells in patients with urothelial cancer, Ann Oncol, 20 (2009) 305–308.

[194] P. Gazzaniga, A. Gradilone, E. de Berardinis, G.M. Busetto, C. Raimondi, O. Gandini, C. Nicolazzo, A. Petracca, B. Vincenzi, A. Farcomeni, V. Gentile, E. Cortesi, L. Frati, Prognostic value of circulating tumor cells in nonmuscle invasive bladder cancer: a CellSearch analysis, Ann Oncol, 23 (2012) 2352–2356.

[195] A. Giordano, M. Giuliano, M. De Laurentiis, G. Arpino, S. Jackson, B.C. Handy, N.T. Ueno, E. Andreopoulou, R.H. Alvarez, V. Valero, S. De Placido, G.N. Hortobagyi, J.M. Reuben, M. Cristofanilli, Circulating tumor cells in immunohistochemical subtypes of metastatic breast cancer: lack of prediction in HER2-positive disease treated with targeted therapy, Ann Oncol, 23 (2012) 1144–1150.

[196] T.J. Hiltermann, M.M. Pore, A. van den Berg, W. Timens, H.M. Boezen, J.J. Liesker, J.H. Schouwink, W.J. Wijnands, G.S. Kerner, F.A. Kruyt, H. Tissing, A.G. Tibbe, L.W. Terstappen, H.J. Groen, Circulating tumor cells in small-cell lung cancer: a predictive and prognostic factor, Ann Oncol, 23 (2012) 2937–2942.

[197] M. Mego, U. De Giorgi, L. Hsu, N.T. Ueno, V. Valero, S. Jackson, E. Andreopoulou, S.W. Kau, J.M. Reuben, M. Cristofanilli, Circulating tumor cells in metastatic inflammatory breast cancer, Ann Oncol, 20 (2009) 1824–1828.

[198] M.J. Sotelo, J. Sastre, M.L. Maestro, S. Veganzones, J.M. Vieitez, V. Alonso, C. Gravalos, P. Escudero, R. Vera, E. Aranda, P. Garcia-Alfonso, J. Gallego-Plazas, C. Lopez, C. Pericay, A. Arrivi, P. Vicente, P. Ballesteros, E. Elez, A. Lopez-Ladron, E. Diaz-Rubio, Role of circulating tumor cells as prognostic marker in resected stage III colorectal cancer, Ann Oncol, 26 (2015) 535–541.

[199] S. Dawood, K. Broglio, V. Valero, J. Reuben, B. Handy, R. Islam, S. Jackson, G.N. Hortobagyi, H. Fritsche, M. Cristofanilli, Circulating tumor cells in metastatic breast cancer: from prognostic stratification to modification of the staging system?, Cancer, 113 (2008) 2422–2430.

[200] W.J. Allard, L.W. Terstappen, CCR 20th anniversary commentary: paving the way for circulating tumor cells, Clin Cancer Res, 21 (2015) 2883–2885.

[201] A. Goldkorn, B. Ely, D.I. Quinn, C.M. Tangen, L.M. Fink, T. Xu, P. Twardowski, P.J. Van Veldhuizen, N. Agarwal, M.A. Carducci, J.P. Monk, 3rd, R.H. Datar, M. Garzotto, P.C. Mack, P. Lara, Jr., C.S. Higano, M. Hussain, I.M. Thompson, Jr., R.J. Cote, N.J. Vogelzang, Circulating tumor cell counts are prognostic of overall survival in SWOG S0421: a phase III trial of docetaxel with or without atrasentan for metastatic castration-resistant prostate cancer, J Clin Oncol, 32 (2014) 1136–1142.

[202] H.I. Scher, M.J. Morris, E. Basch, G. Heller, End points and outcomes in castration-resistant prostate cancer: from clinical trials to clinical practice, J Clin Oncol, 29 (2011) 3695–3704.

[203] C.R. Boland, A. Goel, Prognostic subgroups among patients with stage II colon cancer, N Engl J Med, 374 (2016) 277–278.

[204] A.C. Voogd, K. van Gestel, M.F. Ernst, Circulating epithelial cells in breast cancer, N Engl J Med, 351 (2004) 2452–2454; author reply 2452–2454.

[205] Z. Dombovari, B. Molnar, J. Bocsi, I. Lang, K. Papik, J. Feher, Z. Tulassay, Biologic detection methods in the comparison of circulating tumor cells and micrometastases, Orv Hetil, 139 (1998) 1793–1797.

[206] X.C. Hu, Y. Wang, D.R. Shi, T.Y. Loo, L.W. Chow, Immunomagnetic tumor cell enrichment is promising in detecting circulating breast cancer cells, Oncology, 64 (2003) 160–165.

[207] R. Konigsberg, M. Gneist, D. Jahn-Kuch, G. Pfeiler, G. Hager, M. Hudec, C. Dittrich, R. Zeillinger, Circulating tumor cells in metastatic colorectal cancer: efficacy and feasibility of different enrichment methods, Cancer Lett, 293 (2010) 117–123.

[208] Z.S. Lalmahomed, J. Kraan, J.W. Gratama, B. Mostert, S. Sleijfer, C. Verhoef, Circulating tumor cells and sample size: the more, the better, J Clin Oncol, 28 (2010) e288–289; author reply e290.

[209] T. Yeo, S.J. Tan, C.L. Lim, D.P. Lau, Y.W. Chua, S.S. Krisna, G. Iyer, G.S. Tan, T.K. Lim, D.S. Tan, W.T. Lim, C.T. Lim, Microfluidic enrichment for the single cell analysis of circulating tumor cells, Sci Rep, 6 (2016) 22076.

[210] Y. Deng, Y. Zhang, S. Sun, Z. Wang, M. Wang, B. Yu, D.M. Czajkowsky, B. Liu, Y. Li, W. Wei, Q. Shi, An integrated microfluidic chip system for single-cell secretion profiling of rare circulating tumor cells, Sci Rep, 4 (2014) 7499.

[211] R.L. Eifler, J. Lind, D. Falkenhagen, V. Weber, M.B. Fischer, R. Zeillinger, Enrichment of circulating tumor cells from a large blood volume using leukapheresis and elutriation: proof of concept, Cytometry B Clin Cytom, 80 (2011) 100–111.

[212] H. Kim, H. Terazono, Y. Nakamura, K. Sakai, A. Hattori, M. Odaka, M. Girault, T. Arao, K. Nishio, Y. Miyagi, K. Yasuda, Development of on-chip multi-imaging flow cytometry for identification of imaging biomarkers of clustered circulating tumor cells, PLoS One, 9 (2014) e104372.

[213] L.E. Lowes, D. Goodale, M. Keeney, A.L. Allan, Image cytometry analysis of circulating tumor cells, Methods Cell Biol, 102 (2011) 261–290.

[214] S.K. Lee, G.S. Kim, Y. Wu, D.J. Kim, Y. Lu, M. Kwak, L. Han, J.H. Hyung, J.K. Seol, C. Sander, A. Gonzalez, J. Li, R. Fan, Nanowire substrate-based laser scanning cytometry for quantitation of circulating tumor cells, Nano Lett, 12 (2012) 2697–2704.

[215] S.I. Han, K.H. Han, Electrical detection method for circulating tumor cells using graphene nanoplates, Anal Chem, 87 (2015) 10585–10592.

[216] D.J. Kim, W.Y. Lee, N.W. Park, G.S. Kim, K.M. Lee, J. Kim, M.K. Choi, G.H. Lee, W. Han, S.K. Lee, Drug response of captured BT20 cells and evaluation of circulating tumor cells on a silicon nanowire platform, Biosens Bioelectron, 67 (2015) 370–378.

[217] Z. Liu, A. Fusi, E. Klopocki, A. Schmittel, I. Tinhofer, A. Nonnenmacher, U. Keilholz, Negative enrichment by immunomagnetic nanobeads for unbiased characterization of circulating tumor cells from peripheral blood of cancer patients, J Transl Med, 9 (2011) 70.

[218] B. Naume, New methods for early detection of breast cancer metastasis, Tidsskr Nor Laegeforen, 118 (1998) 354.

[219] P. Balasubramanian, L. Yang, J.C. Lang, K.R. Jatana, D. Schuller, A. Agrawal, M. Zborowski, J.J. Chalmers, Confocal images of circulating tumor cells obtained using a methodology and technology that removes normal cells, Mol Pharm, 6 (2009) 1402–1408.

[220] C. Alix-Panabieres, J.P. Vendrell, M. Slijper, O. Pelle, E. Barbotte, G. Mercier, W. Jacot, M. Fabbro, K. Pantel, Full-length cytokeratin-19 is released by human tumor cells: a potential role in metastatic progression of breast cancer, Breast Cancer Res, 11 (2009) R39.

[221] E. Deneve, S. Riethdorf, J. Ramos, D. Nocca, A. Coffy, J.P. Daures, T. Maudelonde, J.M. Fabre, K. Pantel, C. Alix-Panabieres, Capture of viable circulating tumor cells in the liver of colorectal cancer patients, Clin Chem, 59 (2013) 1384–1392.

[222] S. Kruck, G. Gakis, A. Stenzl, Disseminated and circulating tumor cells for monitoring chemotherapy in urological tumors, Anticancer Res, 31 (2011) 2053–2057.

[223] K. Pantel, E. Deneve, D. Nocca, A. Coffy, J.P. Vendrell, T. Maudelonde, S. Riethdorf, C. Alix-Panabieres, Circulating epithelial cells in patients with benign colon diseases, Clin Chem, 58 (2012) 936–940.

[224] J.M. Ramirez, T. Fehm, M. Orsini, L. Cayrefourcq, T. Maudelonde, K. Pantel, C. Alix-Panabieres, Prognostic relevance of viable circulating tumor cells detected by EPISPOT in metastatic breast cancer patients, Clin Chem, 60 (2014) 214–221.

[225] M.J. Magbanua, E.V. Sosa, R. Roy, L.E. Eisenbud, J.H. Scott, A. Olshen, D. Pinkel, H.S. Rugo, J.W. Park, Genomic profiling of isolated circulating tumor cells from metastatic breast cancer patients, Cancer Res, 73 (2013) 30–40.

[226] C. Alix-Panabieres, J.P. Brouillet, M. Fabbro, H. Yssel, T. Rousset, T. Maudelonde, G. Choquet-Kastylevsky, J.P. Vendrell, Characterization and enumeration of cells secreting tumor markers in the peripheral blood of breast cancer patients, J Immunol Methods, 299 (2005) 177–188.

[227] C. Alix-Panabieres, S. Riethdorf, K. Pantel, Circulating tumor cells and bone marrow micrometastasis, Clin Cancer Res, 14 (2008) 5013–5021.

[228] S. Wu, Z. Liu, S. Liu, L. Lin, W. Yang, J. Xu, Enrichment and enumeration of circulating tumor cells by efficient depletion of leukocyte fractions, Clin Chem Lab Med, 52 (2014) 243–251.

[229] H.C. Lin, H.C. Hsu, C.H. Hsieh, H.M. Wang, C.Y. Huang, M.H. Wu, C.P. Tseng, A negative selection system PowerMag for effective leukocyte depletion and enhanced detection of EpCAM positive and negative circulating tumor cells, Clin Chim Acta, 419 (2013) 77–84.

[230] H.C. Lin, M.J. Liou, H.L. Hsu, J.C. Hsieh, Y.A. Chen, C.P. Tseng, J.D. Lin, Combined analysis of circulating epithelial cells and serum thyroglobulin for distinguishing disease status of the patients with papillary thyroid carcinoma, Oncotarget, 7 (2016) 17242–17253.

[231] J.C. Hsieh, H.C. Lin, C.Y. Huang, H.L. Hsu, T.M. Wu, C.L. Lee, M.C. Chen, H.M. Wang, C.P. Tseng, Prognostic value of circulating tumor cells with podoplanin expression in patients with locally advanced or metastatic head and neck squamous cell carcinoma, Head Neck, 37 (2015) 1448–1455.

[232] F.R. Li, Q. Li, H.X. Zhou, H. Qi, C.Y. Deng, Detection of circulating tumor cells in breast cancer with a refined immunomagnetic nanoparticle enriched assay and nested-RT-PCR, Nanomedicine, 9 (2013) 1106–1113.

[233] S.A. Hosseini, M. Abdolahad, S. Zanganeh, M. Dahmardeh, M. Gharooni, H. Abiri, A. Alikhani, S. Mohajerzadeh, O. Mashinchian, Nanoelectromechanical chip (NELMEC) combination of nanoelectronics and microfluidics to diagnose epithelial and mesenchymal circulating tumor cells from leukocytes, Small, 12 (2016) 883–891.

[234] S. Zhao, Y. Liu, Q. Zhang, H. Li, M. Zhang, W. Ma, W. Zhao, J. Wang, M. Yang, The prognostic role of circulating tumor cells (CTCs) detected by RT-PCR in breast cancer: a meta-analysis of published literature, Breast Cancer Res Treat, 130 (2011) 809–816.

[235] W.J. Janni, B. Rack, L.W. Terstappen, J.Y. Pierga, F.A. Taran, T. Fehm, C. Hall, M.R. de Groot, F.C. Bidard, T.W. Friedl, P.A. Fasching, S.Y. Brucker, K. Pantel, A. Lucci, Pooled analysis of the prognostic relevance of circulating tumor cells in primary breast cancer, Clin Cancer Res, 22 (2016) 2583–2593.

[236] Y. Zhou, B. Bian, X. Yuan, G. Xie, Y. Ma, L. Shen, Prognostic value of circulating tumor cells in ovarian cancer: a meta-analysis, PLoS One, 10 (2015) e0130873.

[237] Q. Lv, L. Gong, T. Zhang, J. Ye, L. Chai, C. Ni, Y. Mao, Prognostic value of circulating tumor cells in metastatic breast cancer: a systemic review and meta-analysis, Clin Transl Oncol, 18 (2016) 322–330.

[238] R. Konigsberg, E. Obermayr, G. Bises, G. Pfeiler, M. Gneist, F. Wrba, M. de Santis, R. Zeillinger, M. Hudec, C. Dittrich, Detection of EpCAM positive and negative circulating tumor cells in metastatic breast cancer patients, Acta Oncol, 50 (2011) 700–710.

[239] I.J. Diel, M. Kaufmann, R. Goerner, S.D. Costa, S. Kaul, G. Bastert, Detection of tumor cells in bone marrow of patients with primary breast cancer: a prognostic factor for distant metastasis, J Clin Oncol, 10 (1992) 1534–1539.

[240] B. Naume, E. Borgen, G. Kvalheim, R. Karesen, H. Qvist, T. Sauer, T. Kumar, J.M. Nesland, Detection of isolated tumor cells in bone marrow in early-stage breast

carcinoma patients: comparison with preoperative clinical parameters and primary tumor characteristics, Clin Cancer Res, 7 (2001) 4122–4129.

[241] R.J. Cote, P.P. Rosen, M.L. Lesser, L.J. Old, M.P. Osborne, Prediction of early relapse in patients with operable breast cancer by detection of occult bone marrow micrometastases, J Clin Oncol, 9 (1991) 1749–1756.

[242] K. Pantel, G. Schlimok, M. Angstwurm, D. Weckermann, W. Schmaus, H. Gath, B. Passlick, J.R. Izbicki, G. Riethmuller, Methodological analysis of immunocytochemical screening for disseminated epithelial tumor cells in bone marrow, J Hematother, 3 (1994) 165–173.

[243] S. Maheswaran, L.V. Sequist, S. Nagrath, L. Ulkus, B. Brannigan, C.V. Collura, E. Inserra, S. Diederichs, A.J. Iafrate, D.W. Bell, S. Digumarthy, A. Muzikansky, D. Irimia, J. Settleman, R.G. Tompkins, T.J. Lynch, M. Toner, D.A. Haber, Detection of mutations in EGFR in circulating lung-cancer cells, N Engl J Med, 359 (2008) 366–377.

[244] J.P. Gleghorn, E.D. Pratt, D. Denning, H. Liu, N.H. Bander, S.T. Tagawa, D.M. Nanus, P.A. Giannakakou, B.J. Kirby, Capture of circulating tumor cells from whole blood of prostate cancer patients using geometrically enhanced differential immunocapture (GEDI) and a prostate-specific antibody, Lab Chip, 10 (2010) 27–29.

[245] S.L. Stott, C.H. Hsu, D.I. Tsukrov, M. Yu, D.T. Miyamoto, B.A. Waltman, S.M. Rothenberg, A.M. Shah, M.E. Smas, G.K. Korir, F.P. Floyd, Jr., A.J. Gilman, J.B. Lord, D. Winokur, S. Springer, D. Irimia, S. Nagrath, L.V. Sequist, R.J. Lee, K.J. Isselbacher, S. Maheswaran, D.A. Haber, M. Toner, Isolation of circulating tumor cells using a microvortex-generating herringbone-chip, Proc Natl Acad Sci USA, 107 (2010) 18392–18397.

[246] S. Wang, A. Thomas, E. Lee, S. Yang, X. Cheng, Y. Liu, Highly efficient and selective isolation of rare tumor cells using a microfluidic chip with wavy-herringbone micropatterned surfaces, Analyst, 141 (2016) 2228–2237.

[247] M. Tang, C.Y. Wen, L.L. Wu, S.L. Hong, J. Hu, C.M. Xu, D.W. Pang, Z.L. Zhang, A chip assisted immunomagnetic separation system for the efficient capture and in situ identification of circulating tumor cells, Lab Chip, 16 (2016) 1214–1223.

[248] J. Chudziak, D.J. Burt, S. Mohan, D.G. Rothwell, B. Mesquita, J. Antonello, S. Dalby, M. Ayub, L. Priest, L. Carter, M.G. Krebs, F. Blackhall, C. Dive, G. Brady, Clinical evaluation of a novel microfluidic device for epitope-independent enrichment of circulating tumour cells in patients with small cell lung cancer, Analyst, 141 (2016) 669–678.

[249] M. Zhao, B. Wei, W.C. Nelson, P.G. Schiro, D.T. Chiu, Simultaneous and selective isolation of multiple subpopulations of rare cells from peripheral blood using ensemble-decision aliquot ranking (eDAR), Lab Chip, 15 (2015) 3391–3396.

[250] Y. Yang, H.S. Rho, M. Stevens, A.G. Tibbe, H. Gardeniers, L.W. Terstappen, Microfluidic device for DNA amplification of single cancer cells isolated from whole blood by self-seeding microwells, Lab Chip, 15 (2015) 4331–4337.

[251] P. Xue, Y. Wu, J. Guo, Y. Kang, Highly efficient capture and harvest of circulating tumor cells on a microfluidic chip integrated with herringbone and micropost arrays, Biomed Microdevices, 17 (2015) 39.

[252] C. Wang, M. Ye, L. Cheng, R. Li, W. Zhu, Z. Shi, C. Fan, J. He, J. Liu, Z. Liu, Simultaneous isolation and detection of circulating tumor cells with a microfluidic silicon-nanowire-array integrated with magnetic upconversion nanoprobes, Biomaterials, 54 (2015) 55–62.

[253] C.E. Nwankire, A. Venkatanarayanan, T. Glennon, T.E. Keyes, R.J. Forster, J. Ducree, Label-free impedance detection of cancer cells from whole blood on an integrated centrifugal microfluidic platform, Biosens Bioelectron, 68 (2015) 382–389.

[254] D. Nieto, R. Couceiro, M. Aymerich, R. Lopez-Lopez, M. Abal, M.T. Flores-Arias, A laser-based technology for fabricating a soda-lime glass based microfluidic device for circulating tumour cell capture, Colloids Surf B Biointerfaces, 134 (2015) 363–369.

[255] N.G. Maremanda, K. Roy, R.K. Kanwar, V. Shyamsundar, V. Ramshankar, A. Krishnamurthy, S. Krishnakumar, J.R. Kanwar, Quick chip assay using locked nucleic acid modified epithelial cell adhesion molecule and nucleolin aptamers for the capture of circulating tumor cells, Biomicrofluidics, 9 (2015) 054110.

[256] D. Issadore, Point-of-care rare cell cancer diagnostics, Methods Mol Biol, 1256 (2015) 123–137.

[257] I. Freitag, C. Matthaus, A. Csaki, J.H. Clement, D. Cialla-May, K. Weber, C. Krafft, J. Popp, Differentiation of MCF-7 tumor cells from leukocytes and fibroblast cells using epithelial cell adhesion molecule targeted multicore surface-enhanced Raman spectroscopy labels, J Biomed Opt, 20 (2015) 55002.

[258] R. Burger, D. Kurzbuch, R. Gorkin, G. Kijanka, M. Glynn, C. McDonagh, J. Ducree, An integrated centrifugo-opto-microfluidic platform for arraying, analysis, identification and manipulation of individual cells, Lab Chip, 15 (2015) 378–381.

[259] X. Zheng, L. Jiang, J. Schroeder, A. Stopeck, Y. Zohar, Isolation of viable cancer cells in antibody-functionalized microfluidic devices, Biomicrofluidics, 8 (2014) 024119.

[260] J.P. Winer-Jones, B. Vahidi, N. Arquilevich, C. Fang, S. Ferguson, D. Harkins, C. Hill, E. Klem, P.C. Pagano, C. Peasley, J. Romero, R. Shartle, R.C. Vasko, W.M. Strauss, P.W. Dempsey, Circulating tumor cells: clinically relevant molecular access based on a novel CTC flow cell, PLoS One, 9 (2014) e86717.

[261] M. Watanabe, M. Serizawa, T. Sawada, K. Takeda, T. Takahashi, N. Yamamoto, F. Koizumi, Y. Koh, A novel flow cytometry-based cell capture platform for the detection,

capture and molecular characterization of rare tumor cells in blood, J Transl Med, 12 (2014) 143.

[262] F.I. Thege, T.B. Lannin, T.N. Saha, S. Tsai, M.L. Kochman, M.A. Hollingsworth, A.D. Rhim, B.J. Kirby, Microfluidic immunocapture of circulating pancreatic cells using parallel EpCAM and MUC1 capture: characterization, optimization and downstream analysis, Lab Chip, 14 (2014) 1775–1784.

[263] Z. Svobodova, J. Kucerova, J. Autebert, D. Horak, L. Bruckova, J.L. Viovy, Z. Bilkova, Application of an improved magnetic immunosorbent in an Ephesia chip designed for circulating tumor cell capture, Electrophoresis, 35 (2014) 323–329.

[264] Y.J. Kim, G.B. Koo, J.Y. Lee, H.S. Moon, D.G. Kim, D.G. Lee, J.Y. Lee, J.H. Oh, J.M. Park, M.S. Kim, H.G. Woo, S.I. Kim, P. Kang, W. Choi, T.S. Sim, W.Y. Park, J.G. Lee, Y.S. Kim, A microchip filter device incorporating slit arrays and 3-D flow for detection of circulating tumor cells using CAV1-EpCAM conjugated microbeads, Biomaterials, 35 (2014) 7501–7510.

[265] B.L. Khoo, M.E. Warkiani, D.S. Tan, A.A. Bhagat, D. Irwin, D.P. Lau, A.S. Lim, K.H. Lim, S.S. Krisna, W.T. Lim, Y.S. Yap, S.C. Lee, R.A. Soo, J. Han, C.T. Lim, Clinical validation of an ultra high-throughput spiral microfluidics for the detection and enrichment of viable circulating tumor cells, PLoS One, 9 (2014) e99409.

[266] S. Jeon, W. Hong, E.S. Lee, Y. Cho, High-purity isolation and recovery of circulating tumor cells using conducting polymer-deposited microfluidic device, Theranostics, 4 (2014) 1123–1132.

[267] K.A. Hyun, H.I. Jung, Advances and critical concerns with the microfluidic enrichments of circulating tumor cells, Lab Chip, 14 (2014) 45–56.

[268] M.L. Hupert, J.M. Jackson, H. Wang, M.A. Witek, J. Kamande, M.I. Milowsky, Y.E. Whang, S.A. Soper, Arrays of high-aspect ratio microchannels for high-throughput isolation of circulating tumor cells (CTCs), Microsyst Technol, 20 (2014) 1815–1825.

[269] C. Huang, J.P. Smith, T.N. Saha, A.D. Rhim, B.J. Kirby, Characterization of microfluidic shear-dependent epithelial cell adhesion molecule immunocapture and enrichment of pancreatic cancer cells from blood cells with dielectrophoresis, Biomicrofluidics, 8 (2014) 044107.

[270] T. Ohnaga, Y. Shimada, K. Takata, T. Obata, T. Okumura, T. Nagata, H. Kishi, A. Muraguchi, K. Tsukada, Capture of esophageal and breast cancer cells with polymeric microfluidic devices for CTC isolation, Mol Clin Oncol, 4 (2016) 599–602.

[271] G. Galletti, M.S. Sung, L.T. Vahdat, M.A. Shah, S.M. Santana, G. Altavilla, B.J. Kirby, P. Giannakakou, Isolation of breast cancer and gastric cancer circulating tumor cells by use of an anti HER2-based microfluidic device, Lab Chip, 14 (2014) 147–156.

[272] M.C. Chang, Y.T. Chang, J.Y. Chen, Y.M. Jeng, C.Y. Yang, Y.W. Tien, S.H. Yang, H.L. Chen, T.Y. Liang, C.F. Wang, E.Y. Lee, Y.C. Chang, W.H. Lee, Clinical significance of

circulating tumor microemboli as a prognostic marker in patients with pancreatic ductal adenocarcinoma, Clin Chem, 62 (2016) 505–513.

[273] R.J. Torphy, C.J. Tignanelli, J.W. Kamande, R.A. Moffitt, S.G. Herrera Loeza, S.A. Soper, J.J. Yeh, Circulating tumor cells as a biomarker of response to treatment in patient-derived xenograft mouse models of pancreatic adenocarcinoma, PLoS One, 9 (2014) e89474.

[274] Z. Zhao, Y. Yang, Y. Zeng, M. He, A microfluidic ExoSearch chip for multiplexed exosome detection towards blood-based ovarian cancer diagnosis, Lab Chip, 16 (2016) 489–496.

[275] J. Li, S.G. Gregory, M.A. Garcia-Blanco, A.J. Armstrong, Using circulating tumor cells to inform on prostate cancer biology and clinical utility, Crit Rev Clin Lab Sci, 52 (2015) 191–210.

[276] J. Coget, F. Borrini, S. Susman, J.C. Sabourin, Colorectal carcinomas in 2013: the search for powerful prognostic markers is still on the go!, Cancer Biomark, 14 (2014) 145–150.

[277] S.H. Lu, W.S. Tsai, Y.H. Chang, T.Y. Chou, S.T. Pang, P.H. Lin, C.M. Tsai, Y.C. Chang, Identifying cancer origin using circulating tumor cells, Cancer Biol Ther, 17 (2016) 430–438.

[278] J. Autebert, B. Coudert, J. Champ, L. Saias, E.T. Guneri, R. Lebofsky, F.C. Bidard, J.Y. Pierga, F. Farace, S. Descroix, L. Malaquin, J.L. Viovy, High purity microfluidic sorting and analysis of circulating tumor cells: towards routine mutation detection, Lab Chip, 15 (2015) 2090–2101.

[279] S.D. Mikolajczyk, L.S. Millar, P. Tsinberg, S.M. Coutts, M. Zomorrodi, T. Pham, F.Z. Bischoff, T.J. Pircher, Detection of EpCAM-negative and cytokeratin-negative circulating tumor cells in peripheral blood, J Oncol, 2011 (2011) 252361.

[280] C. Paoletti, J.M. Larios, M.C. Muniz, K. Aung, E.M. Cannell, E.P. Darga, K.M. Kidwell, D.G. Thomas, N. Tokudome, M.E. Brown, M.C. Connelly, D.A. Chianese, A.F. Schott, N.L. Henry, J.M. Rae, D.F. Hayes, Heterogeneous estrogen receptor expression in circulating tumor cells suggests diverse mechanisms of fulvestrant resistance, Mol Oncol, (2016). DOI: 10.1016/j.molonc.2016.04.006

[281] J. Wang, K. Wang, J. Xu, J. Huang, T. Zhang, Prognostic significance of circulating tumor cells in non-small-cell lung cancer patients: a meta-analysis, PLoS One, 8 (2013) e78070.

[282] C. Bayarri-Lara, F.G. Ortega, A. Cueto Ladron de Guevara, J.L. Puche, J. Ruiz Zafra, D. de Miguel-Perez, A.S. Ramos, C.F. Giraldo-Ospina, J.A. Navajas Gomez, M. Delgado-Rodriguez, J.A. Lorente, M.J. Serrano, Circulating tumor cells identify early recurrence in patients with non-small cell lung cancer undergoing radical resection, PLoS One, 11 (2016) e0148659.

[283] J. Zhang, H.T. Wang, B.G. Li, Prognostic significance of circulating tumor cells in small--cell lung cancer patients: a meta-analysis, Asian Pac J Cancer Prev, 15 (2014) 8429–8433.

[284] M. Yanagita, A.J. Redig, C.P. Paweletz, S.E. Dahlberg, A. O'Connell, N. Feeney, M. Taibi, D. Boucher, G.R. Oxnard, B.E. Johnson, D.B. Costa, D.M. Jackman, P.A. Janne, A prospective evaluation of circulating tumor cells and cell-free DNA in EGFR mutant non-small cell lung cancer patients treated with erlotinib on a phase II trial, Clin Cancer Res, (2016). DOI: 10.1158/1078-0432.CCR-16-0909

[285] E. Pailler, J. Adam, A. Barthelemy, M. Oulhen, N. Auger, A. Valent, I. Borget, D. Planchard, M. Taylor, F. Andre, J.C. Soria, P. Vielh, B. Besse, F. Farace, Detection of circulating tumor cells harboring a unique ALK rearrangement in ALK-positive non-small-cell lung cancer, J Clin Oncol, 31 (2013) 2273–2281.

[286] G. Hamilton, B. Rath, L. Klameth, M.J. Hochmair, Small cell lung cancer: Recruitment of macrophages by circulating tumor cells, Oncoimmunology, 5 (2016) e1093277.

[287] Z.Y. Zhang, Z.L. Dai, X.W. Yin, S.H. Li, S.P. Li, H.Y. Ge, Meta-analysis shows that circulating tumor cells including circulating microRNAs are useful to predict the survival of patients with gastric cancer, BMC Cancer, 14 (2014) 773.

[288] D. Yuan, L. Chen, M. Li, H. Xia, Y. Zhang, T. Chen, R. Xia, Q. Tang, F. Gao, X. Mo, M. Liu, F. Bi, Isolation and characterization of circulating tumor cells from human gastric cancer patients, J Cancer Res Clin Oncol, 141 (2015) 647–660.

[289] S.J. Cohen, C.J. Punt, N. Iannotti, B.H. Saidman, K.D. Sabbath, N.Y. Gabrail, J. Picus, M.A. Morse, E. Mitchell, M.C. Miller, G.V. Doyle, H. Tissing, L.W. Terstappen, N.J. Meropol, Prognostic significance of circulating tumor cells in patients with metastatic colorectal cancer, Ann Oncol, 20 (2009) 1223–1229.

[290] H. Iinuma, T. Watanabe, K. Mimori, M. Adachi, N. Hayashi, J. Tamura, K. Matsuda, R. Fukushima, K. Okinaga, M. Sasako, M. Mori, Clinical significance of circulating tumor cells, including cancer stem-like cells, in peripheral blood for recurrence and prognosis in patients with Dukes' stage B and C colorectal cancer, J Clin Oncol, 29 (2011) 1547–1555.

[291] C. Aggarwal, N.J. Meropol, C.J. Punt, N. Iannotti, B.H. Saidman, K.D. Sabbath, N.Y. Gabrail, J. Picus, M.A. Morse, E. Mitchell, M.C. Miller, S.J. Cohen, Relationship among circulating tumor cells, CEA and overall survival in patients with metastatic colorectal cancer, Ann Oncol, 24 (2013) 420–428.

[292] N.A. Mohamed Suhaimi, Y.M. Foong, D.Y. Lee, W.M. Phyo, I. Cima, E.X. Lee, W.L. Goh, W.Y. Lim, K.S. Chia, S.L. Kong, M. Gong, B. Lim, A.M. Hillmer, P.K. Koh, J.Y. Ying, M.H. Tan, Non-invasive sensitive detection of KRAS and BRAF mutation in circulating tumor cells of colorectal cancer patients, Mol Oncol, 9 (2015) 850–860.

[293] M.E. Buim, M.F. Fanelli, V.S. Souza, J. Romero, E.A. Abdallah, C.A. Mello, V. Alves, L.M. Ocea, N.B. Mingues, P.N. Barbosa, C.J. Tyng, R. Chojniak, L.T. Chinen, Detection of KRAS mutations in circulating tumor cells from patients with metastatic colorectal cancer, Cancer Biol Ther, 16 (2015) 1289–1295.

[294] Q. Li, X. Zhi, J. Zhou, R. Tao, J. Zhang, P. Chen, O.D. Roe, L. Sun, L. Ma, Circulating tumor cells as a prognostic and predictive marker in gastrointestinal stromal tumors: a prospective study, Oncotarget, 7 (2016) 36645-26654.

[295] J.P. Oliveira-Costa, A.F. de Carvalho, G.G. da Silveira da, P. Amaya, Y. Wu, K.J. Park, M.P. Gigliola, M. Lustberg, M.E. Buim, E.N. Ferreira, L.P. Kowalski, J.J. Chalmers, F.A. Soares, D.M. Carraro, A. Ribeiro-Silva, Gene expression patterns through oral squamous cell carcinoma development: PD-L1 expression in primary tumor and circulating tumor cells, Oncotarget, 6 (2015) 20902–20920.

[296] X.L. Wu, Q. Tu, G. Faure, P. Gallet, C. Kohler, C. Bittencourt Mde, Diagnostic and Prognostic Value of Circulating Tumor Cells in Head and Neck Squamous Cell Carcinoma: a systematic review and meta-analysis, Sci Rep, 6 (2016) 20210.

[297] J.L. Fan, Y.F. Yang, C.H. Yuan, H. Chen, F.B. Wang, Circulating tumor cells for predicting the prognostic of patients with hepatocellular carcinoma: a meta analysis, Cell Physiol Biochem, 37 (2015) 629–640.

[298] K. Schulze, C. Gasch, K. Staufer, B. Nashan, A.W. Lohse, K. Pantel, S. Riethdorf, H. Wege, Presence of EpCAM-positive circulating tumor cells as biomarker for systemic disease strongly correlates to survival in patients with hepatocellular carcinoma, Int J Cancer, 133 (2013) 2165–2171.

[299] F. Salvianti, C. Orlando, D. Massi, V. De Giorgi, M. Grazzini, M. Pazzagli, P. Pinzani, Tumor-related methylated cell-free DNA and circulating tumor cells in melanoma, Front Mol Biosci, 2 (2015) 76.

[300] F.C. Bidard, J. Madic, P. Mariani, S. Piperno-Neumann, A. Rampanou, V. Servois, N. Cassoux, L. Desjardins, M. Milder, I. Vaucher, J.Y. Pierga, R. Lebofsky, M.H. Stern, O. Lantz, Detection rate and prognostic value of circulating tumor cells and circulating tumor DNA in metastatic uveal melanoma, Int J Cancer, 134 (2014) 1207–1213.

[301] S. Hoshimoto, M.B. Faries, D.L. Morton, T. Shingai, C. Kuo, H.J. Wang, R. Elashoff, N. Mozzillo, M.C. Kelley, J.F. Thompson, J.E. Lee, D.S. Hoon, Assessment of prognostic circulating tumor cells in a phase III trial of adjuvant immunotherapy after complete resection of stage IV melanoma, Ann Surg, 255 (2012) 357–362.

[302] N. Romero-Laorden, D. Olmos, T. Fehm, J. Garcia-Donas, I. Diaz-Padilla, Circulating and disseminated tumor cells in ovarian cancer: a systematic review, Gynecol Oncol, 133 (2014) 632–639.

[303] K. Kolostova, R. Matkowski, M. Jedryka, K. Soter, M. Cegan, M. Pinkas, A. Jakabova, J. Pavlasek, J. Spicka, V. Bobek, The added value of circulating tumor cells examination in ovarian cancer staging, Am J Cancer Res, 5 (2015) 3363–3375.

[304] K. Kolostova, J. Spicka, R. Matkowski, V. Bobek, Isolation, primary culture, morphological and molecular characterization of circulating tumor cells in gynecological cancers, Am J Transl Res, 7 (2015) 1203–1213.

[305] L. Zeng, X. Liang, Q. Liu, Z. Yang, The predictive value of circulating tumor cells in ovarian cancer: a meta analysis, Int J Gynecol Cancer, (2015). DOI: 10.1097/IGC.0000000000000459

[306] E.M. Matthew, L. Zhou, Z. Yang, D.T. Dicker, S.L. Holder, B. Lim, R. Harouaka, S.Y. Zheng, J.J. Drabick, N.E. Lamparella, C.I. Truica, W.S. El-Deiry, A multiplexed marker-based algorithm for diagnosis of carcinoma of unknown primary using circulating tumor cells, Oncotarget, 7 (2016) 3662–3676.

[307] E. Fina, C. Reduzzi, R. Motta, S. Di Cosimo, G. Bianchi, A. Martinetti, J. Wechsler, V. Cappelletti, M.G. Daidone, Did circulating tumor cells tell us all they could? The missed circulating tumor cell message in breast cancer, Int J Biol Markers, 30 (2015) e429–433.

Chapter 9

Detection of Circulating Tumor Cells and Circulating Tumor Stem Cells in Breast Cancer by Using Flow Cytometry

Yanjie Hu, Jin'e Zheng and Shiang Huang

Additional information is available at the end of the chapter

http://dx.doi.org/10.5772/63423

Abstract

We demonstrated the value of multiparameter flowcytometry in detecting human tumor cells of breast cancer in peripheral blood, which had a sensitivity limit of 10^{-5} and higher specificity compares with real-time polymerase chain reaction (RT-PCR). It was also found that circulating tumor cell (CTC) number was related with TNM stage, metastasis and the overall survival of patients. CTC level was one of the important factors for patients' prognosis. At the same time, we also verified the circulating tumor stem cell (CTSC) was connected with TNM stage by multiparameter cytometry. The detection of CTC and CTSC by multiparameter flowcytometry may be used to diagnose disease at early stage to guide clinical therapy or to predict prognosis. Multiparameter flowcytometry has the potential to be a valuable tool for prognosis assessment among patients with breast cancer in clinical situation in China.

Keywords: circulating tumor cells (CTC), circulating tumor stem cells (CTSC), epithelial-mesenchymal transiton (EMT), multiparameter flow cytometry, subtraction enrichment

1. Introduction

MERGEFORMAT breast cancer is the most common cancer in women in developed countries. In developing countries, such as China, the incidence of breast cancer is currently increasing, particularly in larger cities [1]. It is considered to be a systemeic disease as tumor cell dissemination at early stage. The major problem of recurrence and death is due to the persistence of minimal residual disease [2]. There is great interest in finding biomarkers in peripheral blood, which can be sampled at any stage of the disease. Then, the detection of CTCs for monitoring therapy was highly investigated in breast cancer. Circulating cells with the characteristics of tumor cells can be identified in the peripheral blood that is known as circulating tumor cells (CTCs) in many patients with solid tumors of epithelial origin. These cells are present both in patients with metastasis and in those whose tumors are localized [3]. Tumor cells shed into the circulation intermittently which was corresponding with microinvasive events. The first phase of metastatic consists of lessens of tumor cell adhesion, induction of tumor cell motility and local tumor cell invasion [4]. These steps are followed by either spread to circulation in peripheral blood or regional lymph nodes, and locating in secondary organs [5]. Some of these cells generate metastases eventually that can arise many years after therapy of the primary tumor at earlier phase [2]. CTCs also may be related to a half-life probably 1–2.4 h, which means it cannot always exist in circulating [6]. Some authors argued that these cells were predominantly in G0 phase and thus are not replicating [7]; however, they did not exclude the existence that the proliferation of CTCs can occur, although it was a rare event. Considering the half-life of CTCs, the presence of CTCs in the blood could be maintained by a balance between replication and cell death. While apoptosis contributed to a high rate of circulating tumor cells, only a small part of the cells can adhere in second organs through blood vessels that were named as circulating tumor stem cells (CTSCs) [8].

CTCs can be selected with a monoclonal antibody directed against CD45 for negative selection of leukocytes [9–11]. And from this cluster cells, EpCAM (epithelial-cell adhesion molecule) and cytokeratin-8 (CK-8), CK-18, CK-19 (CK-8, CK-18, CK-19 phycoerythrin staining)-positive cells are the target cells, which were known as the marker of epithelial cells. The characterization of CTCs presents a very hot topic in breast cancer research nowadays [12]. It helped to identify diagnosis and provide individual therapies according to the characterization of CTCs [12–14]. The characterization of CTSCs contributed to the identification and targeted therapy in breast cancer in the near future [15]. Molecularly targeted cancer therapies contributed great help which according to the characterization of CTCs especially on patients whose tumors have a particular mutation [16]. Some of the biological properties and the molecular characteristics of CTCs were connected to CTSCs and the genomic profiles have been completed [15]. Following that, the CD44-positive CD24-negative cells with their tumor-initiating ability had been considered as CTSCs [17]. Hence, from CTC, CD44-positive cell and CD24-negative cell are CTSCs. Molecular characterization of CTCs, which is important for the identification of diagnostically and therapeutically relevant for individual therapies, it is difficult to address since they are very rare and the amount of available sample is very limited. Given the properties of the metastatic CTCs, there should be some opportunities for early identification and therapeutic targeting in breast cancer.

Some immunologic procedures, such as immunohistochemistry-based methods and reverse transcriptase polymerase chain reaction (RT-PCR), have been used to detect CTCs in past time [18–22]. However, current methods of detection do not seem to be sensitive or specific enough to apply in clinical [23–25]. Nowadays, we demonstrate the advent of the flow cytometry in the detection of CTCs, which makes a good balance of sensitivity and specificity. In addition, the procedure of the method was simple and the cost was lower than immunologic technology, which made it possible to apply in clinical.

2. Methods

2.1. Patients

We investigated 45 patients with breast cancer in the Union Hospital in Wuhan during September 2006 and June 2008 with three normal people as negative control. Twenty-five patients had overt metastasis and 20 patients had no sign of overt metastasis. The character-

	All		CTC < 5 (n = 27)		CTC ≥ 5 (n = 18)		*P*-value[a]
	n	%	*n*	%	*n*	%	
Age, years							
Minimum	32	–	32	–	37	–	0.640
Median	50	–	49	–	51	–	
Maximum	74	–	72	–	74	–	
TNM stage							
I	5	13.3	5	100.0	0	0.0	0.033
II	4	8.9	4	100.0	0	0.0	
III	11	24.4	7	63.6	4	36.4	
IV	25	55.6	11	41.7	14	58.3	
Primary tumor sites							
Left breast	24	53.3	14	58.3	10	41.7	0.807
Right breast	21	46.7	13	61.9	8	38.1	
Clinical pathology							
Infiltrating ducta	28	62.2	17	60.7	11	39.3	0.921
Papillary	10	22.2	6	60.0	4	40.0	
Squamous celled	4	8.9	2	50.0	2	50.0	
Mucous cancer	1	2.2	1	100.0	0	0.0	
Medullary	2	4.4	1	50.0	1	50.0	
Diameter of tumor							
≤2.0 cm	13	28.9	9	615	4	30.7	0.522
2.0–5.0 cm	27	60.0	16	59.3	11	40.7	
>5.0 cm	5	11.1	2	40.0	3	60.0	
ALND							
Yes	35	77.8	19	54.3	16	45.7	0.143
No	10	22.2	8	80.0	2	20.0	
Metastasis							
Yes	25	55.6	10	40.0	15	60.0	0.002
No	20	44.4	17	85.0	3	15.0	

ALND, axillary lymph node dissection.

Table 1. Patient characteristics.

istics of the patients are shown in **Table 1**, including mean age, TNM phase, histopathology, lymph node status, metastasis and so on. All these patients were incipient and were treated by systemic therapy, including 12 patients cured by cytokine-induced killer cells therapy (CIK). And all the patients were drawn blood for the detection of CTCs.

2.2. Cell line

Carcinoma cell line SKBR-3 (breast) was used to estimate the sensitivity and specificity of the flow cytometry, which was maintained in RPMI 1640 plus 10% fetal calf serum.

2.3. Antibodies

Antibodies, which were used for multiparameter flow cytometry, were as follows: anti-CD45-PerCP, anti-CD44-APC (allophycocyanin, clone G44-26, catalog number 559942) and anti-CD24-FITC (fluorescein isothiocyanate, clone ML5, catalog number 555427) were from Becton Dickison Crop., USA. Ep-CAM (epithelial-cell adhesion molecule) and CK-8, CK-18, CK-19 (CK-8, CK-18, CK-19 phycoerythrin staining) were from Abcam, USA.

2.4. Preparation of samples

Every patient with breast cancer drew 20 ml blood for CTCs detection and three healthy volunteers. The blood of healthy volunteers was treated as negative control. About 5 ml blood was discarded to avoid contamination with skin cells as previously described [26]. We separated mononucleocytes from 15 ml blood by Ficoll-Paque (Haoyang Biological Production Limited Company, Tianjin, China) for 20 min with 1800 × *g* at 25°C. One half of the mononuclear cells was resuspended in phosphate-buffered saline (PBS) for multiparameter flow cytometry on the account of at least 2–3 × 10^6 cells for each sample and the other half was kept in Trizol reagent (Invitrogen, UK) at -70°C until RNA extraction for RT-PCR.

2.5. Flow cytometry

Mononucleocytes were enriched and washed twice with PBS and then labelled antibodies that target white cell antigens and epithelial cell antigens (CD45-, Ep-CAM$^+$, CK-8, CK-18, CK-19$^+$), kept in dark at 4°C for 30 min. We added 20 μl monoclonal antibodies for each sample. Cell pellets were resuspended in 250 μl PBS and enumerated by FACS Caliber™ (Becton Dickison Crop., USA) at last.

SKBR-3 breast cancer cells were used to evaluate the sensitivity of the flow cytometry (tumor cells recovery). Tumor cells were resuspended and counted. 1, 10, 50, 500 cells were spiked, respectively, into 7.5 ml of blood from healthy person. And then, it was processed as described as earlier and control the preparation for the same volume of the cell suspension and cells were counted to accurately estimate the number of cells spiked into the blood. The average number of Ep-CAM and CK-8, CK-18, CK-19 positive cells on FACS Caliber™ was used to calculate the cells recovery.

The mononuclear cells (MNCs) for FCM were incubated with monoclonal antibodies: anti-CD45-PerCP, anti-EPCAM-PE, anti-CD44-APC and anti-CD24-FITC. About 20 μl of each antibody was needed, and the condition was 4°C for 30 min away from light. Then, the MNCs were washed two times. Finally, cells were resuspended with PBS and analyzed on FACS Calibur™ (BD Bio) using Cell Quest software (BD Bio).

2.6. RT-PCR

We extract RNA with 1 ml trizol from the mononucleocytes, which were separated from 7.5 ml blood and then kept at -70°C. Add 0.2 ml chloroform and then centrifuge the sample at 12,000 × *g* for 15 min at 4°C. The intact RNA, which was contained in the supernatants, was removed into a new tube. RNA was dissolved in 10 μl RNase-free water after precipitating RNA with isopropyl alcohol and washing with 75% ethanol. Then, RNA was transcribed to cDNA by a reverse transcriptase in a total 10 μl RT reaction solution, which was contained of 2 μl 5x Reverse Transcriptase Buffer, 1 μl dNTP (10 mM each), 0.25 μl RNase inhibitor (10 U), 1 μl oligo $(dT)_{15}$ primer (25 pmol), 5.25 μl RNase-free water containing RNA (>0.5 μg), 0.5 μl avian myeloblastosis virus (AMV) reverse transcriptase (5U) (TaKaRa, China). The resulting cDNA was subjected to PCR amplification. PCR was composed of 2 μl cDNA, 10 μl Mix, 2 μl primer of EpCAM, 6 μl H_2O in a total volume of 20 μl. The primer of EpCAM was as follows: 5′-GGACCTGACAGTAAATGGGGAAC-3′; 5′-CTCTTCTTTCTGGAAATAACCAGCAC-3′ [18]. GAPDH mRNA primer detail was as follows: 5′-TGCACCACCAACTGCTTAGC-3′; 5′-GGAGGCAGGGATGATGTTCT-3′ which was designed by Primer 5.0. The reaction condition was 95°C for 2 min to activate Taq DNA polymerase and it finally elongated 72°C for 7 min with 35 cycles. We detected the PCR products by ethidium bromide staining on a 1% agarose gel.

2.7. Statistical analysis

Correlation, regression analysis and a Mann-Whitney rank sum test were performed on titration experiments. Chi-square test was used to compare across CTC groups. Overall survival was performed to describe the condition of CTCs and prognosis and was estimated by the Kaplan-Meier. Comparison of groups used the log-rank test. All statistical tests were two-sided, and P values < 0.05 were considered statistically significant. Analyses above were performed by using the SPSS 13.0.

3. Results

3.1. Sensitivity and specificity

3.1.1. Sensitivity

It is demonstrated that the sensitivity of the method of CTCs detection by using multiparameter flow cytometry was 0.001%, or 10^{-5}, according to the serial dilutions test, which is shown in

Figure 1a–d. It was highly reproducible on recovery and linearity across three separate experiments (**Figure 1e**). The recovery of the tumor events was quite correlated with the tumor events expected based on the serial dilutions ($R^2 = 0.997$). The recovery of the tumor cells was not significantly different from the tumor cells expected according to the serial dilutions ($P > 0.6$, Mann-Whitney rank sum test).

3.1.2. Specificity

The detection of CTCs by multiparameter flow cytometry contributed a higher specificity compared with RT-PCR. We detected the expression of Ep-CAM in three typical advanced breast cancer (ABC) patient (CTCs ≥ 5) and three limited breast cancer (LBC) patients (CTCs < 5). The result showed that the expression of Ep-CAM was positive for both patients with ABC and LBC as shown in **Figure 2**. It was hard to distinguish ABC with LBC by RT-PCR, while the flow cytometry could distinguish them obviously and quantitatively.

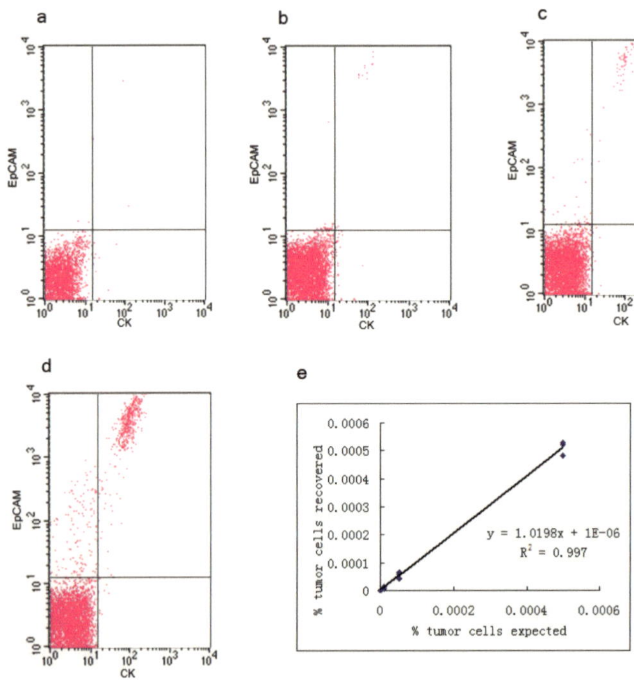

Figure 1. The ability to detect human tumor cells SKBR-3 cells in normal blood by cytomentry is titratable down to a sensitivity of 0.001%.Human tumor cells concentration was normalized adding to the leukocyte count, and serial dilutions (0.0001, 0.001%, 0.005%, 0.05%) using normal mononucleocytes as the diluent. Samples were lysed, incubated with anti-CD45-PerCP (20ul), EpCAM (20ul) and Cytokeratin8, 18, 19 (20ul) at 4°C for 30 minutes, and resuspended in 250ul PBS before multiparameter flow cytometric analysis. For samples with normal blood cells, up to 1000,000 total events were collected. Events that fell within up right region were counted as meeting the criteria for SKBR-3 tumor cells (CD45-EpCAM+CK+). Representative SKBR-3 cells are shown for **(a)** 0.0001% **(b)** 0.001% **(c)** 0.005%, **(d)** 0.05%. **(e)** Correlation and regression analysis of recovered versus expected number of positive tumor events at dilutions significant at the 0.01 level (2-tailed, R^2 =0.997, three separate experiments.). The percentage of tumor cells recovered was not significantly different from the percentage of tumor cells expected based on the serial dilutions (P>0.6, Mann-Whitney rank sum test).

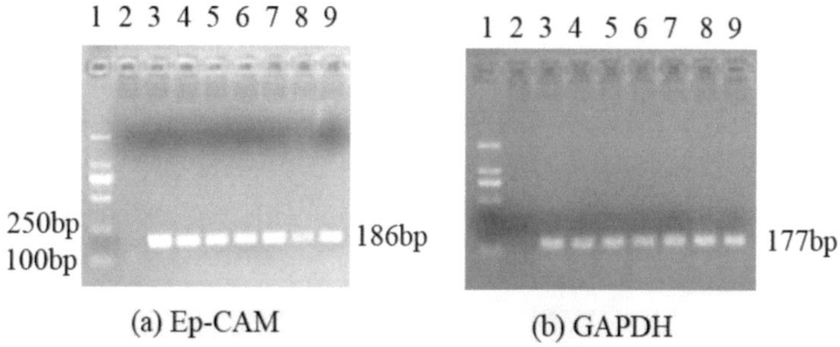

Figure 2. RT-PCR assay for EpCAM mRNA **(a)** and GAPDH mRNA **(b)**. 1. DNA ladder, 2. negative control (H_2O), 3. positive control (SKBR-3 cells), 4.5.6. ABC samples, 7.8.9. LBC samples. All were positive. Size of EpCAM and GAPDH is 186bp and 177bp, respectively.

Patient no.	EPCAM (10^{-5})		CD44	
	CTC <50	CTC≥50	CTSC negative	CTSC positive
1	24.41	97.66	0.38	0.41
2	2.99	72.99	0.36	0.62
3	4.96	48.81	0.48	0.96
4	3.29	1.66	0.92	0.82
5	1.19	3.41	0.75	0.63
6	2.99	24.41	0.66	0.46
7	2.28	24.39	1.04	0.84
8	6.31	48.85	0.44	0.57
9	5.17	39.39	4.20	0.17
10	48.83	5.50	1.01	0.34
11	69.05	48.88	1.17	0.41
12	30.27	2.81	0.84	1.43
13	4.38	11.08	0.06	3.39
14	41.92	6.10	0.63	0.99
15	10.05	5.98	0.58	0.49
16	75.56		0.43	0.47
17	2.62		0.50	
18	29.24			
Control	0.14 ± 0.02	0.59 ± 0.10		

Table 2. Analysis of EPCAM and CD44 gene expression in patients with BC.

We also compared breast cancer (BC) patients with healthy volunteers by QRT-PCR. The expression of Ep-CAM was increased statistically higher in patients with BC (24.29 ± 44.10 vs. $0.14 \pm 0.02 \times 10^{-5}$, $P = 0.000$) than in healthy volunteers, which was shown in **Table 2** and it was calculated by $2^{-\Delta t}$ method. However, there were no obvious differences between BC and health on the expression of CD44. Therefore, we confirmed that Ep-CAM and CD44 cannot be identified by QRT-PCR but can be identified by multiparameter flow cytometry.

3.2. Patient characteristics

Forty-five patients were identified and included in this analysis (detail is shown in **Table 1**); 27 (60.0%) patients had CTCs levels <5 and 18 (40.0%) patients had CTCs levels ≥5, respectively. The age of all the 45 patients ranged from 32 to 74, while the median age of CTCs levels <5 group was 49 years and the median age of CTCs ≥5 was 51 years. There were 25 (55.6%) patients in metastasis including 15 (33.3%) patients had CTCs ≥5. At the same time, there were 20 (44.4%) patients with no metastasis including 17 patients had CTCs <5. It showed that there was statistically significantly differences ($P = 0.002$) on CTCs level between the metastasis group and no metastasis group by chi-square test analyses. And the statistical differences of CTCs level also exist in different TNM stage ($P = 0.033$).

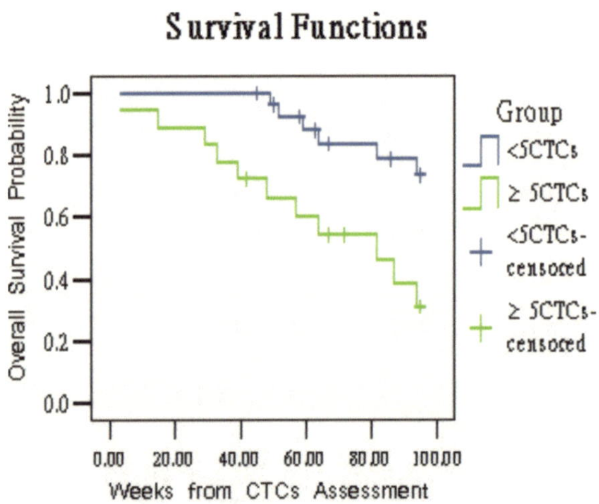

Figure 3. Kaplan-Meier Plots of overall survival are shown for all patients during the follow-up. 27 patients in CTCs <5 group and the median survival is estimated to be 95 weeks. 18 patients in CTCs≥5 group and the median survival is 65.5 weeks. *P* value is 2-tailed. Logrank indicates the *P* value, p=0.004.

3.3. Survival analysis

There were 17 (37.8%) patients who died during the follow-up period including 11 (24.5%) patients in CTCs ≥5 group. The median survival among CTCs <5 group was 95 weeks (standard deviation, 18.67 weeks) and the median survival among CTCs ≥5 was 65.5 weeks (standard deviation, 30.0 weeks). Axillary lymph node dissection (ALND) had correlation with CTCs level ($P = 0.143$) and 45.7% ALND patients got CTCs ≥5. During the follow-up, 11 (24.4%) patients got lost contact with seven (15.6%) in < 5 CTCs and four (8.9%) in ≥ five CTCs group. The results of the patients survival are shown in **Figure 3** by Kaplan-Meier with logrank P=0.004 and Breslow P=0.003, which confirm that the survival of CTCs < 5 and CTCs ≥ 5 group were different statistically. And the overall survival (OS) of CTCs < 5 group was higher than CTCs ≥ 5 group.

Variables	b_j	S_{bj}	P	expb_j	95.0% CI for expb_j	
					Lower	Upper
Age	0.101	0.031	0.001	1.107	1.042	1.176
CTCs	1.204	0.589	0.041	3.333	1.050	10.581
ALND	-1.813	1.111	0.103	0.163	0.018	1.439
Diameter	1.029	0.822	0.211	2.799	.558	14.025
Metastasis	2.825	0.910	0.002	16.855	2.834	100.237

Table 3. Cox regression analysis results.

In addition, we found that the prognosis of patients with breast cancer was statistical significant in CTCs level ($P = 0.041$), age ($P = 0.001$) and metastasis ($P = 0.002$) base on the Cox regression analysis for the follow-up in 45 patients as shown in **Table 3**.

3.4. Circulating tumor stem cells

We also analyzed the expression of CTSCs and the characteristic of clinical data was shown in **Table 4**. There were 21 patients had at least one CTSCs expression among 45 patients with breast cancer. The CTSCs level in different TNM stages was statistically different ($P = 0.020$). It was obvious that stage III and IV patients contributed more CTSCs expression than stage I and II.

Patient characteristics	Number (%)	CTC (%)		P-value	CTSC (%)		P-value
		<50	≥50		Negative	Positive	
Age (years)				0.247			0.168
≤45	24 (53.3)	12 (50)	12 (50)		10 (41.7)	14 (58.3)	
>45	21 (46.7)	15 (71.4)	6 (28.6)		14 (66.7)	7 (33.3)	
TNM stage				0.0272*			0.0202*
0	4 (8.9)	4 (100.0)	0 (0.0)		4 (100.0)	0 (0.0)	
I	6 (13.3)	6 (100.0)	0 (0.0)		4 (66.7)	2 (33.3)	
II	14 (31.1)	8 (57.1)	6 (42.9)		10 (71.4)	4 (28.6)	
III	19 (42.2)	9 (47.4)	10 (52.6)		6 (31.6)	13 (68.4)	
IV	2 (4.4)	0 (0.0)	2 (100.0)		0 (0.0)	2 (100.0)	

Patient characteristics	Number (%)	CTC (%)		*P*-value	CTSC (%)		*P*-value
		<50	≥50		Negative	Positive	
Tumor size				0.155			0.165
Tis	4 (8.9)	4 (100.0)	0 (0.0)		4 (100.0)	0 (0.0)	
T1	10 (22.2)	7 (70.0)	3 (30.0)		7 (70.0)	4 (30.0)	
T2	20 (44.4)	12 (60.0)	8 (40.0)		8 (45.0)	11 (55.0)	
T3	5 (11.1)	1 (20.0)	4 (80.0)		2 (40.0)	3 (60.0)	
T4	6 (13.3)	3 (50.0)	3 (50.0)		2 (33.3)	4 (66.7)	
RLNM				0.075			0.0012*
0	24 (53.3)	16 (66.7)	8 (33.3)		19 (79.2)	5 (20.8)	
1–3	9 (20.0)	7 (77.8)	2 (22.2)		3 (33.3)	6 (66.7)	
>3	12 (26.7)	4 (33.3)	8 (66.7)		2 (16.7)	10 (83.3)	
Clinical pathology				0.264			0.098
CIS	4 (8.9)	4 (100.0)	0 (0.0)		4 (100.0)	0 (0.0)	
Infiltrating duct	36 (80.0)	21 (58.3)	15 (41.7)		16 (44.4)	20 (55.6)	
Mucous	2 (4.4)	1 (50.0)	1 (50.0)		2 (100.0)	0 (0.0)	
Infiltrating lobular	1 (2.2)	1 (100.0)	0 (0.0)		1 (100.0)	0 (0.0)	
Medullar	1 (2.2)	0 (0.0)	1 (100.0)		1 (100.0)	0 (0.0)	
Papillary	1 (2.2)	0 (0.0)	1 (100.0)		0 (0.0)	1 (100.0)	
Histology stage[a]				0.002*			0.919
I	4 (10.5)	3 (75.0)	1 (25.0)		2 (50.0)	2 (50.0)	
II	17 (44.7)	14 (82.4)	3 (17.6)		8 (47.1)	9 (52.9)	
III	17 (44.7)	4 (23.5)	13 (76.5)		7 (41.2)	10 (58.8)	
ER				0.0182*			0.482
-	13 (28.9)	4 (30.8)	9 (69.2)		8 (61.5)	5 (38.5)	
+	32 (71.1)	23 (71.9)	9 (28.1)		16 (50.0)	16 (50.0)	
PR				0.0052*			0.771
-	16 (35.6)	5 (31.3)	11 (68.7)		9 (56.3)	7 (43.7)	
+	29 (64.4)	22 (75.9)	7 (24.1)		15 (51.7)	14 (48.3)	
Her-2				0.405			0.262
1+	14 (31.1)	10 (71.4)	4 (28.6)		10 (71.4)	4 (28.6)	
2+	18 (40.0)	11 (61.1)	7 (38.9)		8 (44.4)	10 (55.6)	
3+	13 (28.9)	6 (46.2)	7 (53.8)		6 (46.2)	7 (53.8)	

CIS, carcinoma *in situ*.
[a]There are missing values.
*$P<0.05$.

Table 4. Patient characteristics in different CTC and CTSC levels.

http://dx.doi.org/10.5772/63423

The CTSC positive was also related with RLNM status (RLNM 0, 20.8%; RLNM 1–2, 66.7%; RLNM >3, 83.3%) and the *P*-value was 0.001. There were no statistical differences in regard to age, diameter of tumor, clinical pathology, histology stage, ER status, PR status and Her-2 status in different CTSC groups.

3.5. Percentages of CD45-cells, CTCs, CTSCs and their clinical relevance

The expression of CD45, CTCs and CTSCs was further explored in different BC groups (**Table 5**). The expression of CTSCs on CD45-C showed a rising tendency in different TNM stage ($P = 0.034$) and also in different RLNM status ($P = 0.001$).

Patient characteristics	$CD45^-$/MNC (%)	CTC/$CD45^-$ (%)	CTSC/$CD45^-$ (%)	CTSC/CTC (%)
TNM stage	a	a	*c	c
0	2.01 ± 1.08	0.11 ± 0.12	0.00 ± 0.00	0.00 ± 0.00
I	1.29 ± 0.92	0.24 ± 0.25	0.03 ± 0.05	5.38 ± 11.46
II	2.72 ± 5.26	0.42 ± 0.51	0.06 ± 0.14	3.72 ± 7.63
III	2.52 ± 2.22	0.48 ± 0.69	0.10 ± 0.09	2.71 ± 3.78
IV	1.94 ± 0.88	1.00 ± 0.53	0.29 ± 0.35	5.45 ± 2.05
RLNM	a	c	*c	a
0	2.43 ± 4.01	0.28 ± 0.28	0.02 ± 0.05	2.49 ± 6.30
1–3	1.99 ± 1.66	0.25 ± 0.21	0.14 ± 0.17	4.77 ± 8.89
≥4	2.46 ± 2.59	0.83 ± 0.90	0.14 ± 0.15	3.67 ± 4.05
Clinical pathology	c	*a	a	a
Carcinoma *in situ*	2.01 ± 1.08	0.12 ± 0.12	0.00 ± 0.00	0.00 ± 0.00
Infiltrating duct	2.00 ± 1.79	0.37 ± 0.38	0.09 ± 0.14	4.07 ± 6.86
Mucous	11.57 ± 13.04	0.21 ± 0.30	0.00 ± 0.00	0.00 ± 0.00
Infiltrating lobular	1.13 ± 0.00	0.24 ± 0.00	0.00 ± 0.00	0.00 ± 0.00
Medullar	0.84 ± 0.00	1.34 ± 0.00	0.00 ± 0.00	0.00 ± 0.00
Papillary	0.47 ± 0.00	3.14 ± 0.00	0.13 ± 0.00	0.42 ± 0.00
Histology stage	a	a	a	c
I	2.56 ± 1.78	0.18 ± 0.16	0.03 ± 0.04	7.43 ± 14.10
II	1.38 ± 0.85	0.34 ± 0.41	0.10 ± 0.14	4.32 ± 7.15
III	2.33 ± 2.29	0.66 ± 0.76	0.10 ± 0.14	2.56 ± 3.31
ER	b	b	b	b
-	1.55 ± 0.78	0.52 ± 0.41	0.08 ± 0.16	2.10 ± 3.03
+	2.67 ± 3.80	0.38 ± 0.61	0.07 ± 0.11	3.73 ± 7.24
PR	b	b	b	b

Patient characteristics	$CD45^-$/MNC (%)	CTC/$CD45^-$ (%)	CTSC/$CD45^-$ (%)	CTSC/CTC (%)
TNM stage	[a]	[a]	*[c]	[c]
-	2.09 ± 2.15	0.51 ± 0.42	0.08 ± 0.15	2.37 ± 3.37
+	2.49 ± 3.76	0.37 ± 0.63	0.07 ± 0.11	3.76 ± 7.49
Her-2	[a]	[a]	[c]	[a]
1+	2.93 ± 5.20	0.33 ± 0.47	0.03 ± 0.05	3.21 ± 7.63
2+	2.45 ± 2.32	0.36 ± 0.35	0.09 ± 0.14	1.68 ± 2.80
3+	1.57 ± 0.99	0.61 ± 0.83	0.11 ± 0.15	5.51 ± 7.96

*$P < 0.05$.
[a]ANOVA test.
[b]Student's *t*-test.
[c]Kruskal-Wallis test.

Table 5. Percentage of $CD45^-$ cells, CTC and CTSC, and their clinical relevance.

The percentages of CTCs on CD45-C with TNM and histology stage increasing. In addition, we found that the percentage of CTCs on CD45-C in ER^- and PR^- groups was higher than that in ER^+ and PR^+ groups. And so was on CTSCs. Above all, we found the relationship between the percentage of CTC on CD45-C and clinical pathology. Then, it was good for evaluate TNM stage and RLNM status according to the percentage of CTSC on CD45-C.

Therefore, multiparameter flow cytometry technique is capable enough to identify patients with breast cancer and assess the progression of disease.

4. Discussion

4.1. The significances of CTCs in breast cancer

The detection of CTCs by using multiparameter flow cytometry relied on the epithelial-specific marker, which was expressed on epithelial cells but not on leukocytes [2, 27, 28]. Some of the CTCs that had higher metastatic potential may lose the expression of epithelial-specific markers during the migration process [29–31]. We also target another epithelial-specific marker—Ep-CAM (epithelial-cell adhesion molecule) to avoid possible false negative [32]. In order to detect the tumor cells that come from epithelium tissue, a monoclonal antibody directed against CD45 for negative selection of leukocytes [9–11]. Therefore, we targeted the dual-positive cells (CD45-$EpCAM^+CK^+$) as a surrogate marker for CTCs. And the serial dilution test was demonstrated to confirm the sensitivity of the assay by adding SKBR-3 into healthy sample. At the same time, we also verified the higher specificity of multiparameter flow cytometry by comparing with RT-PCR, although RT-PCR had a higher sensitivity [10, 11, 33, 34]. However, the detection of CTCs by nucleic acid techniques may overestimate the sensitivity, which resulted from the membrane fragments or nucleic acid of markers because of the crack of tumor cells in circle. CTC detection should be performed on cell level. On the other hand, we came out the result that RT-PCR could not identify the ABC patient (CTCs ≥ 5) from LBC patients (CTCs < 5) because of the high sensitivity of RT-PCR technology. We chose the multiparameter flow cytometry as the way to detect CTCs under considering the balance of sensitivity and specificity. It was important to discard the first few milliliters of sampled blood to make sure that there was no false positive because of the epithelial cell fell off from the skin when punctured.

Some researchers had tried the immunomagnetic combining flow cytometry technique to detect CTCs, which had a higher false negative losing amount of target cells. This technique cost expensive and not brief enough to apply in clinical.

It was common to meet the problem in clinical that it was hard to distinguish the tumor from inflammation by imaging, while we found that there were no more than two CTCs in stage I. Budd et al. [35] proposed that it was more accurately to evaluate the development of disease by CTCs detection than imaging. Both tissue biopsy and marrow biopsy were traumatic, but CTCs detection by multiparameter flow cytomety was atraumatic that can be achieved in clinical. Above all, multiparameter flow cytometry was the appropriate technique for the detection of CTCs to monitor the progression of breast cancer.

We demonstrated that the retrospective study to confirm the CTCs detection by multiparameter flow cytometry technique was a value method to apply in clinical. It suggested the patients who had CTCs ≥5 prompting a poorer median overall survival (65.5 weeks vs. 95 weeks; $P < 0.05$). We also found that the prognosis of the breast cancer was related with CTCs level, age and metastasis but not the clinical pathology and diameter of tumor. Cristofanilli et al. [36] also proposed that the patients with ≥5 CTCs/7.5 ml common had poorer prognosis compared with patients with <5 CTCs. CTCs detection by multiparameter flow cytometry should be a significant method for the evaluation of development and prognosis of cancer, and it also helped to estimate the treatment of target therapy for patients.

4.2. The significances of CTSCs in breast cancer

We chose $CD44^+CD24^-$ as an excellent marker in CTSCs identify. $CD44^+CD24^-$ had been considered as the marker of CSC [17, 37]. While CD133 was much more restricted in expression compared with CD44 that was the reason we did not chose CD133 as the CTSCs marker [38–40]. ALDH1 was another maker to identify CSC from BC. Ginestier et al. reported that the expression of ALDH1 in normal and breast cancer was 3–10%, while expression of $CD44^+CD24^-$ was 31% in contrast [41, 42]. In summary, $CD44^+CD24^-$ was an excellent maker in CSC identify.

CTCs may exist after mastectomy and chemotherapy; even there was no clinical manifestation of breast cancer. It was explained as the theory of "dormancy" in tumor cells [43]. And it was a part of tumor stem cells. Once the balance between proliferation and apoptosis was destroyed by some inducement, the disease progressed. The immune system and angiogenesis was reported, which were correlated closely with tumor cell dormancy [43, 44]. When the tumor stem cells fell off the primary tumor, they came into the peripheral circle and became the circulating tumor stem cells (CTSCs).

We successfully confirmed that the existence of CTSCs and also reveal the relationship between CTSCs level and different TNM stages. The correlation of CTSCs and clinical pathologic features remains unclear before. Previous study had reported that the $CD44^{+}CD24^{-}$ cancer stem cells was not correlated with clinical features such as lymph node status, tumor size, histology grade, ER, and PR, or HER-2 [45, 46].

It was reported that the patients who had high expression of $CD44^{+}CD24^{-}$ tumor stem cells were related with distant metastasis, particularly osseous [45]. And we found the expression of CTSCs was quite related with RLNM status. It was a novel way for treatment targeting at CTSCs to prevent metastasis and to evaluate the prognosis.

Cancer stem cells (CSCs) had been confirmed existed in many kinds of epithelial malignancy [47]. And the CSCs were considered as a subpopulation of tumor cells [48]. The mutation of normal stem cells resulted in the genesis of CSCs, which had been demonstrated by Cariati and Purushotham [49]. Therefore, CTSCs were suggested that it was generated not only from CTCs but also from normal stem cells. Further researches needed to be performed to confirm it.

Detection of CTCs and CTSCs by using multiparameter flow cytometry was considered as an effective technique on monitoring disease development and evaluating prognosis [50, 51]. Using multiparameter flow cytometry to detect CTC and CTSC in peripheral blood may provide new opportunities for the early diagnosis of invasive breast cancer, guide us to select optimal therapeutic regimens and help us to predict the prognosis. Moreover, we wish to isolate the CTSCs that have the marker of $CD44^{+}CD24^{-}ESA^{-}$ expressing. Further researches on CTSCs needed to be demonstrated and we have established a firm basis for following research.

5. Conclusion

Detection of CTCs by using multiparameter flow cytometry was effective and it has the potential to be a valuable method for both prognosis assessment and cancer research in breast cancer.

6. Looking forward

There is no doubt that CTCs would become an important test in clinical in near future. The challenge of the achievement contains the heterogeneity of CTCs and big database of clinical on CTCs. The heterogeneity of CTCs reflected in different tumor related proteins and morphology. However, researchers have pay more and more interesting on EMT phenotype that is common in all kinds of tumors. It will make CTCs detection accessible by decipherment of conundrums underlying EMT phenotype.

Acknowledgements

We thank the Department of oncology and cell therapy in Union Hospital for samples providing.

Author details

Yanjie Hu, Jin'e Zheng and Shiang Huang*

*Address all correspondence to: sa2huang@hotmail.com

Department of Center for Stem Cell Research and Application, Union Hospital, Tongji Medical College, Huazhong University of Science and Technology, Wuhan, China

References

[1] Gao YT, Shu XO, Kushi LH, Ruan Z, Bostick RM, Jin F, Zheng W. Association of menstrual and reproductive factors with breast cancer risk: results from the Shanghai Breast Cancer Study. Int J Cancer 2000; 87:295–300.

[2] Pantel K, Brakenhoff RH. Dissecting the metastastic cascade. Nature Rev Cancer 2004; 4:448–456.

[3] Ring A, Smith IE, Dowsett M. Circulating tumor cells in breast cancer. Lancet Oncol 2004; 5:79 88.

[4] Birchmeier C, Birchmeier W, Gherardi E, Woude GFV. Met, metastasis, motility and more. Nat Rev Mol Cell Biol 2003; 4:915–925.

[5] Uhr JW, Scheuermann RH, Street NE, Vitetta ES. Cancer dormancy: opportunities for newtherapeutic approaches. Nat Med 1997; 3: 505–509.

[6] Liotta LA, Stetler-Stevenson WG. Tumor invasion and metastasis: an imbalance of positive and negative regulation. Cancer Res 1991; 51:S5054–S5059.

[7] Zhao S, Liu Y, Zhang Q, Li H, Zhang M, Ma W, Zhao W, Wang J, Yang M.. The prognostic role of circulating tumor cells (CTC) detected by RT-PCR in breast cancer: a meta-analysis of published literature. Breast Cancer Res Treat 2011; 130:809–816.

[8] Blaqosklonny MV. Target for cancer therapy: proliferating cells or stem cells. Cancer 2006; 20:385–391.

[9] Martin VM, Siewert C, Scharl A, Harms T, Heinze R, Ohl S, Radbruch A, Miltenyi S, Schmitz J. Immunomagnetic enrichment of disseminated epithelial tumor cells from peripheral blood by MACS. Exp Hematol 1998; 26:252–264.

[10] Pachmann K, Heiss P, Demel U, Tilz G. Detection and quantification of small numbers of circulating tumour cells in peripheral blood using laser scanning cytometer (LSC). Clin Chem Lab Med 2001; 39:811–817.

[11] Naume B, Borgen E, Beiske K, Herstad TK, Ravnås G, Renolen A, Trachsel S, Thrane-Steen K, Funderud S, Kvalheim G. Immunomagnetic techniques for the enrichment and detection of isolated breast carcinoma cells in bone marrow and peripheral blood. J Hematother 1997; 6:103–114.

[12] Diamandis EP, Pantel K, Scher HI, Terstappen L, Lianidou E. Circulating cancer cells and their clinical applications. Clin Chem 2011; 57:1478–1484.

[13] de Bono JS, Scher HI, Montgomery RB, Doyle GV, Terstappen LW, Pienta KJ, Raghavan D.. Circulating tumor cells predict survival benefit from treatment in metastatic castration-resistant prostate cancer. Clin Cancer Res 2008; 14:6302–6309.

[14] Scher HI, Jia X, de Bono JS, Fleisher M, Pienta KJ, Raghavan D, Heller G. Circulating tumor cells as prognostic markers in progressive, castration-resistant prostate cancer. A reanalysis of IMMC38 trial data. Lancet Oncol 2009; 10:233–239.

[15] Korkaya H, Wicha MS. HER-2, notch, and breast cancer stem cells: targeting an axis of evil. Clin Cancer Res 2009; 15:1845–1847.

[16] Maheswaran S, Sequist LV, Nagrath S, Ulkus L, Brannigan B, Collura CV, Inserra E, Diederichs S, Iafrate AJ, Bell DW, Digumarthy S, Muzikansky A, Irimia D, Settleman J, Tompkins RG, Lynch TJ, Toner M, Haber DA. Detection of mutations in EGFR in circulating lung-cancer cells. N Engl J Med 2008; 359:366–377.

[17] Al-Hajj M, Wicha MS, Benito-Hemandez A, Morrison SJ, Clarke MF. Prospective identification of tumorigenic breast cancer cells. Proc Natl Acad Sci USA 2003; 100:3983–3988.

[18] Ross AA, Cooper BW, Lazarus HM, Mackay W, Moss TJ, Ciobanu N, Tallman MS, Kennedy MJ, Davidson NE, Sweet et al. Detection and viability of tumor cells in peripheral blood stem cell collections from breast cancer patients using immunocyto-chemical and clonogenic assay techniques. Blood 1993; 82:2605–2610.

[19] Mesker WE, vd Burg JM, Oud PS, Knepfle CF, Ouwerkerk V Velzen MC, Schipper NW, Tanke HJ. Detection of immunocytochemically stained rare events using image analysis. Cytometry 1994; 17:209–215.

[20] Pelkey TJ, Frierson HF Jr, Bruns DE. Molecular and immunological detection of circulating tumor cells and micrometastases from solid tumors. Clin Chem 1996; 42:1369–1381.

[21] Schulze R, Schulze M, Wischnik A, Ehnle S, Doukas K, Behr W, Ehret W, Schlimok G. Tumor cell contamination of peripheral blood stem cell transplants and bone marrow in high-risk breast cancer patients. Bone Marrow Transplant 1997; 19:1223–1228.

[22] Cote RJ, Beattie EJ, Chaiwun B, Beattie EJ. Detection of occult bone marrow micrometastasis in patients with operable lung carcinoma. Ann Surg 1995; 4:415–425.

[23] Allan AL, Vantyghem SA, Tuck AB, Chambers AF, Chin-Yee IH, Keeney M. Detection and quantification of circulating tumor cells in mouse models of human breast cancer using immunomagnetic enrichment and multiparameter flow cytometry. Cytometry Part A 2005; 65A:4–14.

[24] Leather AJ, Gallegos NC, Kocjan G, Savage F, Smales CS, Hu W, Boulos PB, Northover JM, Phillips RK. Detection and enumeration of circulating tumour cell in colorectal cancer. Br J Surg 1993; 80:777–780.

[25] Rosenberg R, Gertler R, Friederichs J, Fuehrer K, Dahm M, Phelps R, Thorban S, Nekarda H, Siewert JR. Comparison of two density gradient centrifugation systems for the enrichment of disseminated tumor cells in blood. Cytometry 2002; 49:150–158.

[26] Sringl J. Detection and analysis of mammaryglalld stem cells. J Pathol 2009; 217:229–241.

[27] Ring A, Smith IE, Dowsett M. Circulating tumour cells in breast cancer. Lancet Oncol 2004; 5:79–88.

[28] Moll R. Cytokeratins in the histological diagnosis of malignant tumors. Int J Biol Markers 1994; 9:63–69.

[29] Schaller G, Fuchs I, Pritze W, Ebert A, Herbst H, Pantel K, Weitzel H, Lengyel E. Elevated keratin 18 protein expression indicates a favorable prognosis in patients with breast cancer. Clin Cancer Res 1996; 2:1879–1885.

[30] Fuchs IB, Lichtenegger W, Buehler H, Henrich W, Stein H, Kleine-Tebbe A, Schaller G. The prognostic significance of epithelial-mesenchymal transition in breast cancer. Anticancer Res 2002; 22:3415–3419.

[31] Gotzmann J, Mikula M, Eger A, Schulte-Hermann R, Foisner R, Beug H, Mikulits W. Molecular aspects of epithelial cell plasticity: implications for local tumor invasion and metastasis. Mutat Res 2004; 566:9–20.

[32] Racila E, Euhus D, Weiss AJ, Rao C, McConnell J, Terstappen LW, Uhr JW. Detection and characterization of carcinoma cells in the blood. Proc Natl Acad Sci USA 1998; 95:4589–4594.

[33] Gross HJ, Verwer B, Houck D, Houck D, Hoffman RA, Recktenwald D. Model study detecting breast cancer cells in peripheral blood mononuclear cells at frequencies as low as 10(–7). Proc Natl Acad Sci USA 1995; 92:537–541.

[34] Palomares MR, Richardson-Lander A, Koehler KM, Gralow JR, Sabath DE. Quantitative real-time RT-PCR for the detection of circulating breast cancer cells: correlation

with stage and treatment. In: Proceedings of 26th Annual San Antonio Breast Cancer Symposium, 2002;217.

[35] Budd GT, Cristofanilli M, Ellis MJ, Stopeck A, Borden E, Miller MC, Matera J, Repollet M, Doyle GV, Terstappen LW, Hayes DF. Circulating tumor cells versus imaging – predicting overall survival in metastatic breast cancer. Clin Cancer Res 2006; 12:6403–6409.

[36] Cristofanilli M, Budd GT, Ellis M, Stopeck A, Miller MC, Matera J, Allard WJ, Doyle GV, Terstappen LW. Circulating tumor cells predict progression free survival and overall survival in metastatic breast cancer. N Engl J Med 2004; 351:781–791.

[37] Saldova R, Reuben JM, Hamid UMA, Rudd PM, Cristofanilli M. Levels of specific serum N-glycans identify breast cancer patients with higher circulating tumor counts. Ann Oncol 2011; 22(5):1113–1119.

[38] Xiao Y, Ye Y, Yearsley K, Jones S, Barsky SH. The lymphovascular embolus of inflammatory breast cancer expresses a stem cell-like phenotype. Am J Pathol 2008; 173:561–574.

[39] Wright MH, Calcagno AM, Salcido CD, Carlson MD, Ambudkar SV, Varticovski L. Brca1 breast tumors contain distinct CD44+/CD24- and CD133+ cells with cancer stem cell characteristics. Breast Cancer Res 2008; 10:R10.

[40] Lorico A, Rappa G. Phenotypic heterogeneity of breast cancer stem cells. J Oncol 2011; 2011:135039.

[41] Ginestier C, Hur MH, Charafe-Jauret E, Monville F, Dutcher J, Brown M, Jacquemier J, Viens P, Kleer CG, Liu S, Schott A, Hayes D, Birnbaum D, Wicha MS, Dontu G. ALDH1 is a marker of normal and malignant human mammary stem cells and a predictor of poor clinical outcome. Cell Stem Cell 2007; 1:555–567.

[42] Honeth G, Bendahl PO, Ringne'r M, Saal LH, Gruvberger-Saal SK, Lövgren K, Grabau D, Fernö M, Borg A, Hegardt C.. The CD44+/CD24- phenotype is enriched in basal-like breast tumors. Breast Cancer Res 2008; 10:R53.

[43] Holmgren L, O'Reilly MS, Folkman J. Dormancy of micrometastases: balanced proliferation and apoptosis in the presence of angiogenesis suppression. Nat Med 1995; 1:149–153.

[44] Schirrmacher V. T-cell immunity in the induction and maintenance of a tumour dormant state. Semin Cancer Biol 2001; 11:285–295.

[45] Abraham BK, Fritz P, McClellan M, Hauptvogel P, Athelogou M, Brauch H. Prevalence of CD44+/CD24-/low cells in breast cancer may not be associated with clinical outcome but may favor distant metastasis. Clin Cancer Res 2005; 11:1154–1159.

[46] Tanei T, Morimoto K, Shimazu K, Kim SJ, Tanji Y, Taguchi T, Tamaki Y, Noguchi S. Association of breast cancer stem cells identified by aldehyde dehydrogenase 1

http://dx.doi.org/10.5772/63423

expression with resistance to sequential paclitaxel and epirubicin-based chemotherapy for breast cancers. Clin Cancer Res 2009; 15:4234–4241.

[47] Gangemi R, Paleari L, Orengo AM, Cesario A, Chessa L, Ferrini S, Russo P. Cancer stem cells: a new paradigm for understanding tumor progression and therapeutic resistance. Curr Med Chem 2009; 16:1688–1703.

[48] Soltanian S, Matin MM. Cancer stem cells and cancer therapy. Tumor Biol 2011; 32:425–440.

[49] Cariati M, Purushotham AD. Stem cells and breast cancer. Histopathology 2008; 52:99–107.

[50] Hu Yanjie, Fan Lingling, Zheng Jin'e, Cui Rui, Liu Wei, He Yanli, Li Xin, Huang Shiang. Detection of circulating tumor cells in breast cancer patients utilizing multiparameter flow cytometry and assessment of the prognosis of patients in different CTCs levels. Cytometry A 2010; 77(3):213–219.

[51] Wang Ningfang, Shi Lan, Li Huiyu, Hu Yanjie, Du Wen, Liu Wei, Zheng Jin'e, Huang Shiang, Qu Xincai. Detection of circulating tumor cells and tumor stem cells in patients with breast cancer by using flow cytometry. Tumor Biol 2012; 33(2):561–569.

Section 3

Epithelial–Mesenchymal Transition

Chapter 10

Epithelial-Mesenchymal Transition and its Regulation in Tumor Metastasis

Tao Sun, Yuan Qin and Wei-long Zhong

Additional information is available at the end of the chapter

http://dx.doi.org/10.5772/64497

Abstract

Epithelial-mesenchymal transition (EMT) plays a key role in cancer metastasis. This process is a complex, multi-functional, and tightly regulated developmental program. EMT has been extensively investigated, but the molecular regulation of its signaling pathway is highly complex. In this study, the different elements of EMT cascades that could be targeted were determined. Difficulties in translating the preclinical findings in routine clinic were also distinguished. Future research will provide insights into the activation and regulation of various EMT programs in different tumor types and at distinct stages of tumor development. These results will likely facilitate the development of early detection strategies and improve the therapeutic targeting of malignant solid tumors.

Keywords: tumor, tumor metastasis, EMT, regulation of EMT

1. Introduction

Cancer metastasis is the major cause of cancer morbidity and mortality. This process accounts for approximately 90% of cancer deaths. Epithelial-mesenchymal transition (EMT) is a characteristic of the majority of metastatic cells. EMT is a natural transdifferentiation mechanism that governs changes in cell states along the epithelial versus mesenchymal axes and confers epithelial-mesenchymal plasticity upon epithelial cells. In particular, epithelial cells are transformed from highly differentiated, polarized, and organized cells into undifferentiated, isolated, and mesenchymal-like cells with migratory and invasive properties. In this chapter, we summarize evidence supporting the widespread involvement of EMT in tumor pathogenesis and the regulation of cancer metastasis.

2. EMT: a naturally occurring transdifferentiation program

Normal adult tissues in terminally differentiated cells have been reprogrammed into pluripotent stem cells in the past 10 years [1, 2]. This process has resulted in the wide acceptance of the initial hypothesis that nearly any type of dedifferentiation or transdifferentiation is possible if the ectopic expression of a transcription factor is properly combined into adult cells. The successful experiments on reprogramming have led to the exploration of the factors that change the state of cells in nature rather than forced to ectopic gene expression.

EMT is the most important cell biology program among naturally occurring transdifferentiation programs. This process converts epithelial cells into mesenchymal derivatives, which is the reverse process of mesenchymal-epithelial transformation (MET) [3]. Accumulated evidence for the past two decades has suggested that EMT occurs during development to ensure the interconversions of cells utilized in the formation of different types of cells, thereby forming the organs of organization and complex multicellular organisms [3, 4]. This cell biological program is orchestrated by a group of transcription factors (EMT-TFs), such as the Snail, Twist, and Zeb families [4, 5].

Two other aspects of EMT are worthy to be discussed in detail. The EMT program in some epithelial tissues is apparently correlated with the residence of cells in stem cell-like states. Moreover, versions of the EMT program are adopted by cancer cells to obtain a series of processes associated with higher levels of malignancy. EMT exhibits the presence of mechanical connections between an individual and the pathogenesis of cancer. These processes prior to EMT are insignificant.

EMT governs changes in cell states along the epithelial versus mesenchymal axes and converts epithelial cells to mesenchymal cells when this program is fully executed. Weinberg described the extreme poles of the epithelial versus mesenchymal axes. Epithelial cells, frequently with polygonal shapes in monolayer culture, are polarized along their apical-basal axis and are tightly connected with one another laterally via adherens and tight junctions in vivo. These lateral ties can ensure the structural integrity of epithelial cell sheets. By contrast, full mesenchymal cells exhibit spindle-like morphology with no sign of apical-basal polarity. These cells are loosely attached to the surrounding extracellular matrix (ECM) through focal adhesions. These features can help improve motility and explain the invasion of mesenchymal cells relative to their epithelial counterparts.

The deep layer of biological contact between epithelial and mesenchymal cells is determined by the differences in their respective transcription programs. These programs also control the expression of other gene products and key structural proteins, including those involved in the maintenance of the cytoskeleton and the strengthening of cell-cell adhesion [3–5]. Thus, epithelial cells express different types of keratin to form intermediate filaments, whereas vimentin constitutes the intermediate filament protein of mesenchymal cells. The expression of cell adhesion molecules and polarized complexes in mesenchymal cells is generally inhibited. EMT is marked by the replacement of E-cadherin by N-cadherin, which leads to the formation of weak cell adhesion between adjacent cells.

EMT can be significantly and rapidly activated in epithelial cells in response to physiological signals in a cell autonomous or non-cell autonomous manner. When gastrulation is used as an example, EMT responds to the induction signal as follows. The program is activated in ectodermal epithelial cells and completely converts epithelial cells into mesoderm mesenchymal cells, such as fibroblast growth factor and Wnt signaling pathway [6]. Similarly, EMT can be rapidly activated in adult tissues; it reacts to wounding and promotes rapid wound healing. This process is necessary to reconstruct the epithelial barrier that is essential for protecting internal organs from external injury [7]. Such rapid conversion between epithelial and mesenchymal states suggests the plasticity of epithelial cells, which facilitates their response to EMT-inducing signals. In addition, this plasticity demonstrates that residence in one of these two states is maintained in a metastable manner, with complex molecular and cellular mechanisms to ensure that a cell is in one or another state for a long period.

The description of EMT as a binary that shifts cells from a fully epithelial state into a fully mesenchymal state misreads the normal actions of this program. EMT is typically only from a fully epithelial state to a partially mesenchymal state, with certain key epithelial markers retained [8, 9]. Nevertheless, obtaining even a subset of mesenchymal traits to endow cells that previously resided in a fully epithelial state with a suite of mesenchymal traits will produce far-reaching effect on their biology.

3. EMT and cancer pathogenesis

Nearly 80% of malignant tumors are derived from epithelial tissues, which produce common cancers, such as tumors of the lung, colon, breast, pancreas, prostate, bladder, ovary, kidney, and liver. The epithelial states of the corresponding normal cells of origin in each determined case sustain the expression of cytokeratin and E-cadherin, which are signs of the epithelial states of early tumor tissues. In addition, tumor cells in early tumors remain the key biological phenotypes of epithelial cells, such as a lack of motility and capability to form a continuous cell sheet. These qualities exhibit a sharp contrast with those of advanced cancer cells, which are products of a complex succession process that is frequently referred to as "tumor progression." Highly invasive tumor cells present mesenchymal features, such as motility and invasion, and the latter is associated with metastasis [10–12]. The acquisition of these malignant features at the mechanism level can be explained by activating EMT, which is previously dormant in tumor cells during tumor progression.

The acquisition of mesenchymal features in breast cancer is positively correlated with tumor progression and an aggressive subtype of the disease [13, 14]. Investigating a large body of loss-of-function and gain-of-function in xenograft tumor models is a direct means to describe the link between the activation of EMT and the degree of malignancy of a tumor. The consumption of EMT-TFS, such as Twist, Snail, and Zinc finger E-box binding homeobox 1 (ZEB1), in both human and mouse breast cancer cell lines significantly inhibits the metastatic dissemination, whether the site is the primary site of tumor formation (e.g., mammary fat pad mass) or after experimental introduction of cancer cells into venous circulation (i.e., tail-vein injection). By contrast, the ectopic activation of EMT can enhance metastatic dissemination of orthotopically implanted human breast cancer cells by forcing the expression of EMT-TFS [15–17].

EMT in patients with breast cancer does not only promote systemic dissemination but also function as a major factor of drug resistance and disease recurrence [18, 19]. A similar phenomenon has been observed in a mouse model of Her2-induced tumors in which Snail EMT-TF can be autoactivated in recurrent malignancy in vivo and make the tumors highly mesenchymal phenotype [20]. The results evidently show an association between EMT activation and tumor relapse. Moreover, the link between EMT activation and enhanced tumorigenicity has been verified in various human cancer cell lines [21]. The inhibition of epithelial-mesenchymal plasticity suppresses the valid transition of carcinoma cells from a weakly tumorigenic into a highly tumorigenic state by blocking the activation of Zeb1 EMT-TF; that is, a state where tumor-initiating cells demonstrate their improved capabilities [22].

Recent studies have associated EMT with the acquisition of immunosuppressive capabilities in various types of cancers. The expression of Snail EMT-TF in melanoma can simultaneously inhibit the differentiation of cytotoxic T cells and induce the immune inhibition of the formation of regulatory T cells; the latter effect is mediated through the production of platelets [23]. Meanwhile, EMT in breast cancer cells enhances the resistance of tumor cells to cytotoxic T cell-mediated lysis, which at least partially induces autophagy [24, 25]. The activation of EMT-TF ZEB1 in lung cancer cells has been linked to the upregulation of programmed death ligand 1 (PD-L1), which is an immunosuppressive molecule that can block tumor-infiltrating lymphocyte attack [26].

EMT activation has a pleiotropic function in driving cancer progression, and an increasing number of reports confirm that invasive cancer is related to various types of aggressive carcinoma cells. Thus, we believe that all carcinomas essentially develop traits that are related with malignancy through the activation of an EMT program in their constituent neoplastic cells. However, the EMT program associated with common cancers has not yet been determined because many clinical pathologists doubt the existence of this program and its role in the production of high-grade cancer [27]. Such reluctance primarily originates from the fact that all markers of clinical biopsy are difficult to score. Although scoring will be possible, cancer cells that underwent EMT are also difficult to distinguish from normal host tissues and adjacent tumor stromal cells. Many fibroblasts and myofibroblasts self-express EMT-related markers. Clear evidence of this program during tumor development can be obtained from cell detection that co-express both mesenchymal and epithelial traits with certain retained epithelial markers inherited from their fully epithelial precursors because cancer cells frequently experience the only part of the EMT program. Recent analysis suggests that all subtypes of invasive breast cancer tumor cells exhibit both epithelial and mesenchymal characteristics as shown by the in situ hybridization in human breast cancer specimens of pooled epithelial and mesenchymal markers [28]. In addition, a part of the circulating tumor cells is isolated from the peripheral blood of patients with advanced prostate and breast cancers, and they also co-express both epithelial and mesenchymal markers [28–30].

4. EMT and tumor metastasis

Through the blood or lymphatic system, tumor cells can migrate far from the primary site and then settle and grow in a remote site to complete tumor metastasis. This process plays a key role in tumor disease, malignance level, and death of over 90% of tumor patients. Several questionnaires have shown the low efficiency of tumor metastasis. The majority of tumor cells can fall off into the blood or lymphatic system, such that only a small portion can form micro metastases, and even fewer can achieve actual metastases and present specific organ affinity. Moreover, the metastatic times of different tumors are not the same [31]. Thus, understanding this process is significant, and the importance of EMT should be discussed from different aspects.

EMT is a characteristic of most metastatic cells [32]. In particular, highly differentiated epithelial cells are converted into undifferentiated and isolated ectomesenchymal cells with migration and invasive properties. Migration is one of the four basic steps in tumor cell metastasis. Various substances, such as secretion factors, growth factors, and ECM components, can stimulate the migration of tumor cells. Cell migration stimulated by these substances can be divided into random and directed migrations. Thus, tumor cells can migrate and metastasize. The migration capability of tumor cells is related to their potential to metastasize. The density of the negative charges that separate from the surface of the tumor cells increases, which enhances electrostatic repulsion between cells. This process facilitates the removal of tumor cells into a free state from the tumor tissue. The adhesion of molecules on the surface of tumor cells is mediated by cell adhesion molecules, namely selectins, integrins, Ig superfamily, and cadherin [33]. Intercellular adhesion capability decreases in the same type, which leads to the detachment of tumor cells from the primary tumor and the abnormal intercellular adhesion contact with the implantation of tumor cells in the vascular wall. Invasion is the important biological characteristic of malignant tumors. Every organization or organ has its own structure. Tumor cells that invade an organ should respond to environmental stress, such as the lack of oxygen and nutrients, low pH, active oxygen free radicals, and inflammation regulatory factor. When the invasive capability is strong, the degree of tumor malignancy will be high. Epithelial cells lose the characteristics of the epithelial cells of ectomesenchymal cells, and the phenotype EMT process is the molecular basis of cancer stem cell invasion and metastasis. In addition, during tumor development, many tumor cells exhibit changes in good plasticity through morphology and phenotype transformation, such as collective amoeboid transition (CAT) and mesenchymal-to-amoeboid transition (MAT) [34]. EMT is a transient dynamic process that is influenced by the microenvironment. Furthermore, in vitro studies are necessary to build an improved genetic mouse model and reliable marker for EMT to realize real-time monitoring of the body, understand the mechanism of tumor evolution and EMT, establish new EMT signs, and to explore the role of transcription factors in the induction of EMT [35]. The loss of epithelial cell polarity during EMT reduces contact between the environment and stromal cells. This process enhances cell migration and mobility, which results in mesenchymal phenotypes. Moreover, changes in cell phenotype, coupled with an alteration in the expression levels of E-cadherin, vimentin, N-cadherin, and α-SMA, among others, in particular, a drop in E-cadherin level, can reduce the adhesion of cells, which facilitates the invasion and metastasis of cells. The loss of E-cadherin expression has been considered the most notable feature of EMT [36]. EMT presents increased opportunities for cell metastasis during tumorigenesis, probably because of its loose cell characteristics. EMT can promote the transfer of various tumor cells. Tumor metastasis includes several steps, such as attacks that are the precondition for cell transfer. EMT plays an important role during tumor invasion. Non-invasive tumors are turned into highly invasive tumors when the E-cadherin protein of tumor cells is cut. Experiments have established EMT marks in some tumor cells in metastases.

Snail, Twist, and ZEBl transcription factors closely linked with EMT can enhance invasion and promote the degradation of E-cadherin. EMT is the interaction between tumor cells and adjacent tumor-associated stromal cells caused by the induction of the transcription factor in the tumor cells. The activation of tumor EMT typically occurs during signal swaps between tumor cells and adjacent stromal cells. The progression of primary tumor cells can raise each model into the surrounding stroma. The recruitment of cells form a "reactive" matrix, induce the release of EMT signals, and start tumor cells by activating the EMT transcription factors [37]. **Figure 1** shows the tumor metastasis and EMT.

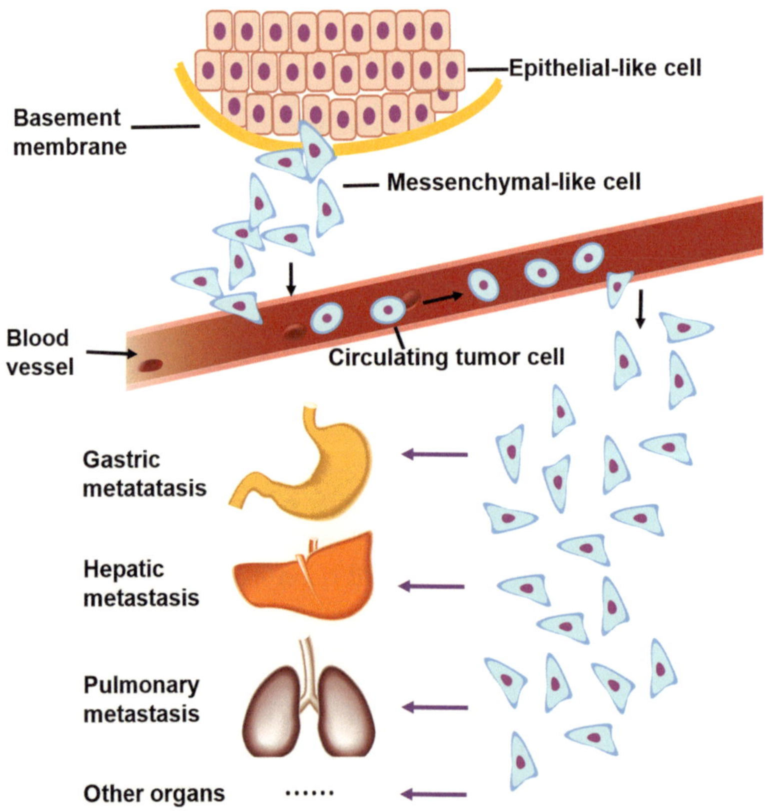

Figure 1. In EMT processes, tumor cells change from epithelial-like cells to mesenchymal-like cells and get the ability to metastasis.

5. EMT-activating transcription factors in cancer

Many transcription factors can induce EMT. Molecular reprogramming during an EMT is caused by three groups of transcription factors, namely the Snail, Twist, and ZEB families [38].

The Snail family includes Snail1, Snail2 (Slug), and Snail3 (Smuc). These factors regulate epithelial and mesenchymal markers [39, 40]. Snail1 induces signal to initiate EMT [41, 42]. These factors inhibit other epithelial markers that affect E-cadherin and bind to the E-cadherin promoter to inhibit its transcription. The Snail factors activate the expression of mesenchymal-like and pro-invasive genes that promote cell migration [43].

Snail factors are absent in normal epithelial cells. Snail1 is expressed higher than Snail2 and Snail3. An upregulated nuclear Snail1 expression is associated with tumor progression and can be found in the cytoplasm of several carcinomas. Snail1 staining is found among fibroblast-like cells, endothelial cells at the peritumoral stroma, and inflammation of colorectal carcinomas [44]. Snail1 promotes the recurrence of Her2/neu-induced breast tumors in mice, and its mesenchymal-like characteristics are exhibited in recurrent human carcinomas [45]. Therefore, recurrent breast carcinomas are induced by Snail1 spontaneously. High level of Snail1 is an independent predictor for reduced relapse-free survival in breast cancer patients. This factor is considered an independent prognostic factor for worst evolution and poor survival in many carcinomas [43].

Twist factor induces EMT by influencing other EMT-ATFs. Twist1 represses E-cadherin by inducing Snail1 or Snail2 and then binding to its promoter [46–48]. The knockdown of Twist1 in breast cancer cells represses the metastasis in xenograft models, but does not influence the formation of primary tumors [49]. Twist1 induces N-cadherin by driving its transcription and the mechanisms of post-transcription [50, 51]. Twist1 promotes the expression of mesenchymal markers without eliciting an N-cadherin/E-cadherin switch in glioblastoma cells [52]. In cell motility, the excessive expression of Twist1 upregulates the expression of cytoskeletal and ECM genes.

Twist1 and Twist2 are upregulated at the invasive front of carcinomas in cancer and stromal cells [53–55]. These factors are absent in normal epithelium but are induced in many human carcinomas, such as those of the digestive tract, liver, breast, ovary endometrium, and prostate [43]. Twist factors are upregulated in the cytoplasm and nuclei of cancer cells. Twist factors are independent prognostic factors for increased tumor recurrence, tumor aggressiveness, and the low survival rate of patients [49, 53, 56]. Twist and Snail factors play distinct but collaborative roles among EMT-ATFs.

The ZEB family includes zinc finger/homeodomain proteins, namely ZEB1 and ZEB2. The expression of ZEB factors drives an EMT by activating mesenchymal properties and repressing epithelial markers [43].

ZEB1 and ZEB2 bind to E-box sequences in the E-cadherin promoter but recruit different sets of co-repressors, namely SWI/SNF and CtBP for ZEB1 and NuRD and CtBP for ZEB2. ZEB proteins bind and repress the promoters of epithelial markers, such as R- and P-cadherins, gap junctions (connexins 26 and 31), cell polarity markers (Crumbs3, Pals1-associated tight junction protein, and lethal giant larvae homologue 2), desmosomes (plakophilin 3, desmoplakin), and components of tight junctions (claudin 7, occludin, junctional adhesion molecule 1, and zonula occludens protein 3). ZEB proteins activate mesenchymal markers, such as N-cadherin and vimentin [43]. ZEB1 and ZEB2 repress epithelial splicing regulatory proteins-1 and 2, the overexpression of which inhibits EMT [57].

ZEB1 inhibits epithelial phenotype, although this factor is found in isolated fibroblasts and immune cells in the interstitial matrix. This factor is not expressed in normal epithelium and well-differentiated carcinomas that express E-cadherin [58, 59]. ZEB1 is highly expressed in invading dedifferentiated cancer cells of many tumors, such as colorectal, breast, liver, endometrial, lung, prostate, and pancreatic carcinomas. ZEB1 and ZEB2 are expressed by stromal cells in epithelial tissues and organs of normal E-cadherin-positive epithelial cells [60]. ZEB-dependent paracrine signaling from the stroma can cooperate in E-cadherin repression in other parts of the tumor [61].

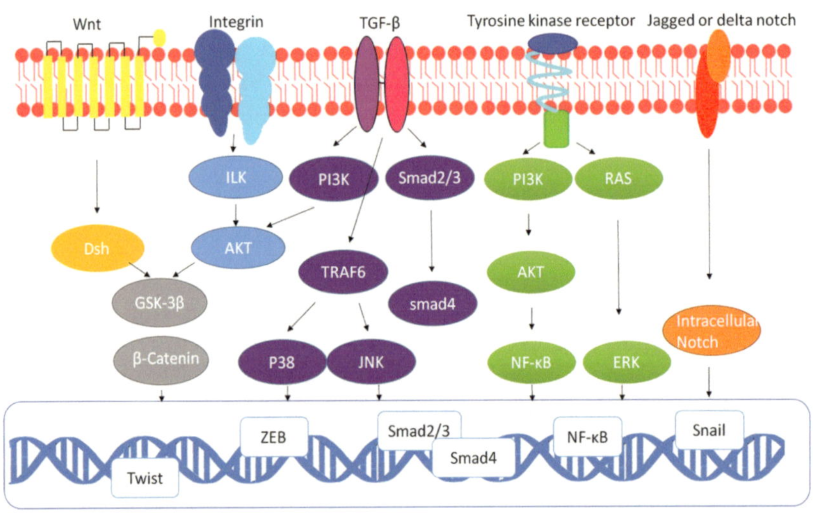

Figure 2. The main signaling pathways involved in EMT.

Other transcription factors also induce EMT and tumor invasiveness. The homeobox factor goosecoid induces EMT by activating mesenchymal genes and repressing epithelial markers [62]. TGF-β induces goosecoid in breast epithelial cells, and goosecoid is overexpressed in ductal breast carcinomas and atypical ductal hyperplasia [62]. **Figure 2** shows the main signaling pathways involved in EMT.

6. EMT in a clinical perspective

EMT significantly affects metastasis in cancers [63]. This process has attracted increasing attention because metastasis is vital in cancer recurrence and in death caused by cancer [64,

65]. In addition, understanding this process is important to determine medical diagnosis and treatment approach. Notably, sufficient information on biomarkers can lead to accurate forecast and precise therapeutic methods for metastases. Hence, proper diagnostic and therapeutic treatment for patients with early-stage cancer can promote good prognosis and prolong survival time to further improve the quality of life of patients [66, 67]. Furthermore, TBLR1, Sam68, SNAI1, Twist 2, etc. have been diagnosed markers or prognostic factors. This information is clinically important to predict survival and provide promising therapeutic targets for patients with early stage cancer [68, 69].

Sulforaphane or salinomycin treatment changes the stemness properties of cancer stem cells (CSCs), which may have been caused by the regulation of the expression of a special gene or protein. Sulforaphane downregulates Twist-1 and vimentin. By contrast, salinomycin treatment does not only significantly reduce vimentin level but also induce and upregulate E-cadherin expression in special cancer cell lines. Various reports have indicated a key role of E-cadherin in EMT. Thus, studying these cadherins can be a promising strategy [70, 71].

Epithelial cancer cells tend to differentiate to acquire invasive and stem cell-like properties. Thus, EMT regulators may function as therapeutic targets of cancer progression and recurrence. EMT-TFs, such as Twist, Snail, and ZEB, will be regarded as potent therapeutic targets for pharmacologic inhibition. Traditionally, EMT regulators are nearly impossible to target; however, evidence suggests that molecular links can offer the possibility for targeting regulation as a therapeutic intervention of EMT among metabolic adaptation, epigenetic alteration, and EMT [4, 72–74].

EMT significantly affects epigenome restructuring. Thus, epigenetic therapies can be used to realize the pharmacologic inhibition of EMT, which makes EMT sensitive to chemotherapy. In recent years, potential EMT inhibitors function as an effective chemotherapeutic sensitive agent, such as HDAC enzymes LBH589 [75]. In addition, histone demethylase LSD1 epigenetic modifiers offer important information on the survival of EMT by reducing invasiveness or inhibiting the transfer function. Thus, inhibiting LSD1 [76] may lead to improved survival because of the inhibition of invasiveness and metastasis [76].

Although epigenetic therapies exhibit considerable potential for clinical applications, the clinical application of epigenetic drugs remains ambiguous because of its unclear mechanism. The mechanism of epigenetic drugs should be investigated further. Therefore, the enhancement of specificity may solve the potential problem on the treatment of particular epigenetic targets in the future [74].

Drugs are likely to become anti-cancer drugs in clinical applications. Further study on the clinical trials of cancer has shown that metformin arouses attention as a promising anti-cancer agent [77, 78]. Metformin involves systemic effects, such as reducing insulin levels and acting on one-carbon metabolism. This metabolism will be explored with epigenetic alterations based on the connection between metabolism and the epigenetic state of cells [79].

Decitabine, which is a DNA methyltransferase (DNMT) inhibitor, suppresses the migration capacities of SDH-mutant cells. This inhibition is evidently displayed by succinate abnormal accumulation in epigenetic dysregulation and the resultant EMT. Mutant enzymes to directly explore the inhibition approach for SDH- and FH-associated cancers are worthy to be explored [80].

7. Epigenetic modification and EMT

EMT is a comprehensive reprogramming during tumor development. This process involves metabolism, epigenetics, and differentiation. In a specific tumor microenvironment, EMT-dedifferentiated cells escape the primary tumor after they acquire migration and invasion capabilities, invade the surrounding tissues, enter into the blood or lymphatic vessels, and settle in distant organs. EMT converts differentiated epithelial cancer cells to an undifferentiated state, thereby expressing stem cell markers and acquiring stem cell-like functions. This process is reversible, and mesenchymal cells can differentiate into epithelial phenotypes. Thus, an important process is developed in the macroscopic metastases in different organs.

DNA methylation, histone modification, and microRNA are the three types of epigenetic modification. Many studies have shown that epigenetic modifications play a key role in tumor metastasis [81]. The downregulation of E-cadherin (a cell adhesion molecule) expression during EMT is an important feature. Therefore, the precise regulation of E-cadherin expression via epigenetic modifications is extremely important to the occurrence of EMT. Several EMT-related transcription factors are recruited as E-cadherin gene promoter, which inhibits transcription [4]. Studies have shown that E-cadherin can be inhibited by the synergy of various histone modification enzymes. The E-cadherin gene promoter is inhibited to different extents to silence E-cadherin expression [82].

The characteristics of EMT are reversible in the type of stem cells and malignant features. Tumor stem cells are unique undifferentiated cells, rather than increasing diffusion, compared with most differentiated epithelial cells. The diffusion of anabolic needs is related to the maintenance of an undifferentiated state, which may be metabolic alterations of the links between EMT and tumor [83]. A change in cell metabolism is an important sign of cancer. The best metabolic phenotype in tumor cell is characterized by the Warburg effect, which proves that ATP is not the only metabolite of tumor cells [84]. Further studies have shown that aerobic glycolysis can better satisfy the basic needs of cell division, known as the post-Warburg model. This process is not only associated with cancer and normal cell proliferation, but also inhibits mitotic cell differentiation. In the same inducers, bunah and inactivated tumor suppressor genes, even oxygen glycolysis capability increased in the EMT, can be attributed to cell undifferentiated state. The appropriate energy level is sufficient for biosynthesis precursor, balancing normal state, and maintaining an undifferentiated state.

Epigenetic modifications are complex, dynamic, and connected with the extracellular environment and nuclear transcription. Energy availability is extremely important. Energy-rich substances, such as carbohydrates and fats, in the human body translate into ATP, along with a large number of metabolites, such as glycolysis and fatty acid oxidation. These metabolites can also drive epigenetic modifications in gene expression. A change in the intermediate metabolites of EMT may not be simple. Metabolic reprogramming plays a role in the energy

http://dx.doi.org/10.5772/64497

crisis causation of cancer cells. This process determines the epigenetic sand by modifying the undifferentiated state of the chromatin structure. Reprogrammed genes and the change in gene expression influence EMT markers and metabolic enzymes to overcome the local restriction to obtain energy in the distant tissues and organs. The microenvironment is significant for the EMT metastasis potential of cancer cells in reprogramming metabolism, epigenetics, and differentiation. Hepatic, epidermal, and fibroblast growth factors activate and maintain the EMT process. The cancer microenvironment growth factor activity generally regulates the interaction between metabolism and EMT to coordinate cell differentiation and metabolism.

The transfer process is the key to the reversibility of EMT based on our previous study, in which EMT regulation is mainly at the transcription level [4]. However, numerous molecular mechanisms cooperate to change the behavior of tumor cells. In particular, the role of the transcription regulation of EMT in the regulation and control of gene expression of the transcription of alternative splicing is extremely important. Spliceosome assembly has experienced gradual, composition, and structure changes required for normal maintenance. The correlation of alternative splicing tumor progression becomes apparent. In fact, all major cell biology deregulations of cancer are related to the changes in the alternative splicing of a specific gene profile. Modifying the splicing expression and activities supervised by SR and hnRNP provides the main source of changes in the stitching program observed in cancer cells [85].

Malignant EMT plays a key role during transfer, and the alternative splicing program affects the cell phenotype, including protein, cell adhesion, and cytoskeleton dynamics, influences tumor microenvironment, and controls tumor metastasis formation. Cancer gene mutations initiate processes, and epigenetic changes will be necessary to promote cancer. The change in the epigenome improves the transfer of cells.

In general, cells, which are affected by external environment signals, satisfy the internal requirements of nutrient and energy metabolism, as well as cooperate actively to promote the occurrence of EMT. Thus, tumor metabolic adaptations and EMT are different mechanisms for the same target cells to survive and grow. A close link and high correlation exist between metabolic reprogramming EMT and the similarity rule and fly mechanism.

8. Regulatory role of microRNAs in EMT

MicroRNAs (miRNAs) are expressed endogenously as small, non-coding RNAs that regulate various biological processes by modulating gene expression at the post-transcriptional level [86]. MiRNAs play an important role in controlling tumor growth and progression. Some miRNAs function as oncogenes and tumor suppressors. Moreover, miRNAs are also master regulators of EMT and dynamically regulate balance between EMT and MET.

The miR-200 family consists of five miRNA sequences, namely miR-200a, miR-200b, miR-200c, miR-141, and miR-429. Aggregated miRNAs that are expressed as two independent polycistronic pri-miRNA transcripts are as follows: miR-200a, miR-200b, and miR-429 (chromosome 1); and miR-200c and miR-141 (chromosome 12) [87].

The autocrine TGF-β/ZEB/miR-200 signaling regulatory networks that control epithelial and mesenchymal states change in the cells. ZEB1/2 and TGF-β exhibit strong correlation, and negative correlations are detected between TGF-β and miR-200, as well as between ZEB1/2 and miR-200, in invasive ductal carcinomas [88]. ZEB1/2 can induce EMT by inhibiting various epithelial genes [89].

Other miRNAs can directly target EMT transcription factors. MiR-205 in mammary cells maintains epithelial differentiation [90–92]. MiR-29b in prostate cancer inhibits metastasis by regulating the EMT signal. MiR-148a in hepatocellular carcinoma (HCC) cells can negatively regulate Met/Snail signaling and prevent EMT and metastasis [93]. Snail and miR-34 form another double feedback loop. EMT is induced by TGF-β, and an increase in Snail expression can be inhibited by miR-34. A novel miR-203/SNAI1 feedback loop has also been reported in breast cancer. These double feedback loops can enhance the balance between EMT activation and control of the two states of the cell (epithelial and mesenchymal). A novel EMT network that integrates the negative feedback loops, miR-203/Snai1, and miR-200/ZEB has been proposed recently as a control epithelial cell plasticity switches during differentiation and cancer [94]. The expression of miR-10b in metastatic breast cancer cells is shown to be induced by the transcription factor Twist, which binds directly to the putative promoter of miR-10b. Twist-induced miR-10b inhibits the translation of mRNA encoding homeobox D10, which results in an increased expression of RHOC, which is a well-characterized prometastatic gene [95].

Many miRNAs interfere with EMT by targeting the structures of cell components [96–98]. MiR-155 is the direct transcriptional target of TGF-β/Smad 4 signaling [99]. MiR-155 ectopic expression can reduce the RhoA (Ras homolog gene families, member A) protein, a small GTPase protein, to modulate the formation of tight junctions in the formation of stress fibers of the actin cytoskeleton during expression and destruction [100]. The activation of miR-31 in establishing metastases results in the regression of metastasis and the enhancement of the survival of patients. In addition, the induction of miR-31 can reduce the metastatic potential of cancer cells by targeting the RhoA [101]. The upregulation of miR-9 and direct repression of E-cadherin-1 (CDH1) in human breast cancer cells are involved in the regulation of cell-cell adhesion, migration, and the epithelial cell proliferation mechanism of calcium-dependent protein. CDH1 repression results in increased cell motility and invasion [102].

9. Inhibitors of EMT

Numerous tumor EMT inhibitors have been found in this study, and many of which are difficult to apply clinically because of stability and targeting isssues. TGF-β is an important factor in regulating EMT.

Various EMT inhibitors have been found in the TGF-β signaling pathway. Thyroid transcription factor-1 is a protein encoded by the NKX2-1 gene in normal tissues that can inhibit the secretion of TGF-β, which increases the expression of E-cadherin in lung cancer cells.

MMPs are other key factors in the induction of EMT. The inhibitors of MMPs play an important role in blocking EMT development in tumor cells. Several MMP inhibitors, which have been tested in clinical trials, can prevent EMT in cell experiments in vitro and inhibit tumor progression in in vivo animal experiments. Orlistat Plymouth, one of the MMP inhibitors, has a relatively significant effect on non-small cell lung cancer, colorectal cancer, and glioma, both in in vitro cell experiments and in vivo animal experiments. Conducting combination chemotherapy with marimastat, captopril, and Fragmin exerts a certain effect on the treatment of advanced kidney cancer. The human body itself can also synthesize a special kind of MMP inhibitor, a tissue inhibitor of metalloproteinase (tissue inhibitors of metalloproteinases, TIMPs). TIMPs, which are produced using genetic engineering technology, can also be used as targeted drugs to treat tumors caused by the imbalance among MMPs and inhibit the progression of EMT in tumor cells.

Certain phytochemicals or food substances exhibit anti-cancer [103, 104] and anti-EMT properties [105]. For example, AIMs (anthocyanidins) and Morusin (a prenylated flavonoid), which are isolated from the fruits of *Vitis coignetiae* Pulliat (known as meoru in Korea) and the root bark of *Morus australis* (Moraceae), respectively, demonstrate anti-cancer activities by inhibiting EMT through the suppression of nuclear factor (NF)-κB activity [106–108].

AIMs can inhibit NF-κB in a dose-dependent manner, and MMP-9 (EMT marker) can be regulated by NF-κB preferentially [109]. IκBα phosphorylation and GSK-3 activity can also be suppressed by increasing the levels of AIMs [110]. Moreover, AIM downregulates mesenchymal markers, such as Vim1, N-cadherin, and SNAI, as well as upregulates epithelial markers, such as E-cadherin [110]. The morphological changes induced by TNF-α [110] are also inhibited by AIM. The suppression of the migratory and invasive properties of cervical cells by AIM has also been reported. Cervical cancer contains a heterogeneous population of cells called CSCs. CSCs are cells with chemotherapy- and radiotherapy resistant properties and are involved in tumor recurrence, metastasis, and high mortality [111, 112]. Morusin, however, are reported to be cytotoxic to several cancer cell lines, including cervical cells. Morusin can inhibit migration and proliferation by inhibiting tumor sphere formation through the inhibition of the NF-kB pathway.

Recent studies in our laboratory have found several EMT inhibitors, including tetracycline and some natural products. The gelatinase inhibitor doxycycline is the prototypical anti-tumor antibiotic. We have investigated the effects of doxycycline on the migration, invasion, and metastasis of human lung cancer cell lines and in a mouse model. We have also measured the effect of doxycycline on the transcription of EMT markers and used immunohistochemistry to determine whether EMT reversal is associated with doxycycline inhibition. Doxycycline dose-dependently inhibits the proliferation, migration, and invasion of NCI-H446 human small cell lung cancer cells. It also suppresses tumor growth from NCI-H446 and A549 lung cancer cell xenografts without altering body weight, inhibits Lewis lung carcinoma cell migration, and prolongs survival. The activities of the transcription factors Twist1/2, SNAI1/2, AP1, NF-κB, and Stat3 are suppressed by doxycycline, which reverses EMT and inhibits signal transduction, thereby suppressing tumor growth and metastasis. Our data demonstrate functional targeting of transcription factors by doxycycline to reverse EMT and suppress tumor proliferation and metastasis. Thus, doxycycline selectively targets malignant tumors and reduces their metastatic potential with less cytotoxicity in lung cancer patients.

Apigenin is a naturally occurring compound with anti-inflammatory, antioxidant, and anticancer properties. We have investigated the effects of apigenin on migration and metastasis in experimental HCC cell lines in vitro and in vivo. Apigenin dose-dependently inhibits the proliferation, migration, and invasion of PLC and Bel-7402 human HCC cells. It also suppresses tumor growth in PLC cell xenografts without altering body weight, thereby prolonging survival. Apigenin reduces Snail and NF-κB expression, reversed increases in EMT marker levels, increases cellular adhesion, regulates actin polymerization and cell migration, and inhibits invasion and migration of HCC cells. Therefore, apigenin may inhibit EMT by inhibiting the NF-κB/Snail pathway in human HCC. **Table 1** shows some EMT inhibitors found in the last 3 years.

Molecules	Tumor types	Pathway	References
Cyclin G2	Ovarian cancer	Wnt/β-catenin	Bernaudo et al. [113]
FOXO3a	Prostate cancer	Wnt/β-catenin	Liu et al. [114]
sFRP4	Head and neck squamous cell carcinoma	Wnt/β-catenin	Warrier et al. [115]
sophocarpine	Hepatocellular carcinoma	AKT/GSK-3β/β-catenin	Zhang et al. [116]
Bisdemethoxycurcumin	Lung cancer	TGF-β	Xu et al. [117]
Ski	Lung cancer	TGF-β	Yang et al. [118]
GRP78	Colon cancer	TGF-β	Zhang et al. [119]
Thymoquinone	Breast cancer	TGF-β	Rajput et al. [120]
BMP-7	Cholangiocarcinoma	TGF-β	Duangkumpha et al. [121]
NDRG2	Colon cancer	TGF-β	Shen et al. [122]
Myrtucommulone-A and thymoquinone	Bladder cancer and breast cancer	PI3K	Iskender et al. [123]
ING5	Breast cancer	PI3K	Zhao et al. [124]
α-Mangostin	Pancreatic cancer	PI3K	Xu et al. [125]
NVP-BEZ235	Ovarian cancer	PI3K	Lin et al. [126]
IL-32θ	Colon cancer	STAT3	Bak et al. [127]
Luteolin	Pancreatic cancer	STAT3	Huang et al. [128]
FTY720	Cholangiocarcinoma	STAT3	Lu et al. [129]
NDRG2	Breast cancer	STAT3	Kim et al. [130]

Table 1. Some EMT inhibitors.

http://dx.doi.org/10.5772/64497

Author details

Tao Sun*, Yuan Qin and Wei-long Zhong

*Address all correspondence to: sunrockmia@hotmail.com

State Key Laboratory of Medicinal Chemical Biology and College of Pharmacy, Nankai University , Tianjin, People's Republic of China

References

[1] Yamanaka, S. and K. Takahashi, *Induction of pluripotent stem cells from mouse fibroblast cultures*. Tanpakushitsu Kakusan Koso, 2006. 51(15): p. 2346–51.

[2] Yu, J., et al., *Induced pluripotent stem cell lines derived from human somatic cells*. Science, 2007. 318(5858): p. 1917–20.

[3] Nieto, M.A., *Epithelial plasticity: a common theme in embryonic and cancer cells*. Science, 2013. 342(6159): p. 1234850.

[4] Thiery, J.P., et al., *Epithelial-mesenchymal transitions in development and disease*. Cell, 2009. 139(5): p. 871–90.

[5] Nieto, M.A., *The ins and outs of the epithelial to mesenchymal transition in health and disease*. Annu Rev Cell Dev Biol, 2011. 27: p. 347–76.

[6] Tam, P.P. and R.R. Behringer, *Mouse gastrulation: the formation of a mammalian body plan*. Mech Dev, 1997. 68(1–2): p. 3–25.

[7] Savagner, P., et al., *Developmental transcription factor slug is required for effective re-epithelialization by adult keratinocytes*. J Cell Physiol, 2005. 202(3): p. 858–66.

[8] Grunert, S., M. Jechlinger, and H. Beug, *Diverse cellular and molecular mechanisms contribute to epithelial plasticity and metastasis*. Nat Rev Mol Cell Biol, 2003. 4(8): p. 657–65.

[9] Theveneau, E., et al., *Collective chemotaxis requires contact-dependent cell polarity*. Dev Cell, 2010. 19(1): p. 39–53.

[10] Morel, A.P., et al., *EMT inducers catalyze malignant transformation of mammary epithelial cells and drive tumorigenesis towards claudin-low tumors in transgenic mice*. PLoS Genet, 2012. 8(5): p. e1002723.

[11] Rhim, A.D., et al., *EMT and dissemination precede pancreatic tumor formation*. Cell, 2012. 148(1–2): p. 349–61.

[12] Sarrio, D., et al., *Epithelial-mesenchymal transition in breast cancer relates to the basal-like phenotype*. Cancer Res, 2008. 68(4): p. 989–97.

[13] Aleskandarany, M.A., et al., *Epithelial mesenchymal transition in early invasive breast cancer: an immunohistochemical and reverse phase protein array study*. Breast Cancer Res Treat, 2014. 145(2): p. 339–48.

[14] Choi, Y., et al., *Epithelial-mesenchymal transition increases during the progression of in situ to invasive basal-like breast cancer*. Hum Pathol, 2013. 44(11): p. 2581–9.

[15] Guo, W., et al., *Slug and Sox9 cooperatively determine the mammary stem cell state*. Cell, 2012. 148(5): p. 1015–28.

[16] Roy, S.S., et al., *Significance of PELP1/HDAC2/miR-200 regulatory network in EMT and metastasis of breast cancer*. Oncogene, 2014. 33(28): p. 3707–16.

[17] Tran, H.D., et al., *Transient SNAIL1 expression is necessary for metastatic competence in breast cancer*. Cancer Res, 2014. 74(21): p. 6330–40.

[18] Cheng, Q., et al., *A signature of epithelial-mesenchymal plasticity and stromal activation in primary tumor modulates late recurrence in breast cancer independent of disease subtype*. Breast Cancer Res, 2014. 16(4): p. 407.

[19] Oliveras-Ferraros, C., et al., *Epithelial-to-mesenchymal transition (EMT) confers primary resistance to trastuzumab (Herceptin)*. Cell Cycle, 2012. 11(21): p. 4020–32.

[20] Moody, S.E., et al., *The transcriptional repressor Snail promotes mammary tumor recurrence*. Cancer Cell, 2005. 8(3): p. 197–209.

[21] Creighton, C.J., J.C. Chang, and J.M. Rosen, *Epithelial-mesenchymal transition (EMT) in tumor-initiating cells and its clinical implications in breast cancer*. J Mammary Gland Biol Neoplasia, 2010. 15(2): p. 253–60.

[22] Chaffer, C.L., et al., *Poised chromatin at the ZEB1 promoter enables breast cancer cell plasticity and enhances tumorigenicity*. Cell, 2013. 154(1): p. 61–74.

[23] Kudo-Saito, C., et al., *Cancer metastasis is accelerated through immunosuppression during Snail-induced EMT of cancer cells*. Cancer Cell, 2009. 15(3): p. 195–206.

[24] Akalay, I., et al., *Epithelial-to-mesenchymal transition and autophagy induction in breast carcinoma promote escape from T-cell-mediated lysis*. Cancer Res, 2013. 73(8): p. 2418–27.

[25] Akalay, I., et al., *Targeting WNT1-inducible signaling pathway protein 2 alters human breast cancer cell susceptibility to specific lysis through regulation of KLF-4 and miR-7 expression*. Oncogene, 2015. 34(17): p. 2261–71.

[26] Chen, L., et al., *Metastasis is regulated via microRNA-200/ZEB1 axis control of tumour cell PD-L1 expression and intratumoral immunosuppression*. Nat Commun, 2014. 5: p. 5241.

[27] Tarin, D., E.W. Thompson, and D.F. Newgreen, *The fallacy of epithelial mesenchymal transition in neoplasia*. Cancer Res, 2005. 65(14): p. 5996–6000; discussion 6000–1.

[28] Yu, M., et al., *Circulating breast tumor cells exhibit dynamic changes in epithelial and mesenchymal composition*. Science, 2013. 339(6119): p. 580–4.

[29] Husemann, Y., et al., *Systemic spread is an early step in breast cancer*. Cancer Cell, 2008. 13(1): p. 58–68.

[30] Raimondi, C., et al., *Epithelial-mesenchymal transition and stemness features in circulating tumor cells from breast cancer patients*. Breast Cancer Res Treat, 2011. 130(2): p. 449–55.

[31] Alonso, D.F., et al., *Metastasis: recent discoveries and novel perioperative treatment strategies with particular interest in the hemostatic compound desmopressin*. Curr Pharm Biotechnol, 2011. 12(11): p. 1974–80.

[32] Alizadeh, A.M., S. Shiri, and S. Farsinejad, *Metastasis review: from bench to bedside*. Tumour Biol, 2014. 35(9): p. 8483–523.

[33] Fridman, R., et al., *The role of cell adhesion and migration in the in vitro invasiveness of mouse adrenal carcinoma cells*. Invasion Metastasis, 1990. 10(4): p. 208–24.

[34] Spano, D., et al., *Molecular networks that regulate cancer metastasis*. Semin Cancer Biol, 2012. 22(3): p. 234–49.

[35] Gavert, N. and A. Ben-Ze'ev, *Epithelial-mesenchymal transition and the invasive potential of tumors*. Trends Mol Med, 2008. 14(5): p. 199–209.

[36] Peinado, H., D. Olmeda, and A. Cano, *Snail, Zeb and bHLH factors in tumour progression: an alliance against the epithelial phenotype?*? Nat Rev Cancer, 2007. 7(6): p. 415–28.

[37] Chaffer, C.L. and R.A. Weinberg, *A perspective on cancer cell metastasis*. Science, 2011. 331(6024): p. 1559–64.

[38] Garg, M., *Epithelial-mesenchymal transition - activating transcription factors – multifunctional regulators in cancer*. World J Stem Cells, 2013. 5(4): p. 188–95.

[39] Peinado, H., et al., *Snail and E47 repressors of E-cadherin induce distinct invasive and angiogenic properties in vivo*. J Cell Sci, 2004. 117(13): p. 2827–39.

[40] Bolós, V., et al., *The transcription factor Slug represses E-cadherin expression and induces epithelial to mesenchymal transitions: a comparison with Snail and E47 repressors*. J Cell Sci, 2003. 116(3): p. 499–511.

[41] Dave, N., et al., *Functional cooperation between Snail1 and twist in the regulation of ZEB1 expression during epithelial to mesenchymal transition*. Journal of Biol Chem, 2011. 286(14): p. 12024–32.

[42] Tran, D.D., et al., *Temporal and spatial cooperation of Snail1 and Twist1 during epithelial–mesenchymal transition predicts for human breast cancer recurrence*. Mol Cancer Res, 2011. 9(12): p. 1644–57.

[43] Sanchez-Tillo, E., et al., *EMT-activating transcription factors in cancer: beyond EMT and tumor invasiveness*. Cell Mol Life Sci, 2012. 69(20): p. 3429–56.

[44] Francí, C., et al., *Snail1 protein in the stroma as a new putative prognosis marker for colon tumours*. PLoS One, 2009. 4(5): p. e5595.

[45] Moody, S.E., et al., *The transcriptional repressor Snail promotes mammary tumor recurrence*. Cancer cell, 2005. 8(3): p. 197–209.

[46] Yang, J., et al., *Twist, a master regulator of morphogenesis, plays an essential role in tumor metastasis*. Cell, 2004. 117(7): p. 927–39.

[47] Smit, M.A., et al., *A Twist-Snail axis critical for TrkB-induced epithelial-mesenchymal transition-like transformation, anoikis resistance, and metastasis*. Mol Cell Biol, 2009. 29(13): p. 3722–37.

[48] Casas, E., et al., *Snail2 is an essential mediator of Twist1-induced epithelial mesenchymal transition and metastasis*. Cancer Res, 2011. 71(1): p. 245–54.

[49] Terauchi, M., et al., *Possible involvement of TWIST in enhanced peritoneal metastasis of epithelial ovarian carcinoma*. Clin Exp Metastasis, 2007. 24(5): p. 329–39.

[50] Alexander, N.R., et al., *N-cadherin gene expression in prostate carcinoma is modulated by integrin-dependent nuclear translocation of Twist1*. Cancer Res, 2006. 66(7): p. 3365–69.

[51] Yang, Z., et al., *Up-regulation of gastric cancer cell invasion by Twist is accompanied by N-cadherin and fibronectin expression*. Biochem Biophys Res Commun, 2007. 358(3): p. 925–30.

[52] Mikheeva, S.A., et al., *TWIST1 promotes invasion through mesenchymal change in human glioblastoma*. Mol Cancer, 2010. 9(1): p. 1.

[53] Song, L.-B., et al., *The clinical significance of twist expression in nasopharyngeal carcinoma*. Cancer Lett, 2006. 242(2): p. 258–65.

[54] Yuen, H.-F., et al., *Upregulation of Twist in oesophageal squamous cell carcinoma is associated with neoplastic transformation and distant metastasis*. J Clin Pathol, 2007. 60(5): p. 510–14.

[55] Fang, X., et al., *Twist2 contributes to breast cancer progression by promoting an epithelial–mesenchymal transition and cancer stem-like cell self-renewal*. Oncogene, 2011. 30(47): p. 4707–20.

[56] Yang, M.H., et al., *Comprehensive analysis of the independent effect of twist and snail in promoting metastasis of hepatocellular carcinoma*. Hepatology, 2009. 50(5): p. 1464–74.

[57] Horiguchi, K., et al., *TGF-β drives epithelial-mesenchymal transition through δEF1-mediated downregulation of ESRP*. Oncogene, 2012. 31(26): p. 3190–201.

[58] Brabletz, T., et al., *Variable β-catenin expression in colorectal cancers indicates tumor progression driven by the tumor environment*. Proc Natl Acad Sci, 2001. 98(18): p. 10356–61.

[59] Spaderna, S., et al., *A transient, EMT-linked loss of basement membranes indicates metastasis and poor survival in colorectal cancer*. Gastroenterology, 2006. 131(3): p. 830–40.

[60] Oztas, E., et al., *Novel monoclonal antibodies detect Smad-interacting protein 1 (SIP1) in the cytoplasm of human cells from multiple tumor tissue arrays*. Exp Mol Pathol, 2010. 89(2): p. 182–9.

[61] Gemmill, R.M., et al., *ZEB1-responsive genes in non-small cell lung cancer*. Cancer Lett, 2011. 300(1): p. 66–78.

[62] Hartwell, K.A., et al., *The Spemann organizer gene, goosecoid, promotes tumor metastasis*. Proc Natl Acad Sci, 2006. 103(50): p. 18969–74.

[63] Noordhuis, M.G., et al., *Involvement of the TGF-beta and beta-catenin pathways in pelvic lymph node metastasis in early-stage cervical cancer*. Clin Cancer Res, 2011. 17(6): p. 1317–30.

[64] Chen, Y., et al., *Significance of the absolute number and ratio of metastatic lymph nodes in predicting postoperative survival for the International Federation of Gynecology and Obstetrics Stage IA2 to IIA Cervical Cancer*. Int J Gynecol Cancer, 2013. 23(1): p. 157–163.

[65] Kodama, J., et al., *Prognostic factors in stage IB-IIB cervical adenocarcinoma patients treated with radical hysterectomy and pelvic lymphadenectomy*. J Surg Oncol, 2010. 101(5): p. 413–7.

[66] Wang, J., et al., *TBLR1 is a novel prognostic marker and promotes epithelial-mesenchymal transition in cervical cancer*. British Journal Of Cancer, 2014. 111(1): p. 112–24.

[67] Gao, Q., et al., *EphB2 promotes cervical cancer progression by inducing epithelial-mesenchymal transition*. Hum Pathol, 2014. 45(2): p. 372–81.

[68] Chen, Z., et al., *The nuclear protein expression levels of SNAI1 and ZEB1 are involved in the progression and lymph node metastasis of cervical cancer via the epithelial-mesenchymal transition pathway*. Hum Pathol, 2013. 44(10): p. 2097–105.

[69] Li, Y., et al., *Correlation of TWIST2 up-regulation and epithelial-mesenchymal transition during tumorigenesis and progression of cervical carcinoma*. Gynecol Oncol, 2012. 124(1): p. 112–8.

[70] Srivastava, R.K., et al., *Sulforaphane synergizes with quercetin to inhibit self-renewal capacity of pancreatic cancer stem cells*. Front Biosci (Elite Ed), 2011. 3: p. 515–28.

[71] Han, S.P., et al., *SNAI1 is involved in the proliferation and migration of glioblastoma cells*. Cell Mol Neurobiol, 2011. 31(3): p. 489–96.

[72] Kiesslich, T., M. Pichler, and D. Neureiter, *Epigenetic control of epithelial-mesenchymal-transition in human cancer*. Mol Clin Oncol, 2013. 1(1): p. 3–11.

[73] Sabbah, M., et al., *Molecular signature and therapeutic perspective of the epithelial-to-mesenchymal transitions in epithelial cancers*. Drug Resist Updat, 2008. 11(4–5): p. 123–51.

[74] Li, L. and W. Li, *Epithelial-mesenchymal transition in human cancer: comprehensive reprogramming of metabolism, epigenetics, and differentiation*. Pharmacol Ther, 2015. 150: p. 33–46.

[75] Di Fazio, P., et al., *The pan-deacetylase inhibitor panobinostat inhibits growth of hepatocellular carcinoma models by alternative pathways of apoptosis*. Cell Oncol, 2010. 32(4): p. 285–300.

[76] Wang, Y., et al., *LSD1 is a subunit of the NuRD complex and targets the metastasis programs in breast cancer*. Cell, 2009. 138(4): p. 660–72.

[77] Aljada, A. and S.A. Mousa, *Metformin and neoplasia: implications and indications*. Pharmacol Ther, 2012. 133(1): p. 108–15.

[78] Pierotti, M.A., et al., *Targeting metabolism for cancer treatment and prevention: metformin, an old drug with multi-faceted effects*. Oncogene, 2013. 32(12): p. 1475–87.

[79] Locasale, J.W., *Serine, glycine and one-carbon units: cancer metabolism in full circle*. Nat Rev Cancer, 2013. 13(8): p. 572–83.

[80] Letouze, E., et al., *SDH mutations establish a hypermethylator phenotype in paraganglioma*. Cancer Cell, 2013. 23(6): p. 739–52.

[81] Bedi, U., et al., *Epigenetic plasticity: a central regulator of epithelial-to-mesenchymal transition in cancer*. Oncotarget, 2014. 5(8): p. 2016–29.

[82] Wu, C.Y., et al., *Epigenetic reprogramming and post-transcriptional regulation during the epithelial-mesenchymal transition*. Trends Genet, 2012. 28(9): p. 454–63.

[83] Agathocleous, M. and W.A. Harris, *Metabolism in physiological cell proliferation and differentiation*. Trends Cell Biol, 2013. 23(10): p. 484–92.

[84] Warburg, O., *Origin of cancer cells*. Oncologia, 1956. 9(2): p. 75–83.

[85] Ghigna, C., et al., *Pro-metastatic splicing of Ron proto-oncogene mRNA can be reversed: therapeutic potential of bifunctional oligonucleotides and indole derivatives*. RNA Biol, 2014. 7(4): p. 495–503.

[86] Bartel, D.P., *MicroRNAs: genomics, biogenesis, mechanism, and function*. Cell, 2004. 116(2): p. 281–97.

[87] Teague, E.M., C.G. Print, and M.L. Hull, *The role of microRNAs in endometriosis and associated reproductive conditions*. Hum Reprod Update, 2010. 16(2): p. 142–65.

[88] Gregory, P.A., et al., *An autocrine TGF-beta/ZEB/miR-200 signaling network regulates establishment and maintenance of epithelial-mesenchymal transition*. Mol Biol Cell, 2011. 22(10): p. 1686–98.

[89] Vandewalle, C., F. Van Roy, and G. Berx, *The role of the ZEB family of transcription factors in development and disease*. Cell Mol Life Sci, 2009. 66(5): p. 773–87.

[90] Gregory, P.A., et al., *MicroRNAs as regulators of epithelial-mesenchymal transition.* Cell Cycle, 2008. 7(20): p. 3112–8.

[91] Sempere, L.F., et al., *Altered MicroRNA expression confined to specific epithelial cell subpopulations in breast cancer.* Cancer Res, 2007. 67(24): p. 11612–20.

[92] Kato, M., et al., *MicroRNA-192 in diabetic kidney glomeruli and its function in TGF-beta-induced collagen expression via inhibition of E-box repressors.* Proc Natl Acad Sci U S A, 2007. 104(9): p. 3432–7.

[93] Zhang, J.P., et al., *MicroRNA-148a suppresses the epithelial-mesenchymal transition and metastasis of hepatoma cells by targeting Met/Snail signaling.* Oncogene, 2014. 33(31): p. 4069–76.

[94] Moes, M., et al., *A novel network integrating a miRNA-203/SNAI1 feedback loop which regulates epithelial to mesenchymal transition.* PLoS One, 2012. 7(4): p. e35440.

[95] Ma, L., J. Teruya-Feldstein, and R.A. Weinberg, *Tumour invasion and metastasis initiated by microRNA-10b in breast cancer.* Nature, 2007. 449(7163): p. 682–8.

[96] Turcatel, G., et al., *MIR-99a and MIR-99b modulate TGF-beta induced epithelial to mesenchymal plasticity in normal murine mammary gland cells.* PLoS One, 2012. 7(1): p. e31032.

[97] Eades, G., et al., *miR-200a regulates SIRT1 expression and epithelial to mesenchymal transition (EMT)-like transformation in mammary epithelial cells.* J Biol Chem, 2011. 286(29): p. 25992–6002.

[98] Gebeshuber, C.A., K. Zatloukal, and J. Martinez, *miR-29a suppresses tristetraprolin, which is a regulator of epithelial polarity and metastasis.* EMBO Rep, 2009. 10(4): p. 400–5.

[99] Eis, P.S., et al., *Accumulation of miR-155 and BIC RNA in human B cell lymphomas.* Proc Natl Acad Sci U S A, 2005. 102(10): p. 3627–32.

[100] Kong, W., et al., *MicroRNA-155 is regulated by the transforming growth factor beta/Smad pathway and contributes to epithelial cell plasticity by targeting RhoA.* Mol Cell Biol, 2008. 28(22): p. 6773–84.

[101] Valastyan, S., et al., *Activation of miR-31 function in already-established metastases elicits metastatic regression.* Genes Dev, 2011. 25(6): p. 646–59.

[102] Ma, L., et al., *miR-9, a MYC/MYCN-activated microRNA, regulates E-cadherin and cancer metastasis.* Nat Cell Biol, 2010. 12(3): p. 247–56.

[103] Pluciennik, E., et al., *The role of WWOX tumor suppressor gene in the regulation of EMT process via regulation of CDH1-ZEB1-VIM expression in endometrial cancer.* Int J Oncol, 2015. 46(6): p. 2639–48.

[104] Hatcher, H., et al., *Curcumin: from ancient medicine to current clinical trials.* Cell Mol Life Sci, 2008. 65(11): p. 1631–52.

[105] Chen, C.L., et al., *E-cadherin expression is silenced by DNA methylation in cervical cancer cell lines and tumours*. Eur J Cancer, 2003. 39(4): p. 517–523.

[106] Aggarwal, S., et al., *Curcumin (diferuloylmethane) down-regulates expression of cell proliferation and antiapoptotic and metastatic gene products through suppression of Ikappa-Balpha kinase and Akt activation*. Mol Pharmacol, 2006. 69(1): p. 195–206.

[107] Schmidt, E.V., *The role of c-myc in regulation of translation initiation*. Oncogene, 2004. 23(18): p. 3217–21.

[108] Wu, Y. and B.P. Zhou, *TNF-alpha/NF-kappaB/Snail pathway in cancer cell migration and invasion*. Br J Cancer, 2010. 102(4): p. 639–44.

[109] Rangaswami, H., A. Bulbule, and G.C. Kundu, *Nuclear factor-inducing kinase plays a crucial role in osteopontin-induced MAPK/IkappaBalpha kinase-dependent nuclear factor kappaB-mediated promatrix metalloproteinase-9 activation*. J Biol Chem, 2004. 279(37): p. 38921–35.

[110] Lu, J.N., et al., *Anthocyanins from vitis coignetiae pulliat inhibit cancer invasion and epithelial-mesenchymal transition, but these effects can be attenuated by tumor necrosis factor in human uterine cervical cancer HeLa cells*. Evid Based Complement Alternat Med, 2013. 2013: p. 503043.

[111] Li, X., et al., *Negative feedback loop between p66Shc and ZEB1 regulates fibrotic EMT response in lung cancer cells*. Cell Death Dis, 2015. 6: p. e1708.

[112] Clarke, M.F., et al., *Cancer stem cells – perspectives on current status and future directions: AACR Workshop on cancer stem cells*. Cancer Res, 2006. 66(19): p. 9339–44.

[113] Bernaudo, S., et al., *Cyclin G2 inhibits epithelial-to-mesenchymal transition by disrupting Wnt/beta-catenin signaling*. Oncogene, 2016.

[114] Liu, H., et al., *FOXO3a modulates WNT/beta-catenin signaling and suppresses epithelial-to-mesenchymal transition in prostate cancer cells*. Cell Signal, 2015. 27(3): p. 510–8.

[115] Warrier, S., et al., *Cancer stem-like cells from head and neck cancers are chemosensitized by the Wnt antagonist, sFRP4, by inducing apoptosis, decreasing stemness, drug resistance and epithelial to mesenchymal transition*. Cancer Gene Ther, 2014. 21(9): p. 381–8.

[116] Zhang, P.P., et al., *Differentiation therapy of hepatocellular carcinoma by inhibiting the activity of AKT/GSK-3beta/beta-catenin axis and TGF-beta induced EMT with sophocarpine*. Cancer Lett, 2016. 376(1): p. 95–103.

[117] Xu, J.H., et al., *Role of Wnt inhibitory factor-1 in inhibition of bisdemethoxycurcumin mediated epithelial-to-mesenchymal transition in highly metastatic lung cancer 95D cells*. Chin Med J (Engl), 2015. 128(10): p. 1376–83.

[118] Yang, H., et al., *Ski prevents TGF-beta-induced EMT and cell invasion by repressing SMAD-dependent signaling in non-small cell lung cancer*. Oncol Rep, 2015. 34(1): p. 87–94.

[119] Zhang, L., et al., *Overexpressed GRP78 affects EMT and cell-matrix adhesion via autocrine TGF-beta/Smad2/3 signaling*. Int J Biochem Cell Biol, 2015. 64: p. 202–11.

[120] Rajput, S., et al., *Thymoquinone restores radiation-induced TGF-beta expression and abrogates EMT in chemoradiotherapy of breast cancer cells*. J Cell Physiol, 2015. 230(3): p. 620–9.

[121] Duangkumpha, K., et al., *BMP-7 blocks the effects of TGF-beta-induced EMT in cholangiocarcinoma*. Tumour Biol, 2014. 35(10): p. 9667–76.

[122] Shen, L., et al., *Tumor suppressor NDRG2 tips the balance of oncogenic TGF-beta via EMT inhibition in colorectal cancer*. Oncogenesis, 2014. 3: p. e86.

[123] Iskender, B., K. Izgi, and H. Canatan, *Novel anti-cancer agent myrtucommulone-A and thymoquinone abrogate epithelial-mesenchymal transition in cancer cells mainly through the inhibition of PI3K/AKT signalling axis*. Mol Cell Biochem, 2016. 416(1–2): p. 71–84.

[124] Zhao, Q.Y., et al., *ING5 inhibits epithelial-mesenchymal transition in breast cancer by suppressing PI3K/Akt pathway*. Int J Clin Exp Med, 2015. 8(9): p. 15498–505.

[125] Xu, Q., et al., *alpha-Mangostin suppresses the viability and epithelial-mesenchymal transition of pancreatic cancer cells by downregulating the PI3K/Akt pathway*. Biomed Res Int, 2014. 2014: p. 546353.

[126] Lin, G., et al., *The dual PI3K/mTOR inhibitor NVP-BEZ235 prevents epithelial-mesenchymal transition induced by hypoxia and TGF-beta1*. Eur J Pharmacol, 2014. 729: p. 45–53.

[127] Bak, Y., et al., *IL-32theta inhibits stemness and epithelial-mesenchymal transition of cancer stem cells via the STAT3 pathway in colon cancer*. Oncotarget, 2016. 7(6): p. 7307–17.

[128] Huang, X., et al., *Luteolin decreases invasiveness, deactivates STAT3 signaling, and reverses interleukin-6 induced epithelial-mesenchymal transition and matrix metalloproteinase secretion of pancreatic cancer cells*. Onco Targets Ther, 2015. 8: p. 2989–3001.

[129] Lu, Z., et al., *FTY720 inhibits proliferation and epithelial-mesenchymal transition in cholangiocarcinoma by inactivating STAT3 signaling*. BMC Cancer, 2014. 14: p. 783.

[130] Kim, M.J., et al., *N-myc downstream-regulated gene 2 (NDRG2) suppresses the epithelial-mesenchymal transition (EMT) in breast cancer cells via STAT3/Snail signaling*. Cancer Lett, 2014. 354(1): p. 33–42.

Chapter 11

Importance and Detection of Epithelial-to-Mesenchymal Transition (EMT) Phenotype in CTCs

Joseph W. Po, David Lynch, Paul de Souza and
Therese M. Becker

Additional information is available at the end of the chapter

http://dx.doi.org/10.5772/64342

Abstract

The current dogma is that epithelial-to-mesenchymal transition (EMT) promotes circulating tumour cell (CTC) formation and is ultimately a driver of metastasis. There is also accumulating evidence that EMT-phenotype changes are commonly associated with therapy resistance. Thus, capturing EMT-phenotype CTCs is expected to yield important clinical information in regard to prognosis and response to therapy as well as allowing the study of metastatic processes. However, the isolation and identification of EMT-phenotype CTCs with commonly used isolation/detection methods are suboptimal, and current efforts on improving the isolation of EMT-phenotype CTCs are associated with pitfalls that need to be overcome. This chapter explores the significance of EMT in CTC formation and the role of EMT in cancer metastasis and resistance to therapy. We also comprehensively review the past and current limitations of evaluating EMT phenotypes in CTC isolation and analysis and discuss how CTCs can be seen in a more holistic fashion as important biomarkers for clinical management.

Keywords: CTC, EMT, vimentin, immunomagnetic cell isolation, metastatic disease

1. Introduction

Circulating tumour cells (CTCs) were first discovered by the Australian pathologist Thomas Ashworth in 1869, who described single cells and cell clusters in a patient's blood and proposed a role for CTCs in the metastatic process [1]. Recently, due to improved CTC detection techniques, these cells, together with circulating tumour nucleic acids (ctNA), are emerging as attractive, accessible, non-invasive biopsies to guide the best therapy for a patient's cancer. CTC counts are closely related to cancer progression and stage, and there is mounting evidence from studies on prostate-, breast-, colorectal- and other cancers that CTCs have prognostic value (reviewed by Caixeiro et al. [2]).

In essence, CTCs are very rare cells, and usually only between 0 and 30 CTCs can be isolated from a 5–10-ml blood sample of a cancer patient; although for some patients, CTC counts can be considerably higher. Isolation technologies allow enrichment and separation of CTCs from the millions of surrounding blood cells by initial gradient centrifugation or red blood cell lysis followed by further enrichment of CTCs due to their physical properties or by employing antibody-based negative or positive enrichment techniques (reviewed by Yu et al. [3]). Enrichment steps are followed by CTC identification primarily by immunocytostaining. The most common CTC identification pattern relies on positive staining for nucleated cells (4',6-diamidino-2-phenylindole (DAPI) or Hoechst staining) and cytokeratin (CK; positive CTC marker) associated with a lack of CD45 staining (negative CTC marker, expressed on leucocytes). Advances in single cell analysis technology have contributed to maximise the information that can be gained from CTCs isolated from a single blood sample. Tumour biomarkers such as gene amplification, mutation, rearrangement and expression can be successfully analysed while CTC protein levels can be determined. There are high expectations that CTC-based assays will find utility for clinical testing, guiding therapy and monitoring treatment in the not-too-distant future (reviewed by Becker et al. [4]). However, cancer cells, including CTCs, are extremely heterogeneous, and therefore, isolating a representative range of CTCs remains difficult.

A particular challenge is the capture of CTCs that have undergone epithelial-to-mesenchymal transition (EMT) [5, 6]. EMT and its reverse, the mesenchymal-to-epithelial transition (MET), are reversible phenotypical changes that allow a cell to form either dense epithelial structures with tight interaction to neighbouring epithelial cells or, by undergoing EMT, to loosen interactions with other cells and become more mesenchymal and migratory. The ability to undergo these changes is important for cells during development to allow the migration of cells and the formation of different tissues. Cancer cells that are able to take advantage of these processes and undergo EMT are proposed to be more motile and consequently are more likely to become CTCs by entering the blood stream [7]. Not surprisingly, EMT-phenotype cancer cells are linked to the presence of metastases. Additionally, cancer cells that have undergone EMT tend to be distinctly more resistant to chemo and radiation therapy [8]. Consequently, the detection and analysis of EMT-phenotype CTCs appear necessary to fully harness CTC information about a given cancer and monitor disease evolution; yet, we are still poorly equipped to detect these cells. Currently, most methods to isolate CTCs, and nearly all current approaches to identify CTCs, rely on the presence of epithelial cell markers. CTC isolation predominantly relies on immunomagnetic targeting of the epithelial cell adhesion molecule (EpCAM), but this epithelial glycoprotein diminishes during EMT, thereby compromising the effectiveness of this strategy [5, 6]. The identification of CTCs usually involves immunocytostaining for epithelial proteins of the cytokeratin protein family, which are similarly downregulated during EMT [9]. Equally problematic is the method of probing for EpCAM, which is frequently used to identify CTCs after size exclusion enrichment [10].

http://dx.doi.org/10.5772/64342

In this chapter, we summarise the current understanding of EMT in CTC formation, detection of EMT markers in CTCs isolated by common methods and their limitations, and new approaches to better isolate and identify EMT-phenotype CTCs (EMT-CTCs). The clinical relevance of detecting EMT-CTCs is also discussed.

2. EMT in CTC formation

The role of EMT in the metastatic process has been controversial mainly because cells in metastatic tumours often display epithelial rather than mesenchymal characteristics, despite the presence of cells with mesenchymal features in the primary cancer. The recognition that EMT is a reversible process has led to a model adaptation, which postulates that EMT reversal, termed MET, has to occur after extravasation to allow motile cancer cells to resettle and form metastases [11] (**Figure 1**). Regardless of robust *in vivo* data that show increased metastasis associated with an EMT phenotype in the primary tumour, experimentally tracking EMT or MET in the metastatic process remains challenging [12].

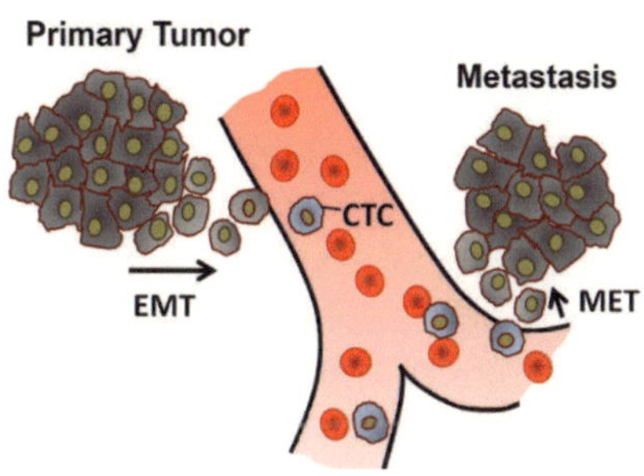

Figure 1. EMT in CTC formation. Simplified illustration of cells in a primary tumour undergoing EMT changes, which enable them to disseminate from the primary cancer, intravasate into the blood stream and travel as CTCs before extravasating the vascular system and, by undergoing MET, regain the ability to form a metastatic tumour.

Several elegant studies and *in vivo* evidence (mainly from mouse models) show that EMT aids tumour cell dissemination and promotes intravasation into the vascular system (CTC formation). MDA-MB-468 breast cancer cells that can be driven to undergo EMT by epidermal growth factor (EGF) exposure were used in a severely compromised immunodeficient (SCID) mouse xenograft model. Xenografts in this model lead to lung and liver metastases, and a peak in CTC counts coincided with the appearance of cells strongly staining for the EMT marker vimentin in the initial xenograft. Vimentin was also expressed in CTCs and CTC clusters, suggesting that EMT promoted CTC formation [13]. Another study, in which KRAS-pancreatic tumour model mice were treated with cerulein to induce pancreatitis and EMT changes in the cancer cells, showed significant increases in CTC counts [14]; however, this finding was not corroborated in a more recent study involving a similar model [15]. A role for EMT in CTC formation was further substantiated when a squamous cell carcinoma prone mouse model with targeted transcription factor Twist1 induction confirmed that Twist1 caused tumour cells to undergo EMT, and this was associated with a doubling of CTC counts as well as increased metastasis [16]. Recently, an innovative model of endothelial cells that form vascular-like structures *in vitro* was used to show that SW620 colorectal cancer cells could migrate into these 'vessels', especially when hypoxia-induced EMT was triggered [17]. A concept supporting the notion that mesenchymal properties afford cancer cells some protection in circulation suggests that any cells shedding from a tumour without undergoing EMT might undergo stressful, traumatic events required for the interruption of the strong epithelial cell-cell interactions resulting in reduced viability [18]. Additionally, EMT-phenotype changes are generally thought to reduce sensitivity to stress signals that would normally lead to apoptosis [8]. Taken together, these observations underpin the emerging opinion that EMT-CTCs may comprise a more viable, aggressive tumour cell population than epithelial CTCs, and go some way to explain the association of EMT-CTCs and increased metastasis. In that regard, it is worth noting that transforming growth factor β (TGFβ), which is commonly released by platelets, may promote or maintain EMT in CTCs while in the circulation and promote extravasation [19]. The current understanding of the role of CTCs in establishing distant metastatic sites was recently reviewed and is beyond the scope of this chapter [2, 20].

3. EMT phenotypes in CTCs isolated by EpCAM targeting

It is important to emphasise that, despite the epithelial nature of EpCAM, CTCs isolated by EpCAM targeting can display markers of EMT. This is due to the fact that changes between epithelial and mesenchymal phenotypes are dynamic, and cells can be found in intermittent stages and express mesenchymal as well as epithelial markers at the same time. Accordingly, mesenchymal markers have been successfully detected in CTCs after EpCAM-based isolation. For instance, intermittent EMT phenotype characterised by co-expression of mesenchymal proteins vimentin, N-cadherin and CD133 with epithelial markers EpCAM, CK and E-cadherin was shown in breast cancer and prostate cancer CTCs isolated by EpCAM targeting [21]. EpCAM-based breast cancer CTC isolation also yielded cells with common gene expression of the EMT markers TGFβ1, FOXC1, CXCR4, NFKB1, VIM and ZEB2 [22]. Moreover, higher breast cancer staging correlated with mesenchymal vimentin and fibronectin expression in EpCAM-enriched CTC samples. Interestingly, vimentin and fibronectin expression was also detected in 31 of 92 (34%) of patient samples, which were CTC negative according to the common CTC definition ($DAPI^+$, CK^+, $CD45^-$) but not in samples from healthy control individuals, suggesting the presence of CTCs lacking CK in some patients [23].

4. EMT phenotype in CTCs isolated with alternate strategies

The inability of EpCAM-based CTC isolation to optimally account for EMT-CTCs with EpCAM loss has led to the targeting of alternative, EMT-associated cell-surface markers, for CTC enrichment, or by avoiding these methods altogether and focussing on CTC enrichment due to physical cancer cell properties, mainly size exclusion. Not surprisingly, when EpCAM-based immunomagnetic CTC isolation was directly compared with size exclusion CTC enrichment of parallel blood samples from 40 NSCLC patients, CTCs were isolated from a higher proportion of patients (80 vs 23%) by size exclusion, and as expected the isolated cells tended to lack EpCAM; however, they expressed CK and had elevated levels of the EMT-associated epithelial growth factor receptor (EGFR) and thus likely were tumour cells [24].

An elegant approach to account for the CTCs missed during EpCAM-based capture in HER2-positive breast cancer patients utilised CD45 immunomagnetic depletion of blood cells after an initial EpCAM-based CTC capture, to further enrich the remaining EpCAM-negative CTCs. The EMT-linked transcription factors SNAI1 and ZEB1 were more commonly expressed in these EpCAM-negative cells that were likely tumour-derived cells compared to the EpCAM-isolated counterparts [25]. Vimentin, best known for its functions as a cytoskeletal support protein, can also be present on the cell surface of mesenchymal cells and has been successfully targeted in immunomagnetic isolation of CTCs from colorectal cancer patients and breast cancer patients. After CD45 immunodepletion, CTCs were positively selected with cell-surface vimentin (CSV) targeting. The authors suggest that CSV expression is restricted to cancer cells, and CSV targeting isolates significantly more CTCs from colorectal cancer patients with progressive disease than those with stable disease; moreover, higher CSV-CTC counts were more commonly found in therapy-resistant patients. In a direct comparison of CSV- and EpCAM-based CTC isolation (CellSearch CTC platform) in breast cancer patients, CTCs isolated with CSV targeting were a more reliable marker for progressive disease compared to stable disease. In both CSV-isolated breast and colorectal cancer CTCs, the EMT markers FOXC2, SNAIL, Twist-1 and Slug tended to be highly expressed while E-cadherin and EpCAM levels were low. The CSV antibody is currently not commercially available, thus limiting its

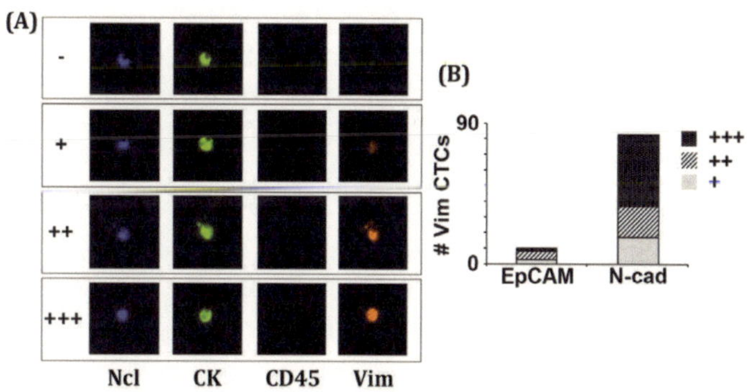

Figure 2. EMT analysis in isolated CTCs. Quadruple staining to detect CTCs with EMT phenotype according to levels of the EMT marker vimentin. (A) CTCs were identified by nuclear Hoechst staining 'Ncl' (blue, Fluxion enumeration kit) and cytokeratin (CK) staining (green; FITC-conjugated anti-cytokeratin antibody: clone c-11, Sigma-Aldrich) as well as exclusion of CD45 expression (red, antibodies: CTC enumeration kit, Fluxion). Vimentin staining, 'Vim' (orange, AF647-conjugated anti-vimentin antibody: clone V9, Abcam), in CTCs, was scored as indicated: Staining of a representative cell for each category, negative (–), weak (+), positive (++) and strongly positive (+++), is depicted. (B) Cell counts for vimentin-positive EMT-CTCs isolated from a representative patient sample using EpCAM- versus N-cadherin- 'N-cad'-based isolation of CTCs using the quadruple staining assay. CTCs were isolated with the IsoFlux CTC isolation platform using EpCAM-based or N-cadherin-based immunomagnetic isolation with the Rare Cell Isolation Kit, Fluxion.

EMT markers	Main finding/clinical correlation [reference]
EpCAM-based immunomagnetic isolation:	
EpCAM, CK, E-cadherin, vimentin, N-cadherin, CD133	CTCs with intermittent EMT phenotype are common in advanced prostate- and breast cancer [21]
CK	Low CK level CTCs were correlated with receptor negative metastatic breast cancer and with poorer OS [30]
Vimentin	Vimentin expression in prostate cancer CTCs is associated with decreased OS [31]
TGFß1, FOXC1, CXCR4, NFKB1, VIM, ZEB2	Gene expression of EMT markers shown in CTCs [22]
HER2, VIM, FN1	Presence of EMT-CTCs correlates to disease stage [23]
CK, VIM, FN1	The presence of EMT-CTCs correlates to shorter PFS [32]
EpCAM-based isolation combined/compared with other methods:	
Cell-surface vimentin (CSV)	EMT-CTC numbers were a more reliable progressive disease marker for breast cancer patients when isolated targeting CSV versus EpCAM [27]
Vimentin, twist, ZEB1, ZEB2, snail, slug and E-cadherin	The expression of both twist and vimentin in CTCs was significantly correlated with portal vein tumor thrombus in liver hepatocellular carcinoma [33].
CK, EpCAM	Most CTCs from metastatic breast cancer patients showed intermittent phenotype while 16% of patients had EpCAM- only CTCs and 33% EpCAM-null CTCs [34]
CK, EpCAM, CDH1, FN1, CDH2	Combined EpCAM/EGFR/Her2-based CTC isolation was linked to increased EMT-CTC numbers in metastatic breast cancer patients with disease progression [35]
TWIST1, SLUG, SNAIL1, ZEB1, FOXC2	EMT-CTCs were more common in primary breast cancer patients with poorer prognostic markers (ie needed neoadjuvant treatment) [36]
Targeted immunomagnetic isolation (non-EpCAM):	
Cell-surface vimentin (CSV)	>5 >5 EMT-CTCs more common in progressive colorectal cancer [26]
CD45-based immunomagnetic blood cell depletion:	
Vimentin, twist, CK	EMT -CTCs more prevalent in CTCs from metastatic breast cancer patients [37]
EpCAM, CK, VIM	CTCs of 'CTC-negative' NSCLC patient by EpCAM based isolation were tumorigenic in mice [29].
Isolation by cell size:	
Vimentin, CK	Pancreatic cancer CTCs without CK or vimentin are more commonly in patients with lymphnode metastasis [38].
CK, EpCAM,VIM, TWIST	Proportion of EMT-CTCS is linked to response to therapy in gastric cancer [39]
EpCAM, CK, VIM, TWIST	Intermittent phenotype and EMT CTCs were predominant in hepatocellular carcinoma and correlated with metastasis [40]

OS: overall survival, PFS: progression-free survival. Dependent on their nature, EMT markers follow protein or gene nomenclature

Table 1. Detection of EMT biomarkers in CTCs.

http://dx.doi.org/10.5772/64342

use and confirmation of the data by others [26, 27]. A study that investigated gene expression in ovarian cancer CTCs showed the expression of EMT markers in most individual CTCs from three patients, while only 30% of these cells also expressed epithelial CK5 or CK7. However, all CTCs expressed epithelial MUC1 [28]. In a patient with non-small cell lung cancer who was CTC-negative according to EpCAM-based (CellSearch) enrichment, it is worth noting that CTCs enriched by CD45 depletion were tumourigenic in mice and CTCs isolated from the same patient by size exclusion showed predominant EMT or intermittent phenotype [29].

In our laboratory, we embarked on the isolation of CTCs from advanced ovarian cancer patients using N-cadherin-based immunomagnetic isolation and captured approximately three times more CTCs$^-$ when using N-cadherin-based versus EpCAM-based CTC isolation (data not shown). We also developed an assay to probe CTCs for vimentin as marker of EMT, which showed that N-cadherin-based CTC isolation from advanced ovarian cancer patients increased the capture of EMT-CTCs (**Figure 2**). Studies that investigated EMT markers in CTCs, isolated by various strategies, are compiled in **Table 1**.

5. The pitfalls of non-EpCAM-based CTC isolation

The clear advantage of EpCAM-based CTC isolation is the observation that EpCAM is only rarely found on cells circulating in the blood stream of healthy individuals, resulting in a limited number of false-positive 'CTCs'. In our hands, using the IsoFlux CTC platform and EpCAM-based enrichment, the average Hoechst$^+$, CK$^+$, CD45$^-$-false positive 'CTCs', obtained from 10 healthy blood donors is 1.8 per 9 ml of blood with a range of 0–5 cells. By contrast, the greatest problem with the use of EMT markers for CTC isolation or CTC identification, or with CTC isolation techniques relying on physical cell properties such as size and plasticity, is the increased risk of detecting false-positive 'CTCs'. This is the case because some rare cells found in normal blood can express a number of epithelial and mesenchymal markers. For instance, circulating endothelial cells (CECs) can be found at varying numbers in blood samples of healthy individuals (0–29/ml blood) [41] and increased numbers in cancer patients [42]. CECs do not only express cytokeratin, but typical EMT markers such as N-cadherin, EGFR, vimentin and fibronectin [43–48]. Moreover, circulating endothelial cells tend to be above 10 μm in diameter [49], and some endothelial cells might therefore not be excluded from size-based CTC enrichment. There are currently limited data evaluating potential CEC contamination in either filter-enriched CTC samples or samples enriched by positive or negative immunotargeting. However, it is likely that the inclusion of CECs in CTC counts in the literature (i.e. false-positive CTCs) has inadvertently led to overestimation.

A particularly interesting approach to avoid the issues surrounding EpCAM is the use of CD146 (MCAM)-based immunomagnetic CTC isolation. Elevated expression of CD146 has been reported for melanoma, breast-, ovarian- and prostate cancer [50], and CD146-based immunomagnetic CTC isolation was reported for breast cancer and melanoma patients [44, 51]. However, CD146 is also an endothelial marker used to define and target CECs [41]. Thus, CD146-based CTC isolation needs to be complemented by cancer-specific CTC identification, such as Melan-A for melanoma CTCs, for example. Alternatively, there is a need to distinguish co-purified CECs from CTCs using specific endothelial markers not expressed on cancer cells. The endothelial marker CD34 has been used to distinguish CD146-enriched breast cancer CTCs from CECs [44]. Whether CD34 is the most reliable or specific marker to distinguish true CTCs from false positives still needs to be confirmed.

Our preliminary data suggest that the accumulation of false positives, most likely endothelial cells, is also an issue when using N-cadherin-based immunomagnetic CTC isolation. While CTC numbers isolated from advanced ovarian cancer patients were approximately four times higher than EpCAM-isolated CTC numbers, we also detected more Hoechst$^+$, CK$^+$, CD45$^-$ false-positive 'CTCs' in the blood from seven individuals without any history of cancer (data not shown). N-cadherin, EGFR and cytokeratin expression of endothelial cells suggest that targeting these proteins in CTC isolation or identification might lead to similar problems. Moreover, other cells in the circulation, such as monocytes, macrophages and neutrophils, also express the EMT markers EGFR, vimentin and N-cadherin. Further, tumour-associated macrophages of breast cancer and prostate cancer patients were also shown to express cytokeratin and therefore could be confused with CTCs [52–55]. Thus, while non-EpCAM-based CTC isolation techniques appear to produce higher CTC counts and favour isolation of CTCs with EMT features, they also may enrich for false-positive cells, and as long as identification solely relies on CK and CD45 staining of nucleated cells, these cannot be sufficiently well discriminated from CTCs. Advances in identifying CTCs and distinguishing them from false positives, in particular endothelial cells, will refine CTC detection and help avoiding diagnostic errors when progressing CTC-based assays into the clinic.

6. EMT-phenotype CTCs, do they have clinical relevance?

Circumstantial evidence linking EMT changes to advanced disease and increased metastasis is strong. EMT phenotype in patient tumour tissue is often prognostic and correlates negatively to overall survival and disease progression. Most notably, a switch from the expression of the epithelial cell-cell adhesion molecule E-cadherin to the mesenchymal N-cadherin is thought to be central to EMT, and it is commonly found in association with disease progression in various cancers including melanoma, pancreatic-, bladder- and colorectal cancer (reviewed by Cavallaro et al. [56]). Other studies found elevated expression of a number of E-cadherin transcriptional repressors such as Twist, Slug, ZEB1/2 and Snail1 linked to poorer prognosis in endometrial-, colorectal-, hepatocellular-, bladder-, gastric- and lung cancer [57–63]. Equally, increased expression of vimentin was associated with poorer outcomes for patients with gastric-, colorectal-, bladder- and breast cancer [58, 64–66]. However, the correlation of EMT with poorer overall or disease-free survival is not universal. A recent study, which established a comprehensive EMT gene expression signature in tumour tissue, found that poorer disease-free survival was associated with an EMT gene expression pattern in ovarian and colorectal cancer but not in breast cancer; therefore, it will be important to better define the context in which EMT gives cancer cells a selective advantage [67]. As detailed above, EMT marker gene or protein expression has also been studied in CTCs, and the overall emerging evidence suggests that increased EMT-phenotype detection in CTCs correlates with more advanced disease stages and is the predominant phenotype found in the blood of patients with metastatic disease (see **Table 1**).

Cancer cells frequently undergo EMT when exposed to stress, and this makes them significantly more resistant to a variety of therapies. However, it is not well understood whether the range of phenotypic EMT changes that cause increased mobility and metastasis is instrumental in resistance or merely associated with it. Mounting *in vitro* evidence suggesting that EMT confers drug resistance has been thoroughly reviewed previously [8]. More recently, *in vivo* data reaffirm the link between EMT and therapy resistance. For instance, the loss of E-cadherin expression in erlotinib-treated non-small cell lung cancer tumour tissues correlated with poorer progression-free patient survival [68], and EMT gene expression signatures in ovarian or prostate cancer patient tissue were associated with resistance to platinum therapy or docetaxel and androgen deprivation, respectively [69, 70]. Interestingly, two recent studies suggested that in breast- and pancreatic cancer mouse models, the majority of cells that metastasised to the lungs did not undergo EMT. Nevertheless, EMT was involved in drug resistance and conditional metastatic outgrowth when mice were treated with the drugs cyclophosphamide and gemcitabine, respectively [15, 71]. These data add to the controversy regarding the role of EMT in the metastatic process and warrant further research. The data do support the survival/therapy resistance functions associated with EMT and it is plausible that cancer cells may 'escape into EMT' to render themselves resistant to drug treatment. Data are starting to emerge suggesting these changes might be detectable by CTC analysis as subtyping CTCs as possessing epithelial, intermittent or mesenchymal characteristics showed that gastric cancer CTCs of a patient progressing on therapy were all of EMT phenotype. However, and confusingly, any remaining CTCs detected in gastric cancer patients that responded to therapy were more epithelial in nature [39].

Regardless, it is possible that therapy inadvertently induces cells that survive drug exposure to change into more mobile, viable and aggressive clones. Due to their EMT phenotype, these cells may be ideally equipped to leave the primary tumour, become CTCs, prevent anoikis and potentially form distant metastases sites. Additionally, the survival advantage of EMT cancer cells might allow time to acquire alternative resistance mechanisms such as mutations. In turn, that would allow EMT-CTCs to undergo MET after extravasation to enable the resettling and formation of proliferating metastases. The underlying mechanisms need to be more thoroughly investigated, and the ability to accurately isolate EMT-CTCs will prove central to clarifying the role of EMT in therapy resistance, disease relapse and metastatic processes. Efficient EMT-CTC isolation and identification may also allow the development of diagnostic tests that monitor escape into EMT as part of therapy response to inform improved patient management.

7. Conclusion

Despite open questions regarding how EMT contributes to cancer progression and drug resistance, there is strong evidence that EMT changes, per se, are useful prognostic markers.

Consequently, EMT-CTC isolation and analysis have the capacity to progress EMT research and importantly allow the development of feasible, non-invasive diagnostic tests to predict and monitor the effectiveness of specific therapies. More reliable identification of these cells will permit the translation of EMT and CTC research into clinically relevant tests to guide therapy.

This work was supported by the Cancer Institute New South Wales through the Centre for Oncology Education and Research Translation (CONCERT). J.P. is recipient of an Australian Rotary Health Gynaecological Oncology PhD Scholarship. D.L. is recipient of an Ingham Research Institute Director's PhD Scholarship. Human ethics approval, HREC/13/LPOOL/158, was obtained and managed by the CONCERT Biobank.

Author details

Joseph W. Po[1,3], David Lynch[1,3], Paul de Souza[1,2,3,4] and Therese M. Becker[1,3,4*]

*Address all correspondence to: t.becker@unsw.edu.au

1 Ingham Institute for Applied Medical Research, Liverpool, NSW, Australia

2 Liverpool Hospital, Liverpool, NSW, Australia

3 Western Sydney University Clinical School, Liverpool, NSW, Australia

4 University of New South Wales, Liverpool, NSW, Australia

References

[1] Ashworth TR. A case of cancer in which cells similar to those in the tumours were seen in the blood after death. Australian Med J. 1869;14:146–7.

[2] Caixeiro NJ, Kienzle N, Lim SH, Spring KJ, Tognela A, Scott KF, et al. Circulating tumour cells—a bona fide cause of metastatic cancer. Cancer Metastasis Rev. 2014;33(2–3):747–56.

[3] Yu M, Stott S, Toner M, Maheswaran S, Haber DA. Circulating tumor cells: approaches to isolation and characterization. J Cell Biol. 2011;192(3):373–82.

[4] Becker TM, Caixeiro NJ, Lim SH, Tognela A, Kienzle N, Scott KF, et al. New frontiers in circulating tumor cell analysis: a reference guide for biomolecular profiling toward translational clinical use. Int J Cancer. 2014;134(11):2523–33.

[5] Punnoose EA, Atwal SK, Spoerke JM, Savage H, Pandita A, Yeh RF, et al. Molecular biomarker analyses using circulating tumor cells. PLoS One. 2010;5(9):e12517.

[6] Gorges TM, Tinhofer I, Drosch M, Rose L, Zollner TM, Krahn T, et al. Circulating tumour cells escape from EpCAM-based detection due to epithelial-to-mesenchymal transition. BMC Cancer. 2012;12:178.

[7] Lim SH, Becker TM, Chua W, Ng WL, de Souza P, Spring KJ. Circulating tumour cells and the epithelial mesenchymal transition in colorectal cancer. J Clin Path. 2014;67(10): 848–53.

[8] Singh A, Settleman J. EMT, cancer stem cells and drug resistance: an emerging axis of evil in the war on cancer. Oncogene. 2010;29(34):4741–51.

[9] Huang RY, Guilford P, Thiery JP. Early events in cell adhesion and polarity during epithelial-mesenchymal transition. J Cell Sci. 2012;125(Pt 19):4417–22.

[10] Hou JM, Krebs M, Ward T, Sloane R, Priest L, Hughes A, et al. Circulating tumor cells as a window on metastasis biology in lung cancer. Am J Pathol. 2011;178(3):989–96.

[11] Thiery JP. Epithelial-mesenchymal transitions in tumour progression. Nat Rev Cancer. 2002;2(6):442–54.

[12] Chui MH. Insights into cancer metastasis from a clinicopathologic perspective: epithelial-mesenchymal transition is not a necessary step. Int J Cancer. 2013;132(7): 1487–95.

[13] Bonnomet A, Syne L, Brysse A, Feyereisen E, Thompson EW, Noel A, et al. A dynamic in vivo model of epithelial-to-mesenchymal transitions in circulating tumor cells and metastases of breast cancer. Oncogene. 2012;31(33):3741–53.

[14] Rhim AD, Mirek ET, Aiello NM, Maitra A, Bailey JM, McAllister F, et al. EMT and dissemination precede pancreatic tumor formation. Cell. 2012;148(1–2):349–61.

[15] Zheng X, Carstens JL, Kim J, Scheible M, Kaye J, Sugimoto H, et al. Epithelial-to-mesenchymal transition is dispensable for metastasis but induces chemoresistance in pancreatic cancer. Nature. 2015;527(7579):525–30.

[16] Tsai JH, Donaher JL, Murphy DA, Chau S, Yang J. Spatiotemporal regulation of epithelial-mesenchymal transition is essential for squamous cell carcinoma metastasis. Cancer Cell. 2012;22(6):725–36.

[17] Ehsan SM, Welch-Reardon KM, Waterman ML, Hughes CC, George SC. A three-dimensional in vitro model of tumor cell intravasation. Integrative Biol. 2014;6(6):603–10.

[18] Grover PK, Cummins AG, Price TJ, Roberts-Thomson IC, Hardingham JE. Circulating tumour cells: the evolving concept and the inadequacy of their enrichment by EpCAM-based methodology for basic and clinical cancer research. Ann Oncol. 2014;25(8):1506–16.

[19] Labelle M, Begum S, Hynes RO. Direct signaling between platelets and cancer cells induces an epithelial-mesenchymal-like transition and promotes metastasis. Cancer Cell. 2011;20(5):576–90.

[20] Pantel K, Speicher MR. The biology of circulating tumor cells. Oncogene. 2015; 35(10): 1216–24.

[21] Armstrong AJ, Marengo MS, Oltean S, Kemeny G, Bitting RL, Turnbull JD, et al. Circulating tumor cells from patients with advanced prostate and breast cancer display both epithelial and mesenchymal markers. M Mol Cancer Res. 2011;9(8):997–1007.

[22] Powell AA, Talasaz AH, Zhang H, Coram MA, Reddy A, Deng G, et al. Single cell profiling of circulating tumor cells: transcriptional heterogeneity and diversity from breast cancer cell lines. PLoS One. 2012;7(5):e33788.

[23] Raimondi C, Gradilone A, Naso G, Vincenzi B, Petracca A, Nicolazzo C, et al. Epithelial-mesenchymal transition and stemness features in circulating tumor cells from breast cancer patients. Breast Cancer Res Treat. 2011;130(2):449–55.

[24] Krebs MG, Hou JM, Sloane R, Lancashire L, Priest L, Nonaka D, et al. Analysis of circulating tumor cells in patients with non-small cell lung cancer using epithelial marker-dependent and -independent approaches. J Thor Oncol. 2012;7(2):306–15.

[25] Giordano A, Gao H, Anfossi S, Cohen E, Mego M, Lee BN, et al. Epithelial-mesenchymal transition and stem cell markers in patients with HER2-positive metastatic breast cancer. Mol Cancer Ther. 2012;11(11):2526–34.

[26] Satelli A, Mitra A, Brownlee Z, Xia X, Bellister S, Overman MJ, et al. Epithelial-mesenchymal transitioned circulating tumor cells capture for detecting tumor progression. Clin Cancer Res. 2015;21(4):899–906.

[27] Satelli A, Brownlee Z, Mitra A, Meng QH, Li S. Circulating tumor cell enumeration with a combination of epithelial cell adhesion molecule- and cell-surface vimentin-based methods for monitoring breast cancer therapeutic response. Clin Chem. 2015;61(1):259–66.

[28] Blassl C, Kuhlmann JD, Webers A, Wimberger P, Fehm T, Neubauer H. Gene expression profiling of single circulating tumor cells in ovarian cancer—establishment of a multi-marker gene panel. Mol Oncol. 2016.PMID:27157930 doi: 10.1016/j.molonc.2016.04.002

[29] Morrow CJ, Trapani F, Metcalf RL, Bertolini G, Hodgkinson CL, Khandelwal G, et al. Tumourigenic non-small-cell lung cancer mesenchymal circulating tumour cells: a clinical case study. Ann Oncol. 2016.PMID:27013395 doi: 10.1093/annonc/mdw122

[30] Polioudaki H, Agelaki S, Chiotaki R, Politaki E, Mavroudis D, Matikas A, et al. Variable expression levels of keratin and vimentin reveal differential EMT status of circulating tumor cells and correlation with clinical characteristics and outcome of patients with metastatic breast cancer. BMC Cancer. 2015;15:399.

[31] Lindsay CR, Le Moulec S, Billiot F, Loriot Y, Ngo-Camus M, Vielh P, et al. Vimentin and Ki67 expression in circulating tumour cells derived from castrate-resistant prostate cancer. BMC Cancer. 2016;16(1):168.

[32] Gradilone A, Raimondi C, Nicolazzo C, Petracca A, Gandini O, Vincenzi B, et al. Circulating tumour cells lacking cytokeratin in breast cancer: the importance of being mesenchymal. Cell Mol Med. 2011;15(5):1066–70.

[33] Li YM, Xu SC, Li J, Han KQ, Pi HF, Zheng L, et al. Epithelial-mesenchymal transition markers expressed in circulating tumor cells in hepatocellular carcinoma patients with different stages of disease. Cell Death Dis. 2013;4:e831.

[34] Hyun KA, Goo KB, Han H, Sohn J, Choi W, Kim SI, et al. Epithelial-to-mesenchymal transition leads to loss of EpCAM and different physical properties in circulating tumor cells from metastatic breast cancer. Oncotarget. 2016.PMID:27013581 doi: 10.18632/oncotarget.8250

[35] Yu M, Bardia A, Wittner BS, Stott SL, Smas ME, Ting DT, et al. Circulating breast tumor cells exhibit dynamic changes in epithelial and mesenchymal composition. Science. 2013;339(6119):580–4.

[36] Mego M, Mani SA, Lee BN, Li C, Evans KW, Cohen EN, et al. Expression of epithelial-mesenchymal transition-inducing transcription factors in primary breast cancer: the effect of neoadjuvant therapy. Int J Cancer. 2012;130(4):808–16.

[37] Kallergi G, Papadaki MA, Politaki E, Mavroudis D, Georgoulias V, Agelaki S. Epithelial to mesenchymal transition markers expressed in circulating tumour cells of early and metastatic breast cancer patients. Breast Cancer Res. 2011;13(3):R59.

[38] Poruk KE, Valero V, 3rd, Saunders T, Blackford AL, Griffin JF, Poling J, et al. Circulating tumor cell phenotype predicts recurrence and survival in pancreatic adenocarcinoma. Ann Surg. 2016.PMID:26756760 DOI:10.1097/SLA.0000000000001600

[39] Li TT, Liu H, Li FP, Hu YF, Mou TY, Lin T, et al. Evaluation of epithelial-mesenchymal transitioned circulating tumor cells in patients with resectable gastric cancer: Relevance to therapy response. World J Gastroenterol. 2015;21(47):13259–67.

[40] Liu YK, Hu BS, Li ZL, He X, Li Y, Lu LG. An improved strategy to detect the epithelial-mesenchymal transition process in circulating tumor cells in hepatocellular carcinoma patients. Hepatol Int. 2016.PMID:27115761 doi: 10.1007/s12072-016-9732-7

[41] Damani S, Bacconi A, Libiger O, Chourasia AH, Serry R, Gollapudi R, et al. Characterization of circulating endothelial cells in acute myocardial infarction. Sci Transl Med. 2012;4(126):126ra33.

[42] Ilie M, Long E, Hofman V, Selva E, Bonnetaud C, Boyer J, et al. Clinical value of circulating endothelial cells and of soluble CD146 levels in patients undergoing surgery for non-small cell lung cancer. Br J Cancer. 2014;110(5):1236–43.

[43] Miettinen M, Fetsch JF. Distribution of keratins in normal endothelial cells and a spectrum of vascular tumors: implications in tumor diagnosis. Hum Pathol. 2000;31(9): 1062–7.

[44] Mostert B, Kraan J, Bolt-de Vries J, van der Spoel P, Sieuwerts AM, Schutte M, et al. Detection of circulating tumor cells in breast cancer may improve through enrichment with anti-CD146. Br Cancer Res Treat. 2011;127(1):33–41.

[45] Ferreri DM, Minnear FL, Yin T, Kowalczyk AP, Vincent PA. N-cadherin levels in endothelial cells are regulated by monolayer maturity and p120 availability. Cell Commun Adhes. 2008;15(4):333–49.

[46] Toby IT, Chicoine LG, Cui H, Chen B, Nelin LD. Hypoxia-induced proliferation of human pulmonary microvascular endothelial cells depends on epidermal growth factor receptor tyrosine kinase activation. Am J Physiol Lung Cell Mol Physiol. 2010;298(4):L600–6.

[47] Tsuruta D, Jones JC. The vimentin cytoskeleton regulates focal contact size and adhesion of endothelial cells subjected to shear stress. J Cell Sci. 2003;116(Pt 24):4977–84.

[48] Daramola OA, Heyderman RS, Klein NJ, Shennan GI, Levin M. Detection of fibronectin expression by human endothelial cells using a enzyme-linked immunosorbent assay (ELISA): enzymatic degradation by activated plasminogen. J Immunol Meth. 1997;202(1):67–75.

[49] Woywodt A, Blann AD, Kirsch T, Erdbruegger U, Banzet N, Haubitz M, et al. Isolation and enumeration of circulating endothelial cells by immunomagnetic isolation: proposal of a definition and a consensus protocol. J Thromb Haemost. 2006;4(3):671–7.

[50] Zeng Q, Li W, Lu D, Wu Z, Duan H, Luo Y, et al. CD146, an epithelial-mesenchymal transition inducer, is associated with triple-negative breast cancer. Proc Natl Acad Sci USA. 2012;109(4):1127–32.

[51] Khoja L, Lorigan P, Zhou C, Lancashire M, Booth J, Cummings J, et al. Biomarker utility of circulating tumor cells in metastatic cutaneous melanoma. J Invest Dermatol. 2012; 133(6):1582-90.

[52] Chan G, Nogalski MT, Yurochko AD. Activation of EGFR on monocytes is required for human cytomegalovirus entry and mediates cellular motility. Proc Natl Acad Sci USA. 2009;106(52):22369–74.

[53] Lanaya H, Natarajan A, Komposch K, Li L, Amberg N, Chen L, et al. EGFR has a tumour-promoting role in liver macrophages during hepatocellular carcinoma formation. Nature Cell Biol. 2014;16(10):972–81, 1–7.

[54] Benes P, Maceckova V, Zdrahal Z, Konecna H, Zahradnickova E, Muzik J, et al. Role of vimentin in regulation of monocyte/macrophage differentiation. Differentiation. 2006;74(6):265–76.

[55] Adams DL, Martin SS, Alpaugh RK, Charpentier M, Tsai S, Bergan RC, et al. Circulating giant macrophages as a potential biomarker of solid tumors. Proc Natl Acad Sci USA. 2014;111(9):3514–9.

[56] Cavallaro U, Schaffhauser B, Christofori G. Cadherins and the tumour progression: is it all in a switch? Cancer Lett. 2002;176(2):123–8.

[57] Tanaka Y, Terai Y, Kawaguchi H, Fujiwara S, Yoo S, Tsunetoh S, et al. Prognostic impact of EMT (epithelial-mesenchymal-transition)-related protein expression in endometrial cancer. Cancer Biol Ther. 2013;14(1):13–9.

[58] Toiyama Y, Yasuda H, Saigusa S, Tanaka K, Inoue Y, Goel A, et al. Increased expression of slug and vimentin as novel predictive biomarkers for lymph node metastasis and poor prognosis in colorectal cancer. Carcinogenesis. 2013;34(11):2548–57.

[59] Kahlert C, Lahes S, Radhakrishnan P, Dutta S, Mogler C, Herpel E, et al. Overexpression of ZEB2 at the invasion front of colorectal cancer is an independent prognostic marker and regulates tumor invasion in vitro. Clin Cancer Res. 2011;17(24):7654–63.

[60] Zhou YM, Cao L, Li B, Zhang RX, Sui CJ, Yin ZF, et al. Clinicopathological significance of ZEB1 protein in patients with hepatocellular carcinoma. Ann Surg Oncology. 2012;19(5):1700–6.

[61] Yun SJ, Kim WJ. Role of the epithelial-mesenchymal transition in bladder cancer: from prognosis to therapeutic target. Korean J Urol. 2013;54(10):645–50.

[62] Ru GQ, Wang HJ, Xu WJ, Zhao ZS. Upregulation of Twist in gastric carcinoma associated with tumor invasion and poor prognosis. Pathol Oncol Res. 2011;17(2):341–7.

[63] Zeng J, Zhan P, Wu G, Yang W, Liang W, Lv T, et al. Prognostic value of Twist in lung cancer: systematic review and meta-analysis. Transl Lung Cancer Res. 2015;4(3):236–41.

[64] Otsuki S, Inokuchi M, Enjoji M, Ishikawa T, Takagi Y, Kato K, et al. Vimentin expression is associated with decreased survival in gastric cancer. Oncol Rep. 2011;25(5):1235–42.

[65] Zhao J, Dong D, Sun L, Zhang G, Sun L. Prognostic significance of the epithelial-to-mesenchymal transition markers e-cadherin, vimentin and twist in bladder cancer. Int Braz J Urol. 2014;40(2):179–89.

[66] Yamashita N, Tokunaga E, Kitao H, Hisamatsu Y, Taketani K, Akiyoshi S, et al. Vimentin as a poor prognostic factor for triple-negative breast cancer. J Cancer Res Clin Oncol. 2013;139(5):739–46.

[67] Tan TZ, Miow QH, Miki Y, Noda T, Mori S, Huang RY, et al. Epithelial-mesenchymal transition spectrum quantification and its efficacy in deciphering survival and drug responses of cancer patients. EMBO Mol Med. 2014;6(10):1279–93.

[68] Yauch RL, Januario T, Eberhard DA, Cavet G, Zhu W, Fu L, et al. Epithelial versus mesenchymal phenotype determines in vitro sensitivity and predicts clinical activity of erlotinib in lung cancer patients. Clin Cancer Res. 2005;11(24 Pt 1):8686–98.

[69] Marchini S, Fruscio R, Clivio L, Beltrame L, Porcu L, Fuso Nerini I, et al. Resistance to platinum-based chemotherapy is associated with epithelial to mesenchymal transition in epithelial ovarian cancer. Eur J Cancer. 2013;49(2):520–30.

[70] Marin-Aguilera M, Codony-Servat J, Reig O, Lozano JJ, Fernandez PL, Pereira MV, et al. Epithelial-to-mesenchymal transition mediates docetaxel resistance and high risk of relapse in prostate cancer. Mol Cancer Ther. 2014;13(5):1270–84.

[71] Fischer KR, Durrans A, Lee S, Sheng J, Li F, Wong ST, et al. Epithelial-to-mesenchymal transition is not required for lung metastasis but contributes to chemoresistance. Nature. 2015;527(7579):472–6.